A Pathophysiological Approach to Mood Disorders

A Pathophysiological Approach to Mood Disorders

Editor: Sean Gunner

FOSTER ACADEMICS
www.fosteracademics.com

www.fosteracademics.com

FOSTER ACADEMICS

Cataloging-in-Publication Data

A pathophysiological approach to mood disorders / edited by Sean Gunner.
p. cm.
Includes bibliographical references and index.
ISBN 978-1-63242-632-1
1. Affective disorders. 2. Psychology, Pathological. 3. Physiology, Pathological.
I. Gunner, Sean.
RC537 .P38 2019
616.852 7--dc23

Foster Academics,
118-35 Queens Blvd., Suite 400,
Forest Hills, NY 11375, USA

ISBN 978-1-63242-632-1 (Hardback)

Printed and bound in China.

Contents

Preface

Mood disorder is a group of conditions in which an individual's mood is affected. It manifests as mania or hypomania, depressive disorders and bipolar disorders. Some psychiatric syndromes or depressive disorders that feature less severe symptoms are cyclothymic disorder and dysthymic disorder. Mood disorders may also be triggered by substance use or may occur as a response to a medical condition. This may be an evolved mechanism of delimiting physical activities for assisting the individual to regain his health. A depressed mood can be a response to life's occurrences, such as death of a child or spouse, divorce, loss of status, etc. Both therapy and medications can work to elevate mental health. Behavioral therapy, interpersonal therapy and cognitive behavioral therapy and drugs such as antidepressants, mood stabilizers, anticonvulsants and antipsychotics have potential benefits. This book explores all the important aspects of mood disorders in the present day scenario. It attempts to understand the varied mood disorders of modern society and their emotional and psychological implications. With state-of-the-art inputs by acclaimed experts of this field, this book targets students and professionals.

The researches compiled throughout the book are authentic and of high quality, combining several disciplines and from very diverse regions from around the world. Drawing on the contributions of many researchers from diverse countries, the book's objective is to provide the readers with the latest achievements in the area of research. This book will surely be a source of knowledge to all interested and researching the field.

In the end, I would like to express my deep sense of gratitude to all the authors for meeting the set deadlines in completing and submitting their research chapters. I would also like to thank the publisher for the support offered to us throughout the course of the book. Finally, I extend my sincere thanks to my family for being a constant source of inspiration and encouragement.

Editor

Influence of the CYP2D6 Isoenzyme in Patients Treated with Venlafaxine for Major Depressive Disorder: Clinical and Economic Consequences

Antoni Sicras-Mainar[1]*, Pablo Guijarro[2], Beatriz Armada[2], Milagrosa Blanca-Tamayo[3], Ruth Navarro-Artieda[4]

1 Directorate of Planning, Badalona Serveis Assistencials, S.A., Badalona, Barcelona, Spain, **2** Pfizer, Madrid, Spain, **3** Department of Psychiatry, Badalona Serveis Assistencials, S.A., Badalona, Barcelona, Spain, **4** Medical Documentation, Hospital Germans Trias i Pujol, Badalona, Barcelona, Spain

Abstract

Background: Antidepressant drugs are the mainstay of drug therapy for sustained remission of symptoms. However, the clinical results are not encouraging. This lack of response could be due, among other causes, to factors that alter the metabolism of the antidepressant drug. Objective: to evaluate the impact of concomitant administration of CYP2D6 inhibitors or substrates on the efficacy, tolerability and costs of patients treated with venlafaxine for major depressive disorder in clinical practice.

Methods: We designed an observational study using the medical records of outpatients. Subjects aged ≥18 years who started taking venlafaxine during 2008–2010 were included. Three study groups were considered: no combinations (reference), venlafaxine-substrate, and venlafaxine-inhibitor. The follow-up period was 12 months. The main variables were: demographic data, comorbidity, remission (Hamilton <7), response to treatment, adverse events and costs. The statistical analysis included logistic regression models and ANCOVA, with p values <0.05 considered significant.

Results: A total of 1,115 subjects were recruited. The mean age was 61.7 years and 75.1% were female. Approximately 33.3% (95% CI: 30.5 to 36.1) were receiving some kind of drug combination (venlafaxine-substrate: 23.0%, and venlafaxine-inhibitor: 10.3%). Compared with the venlafaxine-substrate and venlafaxine-inhibitor groups, patients not taking concomitant drugs had a better response to therapy (49.1% *vs.* 39.9% and 34.3%, p<0.01), greater remission of symptoms (59.9% *vs.* 50.2% and 43.8%, p<0.001), fewer adverse events (1.9% *vs.* 7.0% and 6.1%, p<0.05) and a lower mean adjusted cost (€2,881.7 vs. €4,963.3 and €7,389.1, p<0.001), respectively. All cost components showed these differences.

Conclusions: The patients treated with venlafaxine alone showed a better response to anti-depressant treatment, greater remission of symptoms, a lower incidence of adverse events and lower healthcare costs.

Editor: Fernando de Castro, Hospital Nacional de Parapléjicos - SESCAM, Spain

Funding: This study was funded by Pfizer Inc. All authors had a role in study design, decision to publish and manuscript preparation. A. Sicras was a paid as consultant from Pfizer responsible for data collection and analysis and statistical analysis.

Competing Interests: This study was funded by Pfizer Inc. P. Guijarro and B. Armada are full-time employees of Pfizer, SLU. A. Sicras-Mainar was paid as a consultant from Pfizer, responsible for data collection and analysis and statistical analysis. Venlafaxine is a Pfizer product. There are no further patents, products in development or marketed products to declare.

* Email: asicras@bsa.cat

Introduction

Depression is a major public health issue due to its high frequency, disability and mortality rate, and its impact on healthcare resource use and individual loss of productivity [1,2]. According to the ESEMeD study, major depressive disorder (MDD) has an estimated yearly prevalence of 3.9% and a lifetime prevalence of 10.5% in Spain [3] and 14% of patients seen in primary care in Spain have MDD [4].

Antidepressants (AD) are the mainstay of drug therapy for sustained remission of symptoms [5]. However, although a wide range of AD is available, clinical results are not encouraging. About 38% of patients do not respond to AD treatment, and 54% do not achieve complete remission of symptoms [6]. This lack of response or adverse effects at generally effective and well tolerated doses could be due, among other causes, to factors that alter the metabolism of antidepressant drugs [7].

Many AD in current use are substrates of the cytochrome P450 2D6 enzyme (CYP2D6). This coenzyme has a high degree of polymorphism, resulting in a variety of phenotypes between individuals [8]. Approximately 7–10% of Caucasians are poor metabolizers of CYP2D6 [9,10]. In these individuals, drugs subject to first-pass hepatic metabolism by CYP2D6 have a higher exposure of the parent compound than expected and fewer active metabolites. Furthermore, co-administration of a CYP2D6 inhibitor may also affect the pharmacokinetics of AD in which the metabolism is dependent on CYP2D6 activity (an effect known as phenotypic conversion) [11]. These two phenomena have been associated with lower efficacy and tolerability of AD, depending on the characteristics of the drug [11].

Venlafaxine (VEN) is an antidepressant belonging to the group of serotonin and norepinephrine reuptake inhibitors. According to *in vitro* data, venlafaxine is metabolised primarily by CYP2D6 and, to a lesser extent, by CYP3A4, CYP2C19 and CYP1A2. Given its pharmacodynamic activity, O-desmethylvenlafaxine (ODV) is the main clinically-relevant metabolite and is comparable to the parent compound. Both venlafaxine and ODV are chiral compounds, with a differing pharmacokinetic profile depending on their permeability in the brain (P-glycoprotein) [12].

Studies have shown that venlafaxine has a reduced antidepressant effect in patients with a slow CYP2D6 metabolizing phenotype, which is determined by the ODV/VEN ratio [8,13]. Another recent study reported a prevalence of phenotypic conversion of CYP2D6 of 24% in MDD patients treated with venlafaxine. Phenotypic conversion was associated with the concomitant use of other drugs, especially CYP2D6 inhibitors and substrates [11]. However, to date, no study has evaluated the results of these trials in real life situations. The aim of this study was to evaluate the impact of concomitant administration of CYP2D6 substrates or inhibitors on the efficacy, safety and resource consumption of patients treated with venlafaxine for MDD in daily clinical practice.

Materials and Methods

Design and study population

We conducted a multicentre, observational study through retrospective review of medical records (computerised databases) of outpatients from six primary care centres (Apenins-Montigalà, Morera-Pomar, Montgat-Tiana, Nova Lloreda, Martí-Julià and El Progrés) and the Hospital Municipal de Badalona, all managed by Badalona Serveis Assistencials, S.A., and hospital discharge reports from the Hospital Germans Trias i Pujol, Badalona. The population assigned to these centres is mostly urban, with middle-low socioeconomic status.

Data confidentiality was respected pursuant to the Personal Data Protection Act (Law 15/1999, of 13 December), with encoding of personal data. The study was classified by the Spanish Agency of Medicines and Medical Devices as a Post-Authorisation Study - Other Designs and was subsequently approved by the Independent Ethics Committee of the Hospital Clinic of Barcelona. ORCID: 0000-0002-8975-7303. This study was not interventional. In order to conduct this retrospective study, data was collected anonymously and encrypted, according to the Spanish Organic Law on Personal Data Protection. Patients gave written consent that their information be stored in the hospital database and used for research.

Inclusion and exclusion criteria

Inclusion criteria were: a) age ≥ 18 years, b) patients who presented with an episode of MDD (according to the criteria of the International Classification of Primary Care [ICPC-2] [14] and/or the Diagnostic and Statistical Manual of Mental Disorders - Text Revision [DSM-IV-TR]) [15] and were treated with venlafaxine between 1/1/2008 and 31/12/2010, c) that the prescription complied with the minimum criteria for correct treatment (at least 8 weeks of AD treatment after the first prescription), d) patients who were included in the chronic medication programme (with a record of the daily dose, time interval and duration of each treatment), and e) with a clinical follow-up of ≥12 months. Exclusion criteria were: patients transferred to other primary care centres, death, and patients transferred to other regions.

Study groups

We divided patients into three study groups: a) patients who started treatment with venlafaxine and did not receive substrates or inhibitors, b) patients who started treatment with venlafaxine and received substrates (venlafaxine-substrate group), and c) patients who started treatment with venlafaxine and received inhibitors (venlafaxine-inhibitor group). The potential impact of CYP2D6 inhibitors and substrates was analysed individually and by therapeutic group. Follow-up of the main study variables was for 12 months from start of treatment: frequency of combinations, remission, response to treatment, safety (adverse events) and calculation of healthcare and non-healthcare costs.

Definition of MDD, remission and response to treatment

The Hamilton scale was used to diagnose the severity of MDD (intensity of depressive symptoms; Hamilton scale ≥ 18 points) in adults [16]. A patient was considered to be in symptomatic remission of MDD when the total Hamilton depression scale score was ≤ 7 points after at least 8 weeks of correct AD treatment [17]. No remission was defined as the presence of residual symptoms after dose- and time-appropriate pharmacological treatment. Hamilton scale evaluations were performed by the doctors or nursing staff caring for the patient. Response to treatment was defined as a reduction of ≥ 50% in the initial Hamilton scale score, partial response as a reduction of 25–49% and non-response as a reduction of <25% [18]. Hamilton scale data that could not be obtained from the computerised records were obtained by comprehensive review of the medical history.

Sociodemographic and comorbidity data

The main variables studied were: age (continuous and ranges) and gender, as well as the following comorbidities obtained from the ICPC-2 [14]: hypertension (K86, K87), diabetes mellitus (T89, T90), dyslipidaemia (T93), obesity (T82), smoking (P17), alcoholism (P15, P16), all types of organ failure (heart, liver and kidney), ischaemic heart disease (codes: K74, K76, K75), stroke (K90, K91, K93), chronic obstructive pulmonary disease (R95, chronic airflow obstruction), bronchial asthma (R96), dementia or memory disorders (P70, P20), neurological diseases: Parkinson's disease (N87), epilepsy (N88), multiple sclerosis (N86) and other neurological diseases (N99), and malignancies (all types, A79, B72-75, D74-78, F75, H75, K72, L71, L97, N74-76, R84-86, T71-73, U75-79, W72-73, X75-81, Y77-79).

The general comorbidity summary variables used for each patient treated were: a) the Charlson comorbidity index [19] and b) the individual causality index, obtained from the Adjusted Clinical Groups (ACG), a patient classification system based on iso-resource use [20]. The Grouper ACG Case-mix system algorithm consists of a series of consecutive steps which provide 106 mutually-exclusive ACG groups, one for each patient seen. The ACG application provides resource utilisation bands (RUBs) for each patient, according to general morbidity, in one of five mutually-exclusive categories: 1 (healthy or very low morbidity users), 2 (low morbidity), 3 (moderate morbidity), 4 (high morbidity), and 5 (very high morbidity) (Table 1). The clinical characteristics of the patients were assessed from one year before until the start of treatment with venlafaxine. All study registries were properly validated.

Table 1. Baseline characteristics of the study series according to study group.

Study groups	No combinations	Venlafaxine/substrate	Venlafaxine/inhibitor	Total
Number of patients	**N = 744**	**N = 256**	**N = 115**	**N = 1,115**
Sociodemographic characteristics				
Mean age, years	60.9 (14.1)	62.0 (14.8)	63.0 (12.4)	61.7 (14.1)
Ranges: 18–44 years	13.0%	12.5%	7.3%	11.9%
45–64 years	46.5%	39.7%	44.9%	43.8%
65–74 years	21.4%	25.0%	27.5%	23.7%
≥75 years	19.1%	22.8%	20.2%	20.6%
Gender (female)	75.4%	74.0%	76.4%	75.1%
Pensioner	62.2%	77.5%‡	79.6%‡	71.0%
General comorbidity				
Mean diagnosis	7.1 (3.9)	8.9 (4.3)‡	9.5 (4.4)†	8.1 (4.3)
Mean Charlson index	0.4 (0.7)	0.5 (0.6)	0.4 (0.8)	0.4 (0.7)
Mean RUB	2.9 (0.6)	3.1 (0.6)‡	3.1 (0.6)†	3.0 (0.6)
RUB-1	3.2%	1.0%	2.2%	2.2%
RUB-2	12.5%	7.6%†	6.7%	9.8%
RUB-3	73.2%	72.1%	70.8%	72.4%
RUB-4	9.6%	15.4%‡	18.0%‡	13.1%
RUB-5	1.5%	3.9%*	2.2%	2.5%
Associated comorbidities				
Hypertension	36.5%	51.7%‡	55.1%‡	45.0%
Diabetes	16.8%	21.1%	16.9%	18.4%
Dyslipidaemia	53.7%	57.8%	62.4%	56.6%
Obesity	21.2%	24.0%†	31.5%†	23.9%
Active smoker	22.3%	21.6%	16.3%	21.1%
Alcoholism	3.2%	4.4%	2.2%	3.5%
Ischaemic heart disease	6.4%	7.8%	5.6%	6.8%
Cerebrovascular accident	10.6%	14.7%	14.0%	12.6%
Cardiovascular event	15.1%	19.4%	17.4%	17.0%
Organ failure	9.5%	15.2%‡	21.3%‡	13.5%
Bronchial asthma	7.8%	6.4%	7.3%	7.2%
COPD	2.8%	3.7%	1.7%	3.0%
Neuropathies	2.1%	4.7%‡	1.7%	3.0%
Dementia (all types)	3.2%	11.8%‡	7.3%*	7.0%
Malignant neoplasms	8.9%	14.0%*	11.2%*	11.1%

Values expressed as percentage or mean (SD standard deviation), RUB: resource utilisation band, COPD: chronic obstructive pulmonary disease.
* Paired comparisons using the *No combinations* group as the reference; p value in comparisons between groups: *$p<0.05$, †$p<0.01$, ‡$p<0.001$.

Resource use and cost model

Direct healthcare costs (direct costs) were considered to be those related to medical care (medical visits, diagnostic or therapeutic applications, etc.) carried out by physicians. Non-healthcare costs (indirect costs) were those related to lost productivity (number of sick days and days of disability at work) [21]. The design of the cost system took into account the characteristics of the organisations and the degree of development of the information systems available. The product unit that formed the basis for the final calculation (during the study period) was the patient treated, and the cost was expressed as the mean cost per patient (mean unit cost)3. The rates were obtained from the cost-accounting systems at each centre, except for medications and the days of work disability. Prescriptions (acute, chronic or on demand) were quantified according to the retail price including VAT per container at the time of prescription. The costs of days of work disability were quantified according to the minimum wage (source: National Institute of Statistics) [21].

Medications prescribed (substrates and inhibitors)

The active substances that act as CYP2D6 substrates or inhibitors were defined according to the Anatomical Therapeutic Chemical Classification System (ATC) [22] (Table 2 - adapted from Preskorn) [23]. Patients who could have been included in both the venlafaxine-substrate and venlafaxine-inhibitor groups were included in the latter. The following substrates were not included in the study as they were excluded, withdrawn or not licensed by the Spanish National Health System or were not prescribed during the study period: clozapine, thioridazine, tacrine, aprindine, encainide, mexiletine, procainamide, alprenolol, bupranolol and metoprolol. Administration of CYP2D6 substrates/inhibitors was prior to starting treatment with venlafaxine. For patients who were already receiving drug treatment prior to the administration of venlafaxine, the combined consumption of venlafaxine and substrates/inhibitors was at least 6 months; in the case of venlafaxine alone it was less than 6 months during the time of treatment.

Safety: adverse reactions

Information was obtained from medical records of patients who discontinued treatment with venlafaxine for MDD due to an adverse reaction to the medication. The expected adverse events included: a) gastrointestinal disorders (nausea, anorexia/fatigue, xerostomia), b) nervous system disorders (headache/dizziness/dry mouth, sleep disturbances, sexual dysfunction and/or anxiety/nervousness/sweating), c) circulatory disorders (increased blood pressure, flushing/palpitations), as well as any others documented in the medical record.

Statistical analysis

Descriptive statistics were described using means, standard deviation (SD) and 95% confidence intervals (CI). The Kolmogorov-Smirnov test was used to assess the normality of distribution. A bivariate analysis was performed using analysis of variance (ANOVA) (*a posteriori* contrasts: Scheffé), the chi-square test, Pearson's linear correlation and comparison of means for paired groups. Logistic regression was performed to obtain the variables associated with the drug combinations (venlafaxine-substrate and venlafaxine-inhibitor as dependent variables), using an entry procedure (statistic: Wald). The outpatient cost comparison was performed as recommended by Thompson and Barber [24] by analysis of covariance (ANCOVA), with gender, age, RUB and the Charlson index as covariates (method: estimated marginal means, Bonferroni adjustment). The analysis was performed using the statistical package SPSSWIN version 17.0. Statistical significance was established as $p<0.05$.

Results

Of the 86,628 patients aged ≥ 18 years who were initially selected, 6.7% (N = 5,769, 95% CI: 6.5–6.9%) had a diagnosis of MDD. Of these, 1,115 patients met the inclusion/exclusion criteria and were included in the study.

Table 1 shows the baseline characteristics of patients included according to the study groups. The overall mean age was 61.7 years (SD 14.1) and 75.1% were female, with a mean of 8.1 diagnoses per patient and a RUB of 3.0. 94.8% of the study population had ≥ 1 concomitant condition along with MDD. Dyslipidaemia (56.6%), hypertension (45%) and obesity (23.9%) were the most common comorbidities.

Of the 1,115 patients, 33.3% (95% CI: 30.5 to 36.1%) were administered a combination of drugs that act on the CYP2D6 metabolic pathway: 23% (N = 256, 95% CI: 20.5 to 25.5%) venlafaxine-substrate and 10.3% (N = 115, 95% CI: 7.7–11.1%) venlafaxine-inhibitor. Patients with these combinations had higher overall comorbidity (8.9 and 9.5 *vs.* 7.1 diagnoses, $p<0.01$) and greater resource use (3.1 and 3.1 *vs.* 2.9 RUB/year, $p<0.01$) compared with patients without combinations.

In the logistic regression model, the variables that were significantly associated with the venlafaxine-substrate and venlafaxine-inhibitor groups were dementia [odds ratio (OR) = 3.8 (95% CI: 2.1 to 6.6), $p<0.001$], hypertension [OR = 2.1 (95% CI: 1.6 to 2.8), $p<0.001$], organ failure [OR = 1.6 (95% CI: 1.1 to 2.4), $p<0.001$] and RUB [OR = 1.5 (95%: 1.3 to 1.8), $p<0.001$].

Table 2 shows the ratio of substrates and inhibitors according to the study groups. The therapeutic groups that most-frequently acted as substrates were analgesics (27.3%), AD (23%), beta blockers (16.8%) and antipsychotics (16.4%). The most-frequently prescribed CYP2D6 inhibitors were AD (53%). The most-prescribed active substances were tramadol (16%), amitriptyline (16%), timolol (9.8%) and codeine (7.8%) in the venlafaxine-substrate group and celecoxib (40.0%), duloxetine (35.7%), ranitidine (21.7%) and fluoxetine (15.7%) in the venlafaxine-inhibitor group. In the venlafaxine group, the following CYP2D6 substrates were also administered concomitantly: analgesics (38.3%), antipsychotics (26.1%) and AD (17.4%), of which tramadol (29.6%), risperidone (13.0%), quetiapine (12.2%) and amitriptyline (12.2%) were the most-common active substances.

Table 3 shows the efficacy and safety of venlafaxine in clinical practice. The Hamilton scale score at start of AD was similar in the study groups (15.3 *vs.* 14.9 and 15.3 points, $p = 0.347$). However, compared to the venlafaxine-substrate and venlafaxine-inhibitor groups, the no-combination group had a better response to AD treatment with a reduction of ≥ 50% on the Hamilton scale (49.1% vs. 39.9% and 34.3%, $p<0.01$) and a greater percentage of patients with remission of symptoms (59.9 *vs.* 50.2% and 43.8%, $p<0.001$). Likewise, the no-combination group had fewer adverse drug reactions leading to treatment discontinuation (1.9% *vs.* 7.0% and 6.1%, $p<0.05$).

In the 12-month follow-up, the no-combination group used fewer healthcare resources compared with the other groups: primary care visits (11.4 *vs.* 16.7 and 20.3, $p<0.001$), days of hospitalisation (9.5 and 14.0 *vs.* 15.7, $p = 0.01$), specialist visits (3.2 *vs.* 5.3 and 6.9, $p<0.001$), A&E visits (0.5 *vs.* 1.3 and 1.9, $p<0.001$) and days of temporary work disability (8.7 *vs.* 14.4 and 13.8, $p<0.01$).

The gross cost model is shown in Table 4. The total cost of the patients included in the study was €4.9 million, of which 67.0% were direct medical costs and 33.0% were non-healthcare costs (lost productivity), with a mean unit cost of €4,345. Of the total costs, 44.2% were attributable to primary healthcare and 22.8% to specialist care: of these, 7.9% were attributable to primary care visits and 30.9% to drug prescriptions.

With respect to the mean unit cost adjusted for covariates (ANCOVA), the total cost of patients in the no-combination, venlafaxine-substrate and venlafaxine-inhibitor groups was €2,882, €4,963 and €7,389, respectively ($p<0.001$). All cost components showed these differences. Additionally, differences were found in the cost associated with MDD patients according to the response to treatment in each of the study groups (Figure 1). Patients who did not achieve a response had a higher associated cost than patients who achieved remission or a better response.

Discussion

To our knowledge, this is the first study to assess the impact of concomitant administration of CYP2D6 substrates and inhibitors on the efficacy, safety and resource use of patients treated with venlafaxine for MDD in routine clinical practice.

As reported, the metabolizing profile of CYP2D6 can cause clinically significant differences in drug efficacy when the drug in question is a substrate of CYP2D6 [8,25–27]. In the case of venlafaxine, which is converted into its major active metabolite, ODV, by the action of CYP2D6, the metabolic profile can be determined using the ratio of plasma concentrations of ODV/VEN, which is higher in rapid metabolizers than in slow

Table 2. Distribution of *active substances* metabolised by the CYP2D6 genotype according to study groups.

Study groups*		**Venlafaxine/substrate**
Number of patients		**N = 256**
SUBSTRATES		
Antidepressants		59 (23.0%)
	Clomipramine	16 (6.3%)
	Amitriptyline	41 (16.0%)
	Nortriptyline	5 (2.0%)
	Sertraline	18 (7.0%)
	Mirtazapine	12 (4.7%)
Antipsychotics		42 (16.4%)
	Haloperidol	8 (3.1%)
	Quetiapine	15 (5.9%)
	Risperidone	19 (7.4%)
	Aripiprazole	15 (5.9%)
Antiarrhythmics		5 (2.0%)
	Propafenone	2 (0.8%)
	Flecainide	3 (1.2%)
Oestrogens		3 (1.2%)
	Tamoxifen	3 (1.2%)
Beta-blockers		43 (16.8%)
	Propranolol	10 (3.9%)
	Carvedilol	8 (3.1%)
	Timolol	25 (9.8%)
Anti-dementia drugs		26 (10.2%)
	Nicergoline	6 (2.3%)
	Donepezil	14 (5.5%)
	Galantamine	6 (2.3%)
Analgesics		70 (27.3%)
	Oxycodone	9 (3.5%)
	Codeine	20 (7.8%)
	Tramadol	41 (16.0%)
Study groups*		**Venlafaxine/inhibitor**
Number of patients		**N = 115**
INHIBITORS		
Antidepressants		61 (53.0%)
	Fluoxetine	18 (15.7%)
	Paroxetine	13 (11.3%)
	Bupropion	2 (1.7%)
	Duloxetine	41 (35.7%)
Antipsychotics		3 (2.6%)
	Chlorpromazine	1 (0.9%)
	Levomepromazine	2 (1.7%)
Other drugs		49 (47.8%)
	Ranitidine	25 (21.7%)
	Celecoxib	46 (40.0%)
	Amiodarone	3 (2.6%)

* Patients may consume more than one drug simultaneously.

Table 3. Evaluation of efficacy and safety by study group.

Study groups	No combinations	Venlafaxine/substrate	Venlafaxine/inhibitor
Number of patients	**N = 744**	**N = 256**	**N = 115**
Hamilton scale score			
Mean baseline score	15.3 (4.3)	14.9 (4.2)	15.3 (4.2)
Mean final score	8.1 (3.3)	8.6 (3.3)*	9.1 (3.6)*
Reduction in score	−7.2	−6.3*	−6.2*
Evaluation of initial Hamilton scale score			
Mild depression (8–13 points)	35.5%	37.7%	37.1%
Moderate depression (14–18 points)	37.2%	40.0%	33.1%
Severe/very severe depression (≥19 points)	27.2%	22.3%	29.8%
Evaluation of final Hamilton scale score			
Not depressed (0–7 points)	61.6%	51.5%†	44.6%†
Mild depression (8–13 points)	25.9%	33.9%*	34.3%*
Moderate depression (14–18 points)	12.5%	14.6%*	21.1%†
Response to treatment			
≥ 50%	49.1%	39.9%†	34.3%†
25–49%	19.1%	18.6%	21.7%*
≤24%	31.8%	41.5%†	44.0%†
Remission of symptoms	59.9%	50.2%‡	43.8%‡
Safety/adverse reactions	N = 14 (1.9%)	N = 18 (7.0%)†	N = 7 (6.1%)*

Values expressed as percentages or means (standard deviation).
* Paired comparisons using the *No combination* group as the reference; p value in comparisons between groups: *p<0.05, †p<0.01, ‡p<0.001.

metabolizers. A study that pooled data from four clinical trials of patients with MDD treated with venlafaxine, found lower efficacy in slow metabolizers. Thus, there is a correlation between the CYP2D6 slow metabolizer phenotype and the response to AD treatment [8].

In addition, there are reports of phenotypic conversion in patients who did not have a slow metabolizer profile, according to genotyping, but who became slow metabolizers as a result of concomitant administration of drugs acting on the CYP2D6 pathway. The recent study by Perskorn of 865 patients treated with venlafaxine found phenotypic conversion to a slow profile in

Table 4. Gross cost model per patient/year according to study groups.

Study groups	No combinations	Venlafaxine/substrate	Venlafaxine/inhibitor
Number of patients	**N = 744**	**N = 256**	**N = 115**
Total healthcare costs*	1,894 (1,671)	3,585 (3,424)	4,393 (3,570)
Primary care costs*	1,356 (1,181)	2,292 (1,696)	2,747 (1,625)
Medical visits	263 (217)	387 (289)	472 (345)
Laboratory tests	109 (77)	149 (90)	159 (90)
Conventional radiology	53 (50)	59 (57)	70 (54)
Complementary tests	39 (59)	57 (77)	56 (69)
Pharmaceutical prescriptions	891 (1,044)	1,640 (1,572)	1,991 (1,449)
Specialist care costs*	538 (964)	1,293 (2,646)	1,646 (2,722)
Medical visits	148 (704)	595 (2,234)	694 (2,261)
Hospitalisation	330 (414)	549 (626)	721 (658)
A&E	60 (124)	150 (325)	231 (415)
Non-healthcare costs*	883 (3,984)	1,457 (6,130)	3,018 (9,426)
Total costs (healthcare/non-healthcare)*	2,777 (4,372)	5,041 (6,890)	7,412 (10,185)

Values expressed as means (standard deviation), in euros; CI: 95% confidence interval. * p<0.05 in all between-group comparisons. Paired comparisons using the *No combination* group as the reference; p value in comparisons between groups: *p<0.05, †p<0.01, ‡p<0.001.

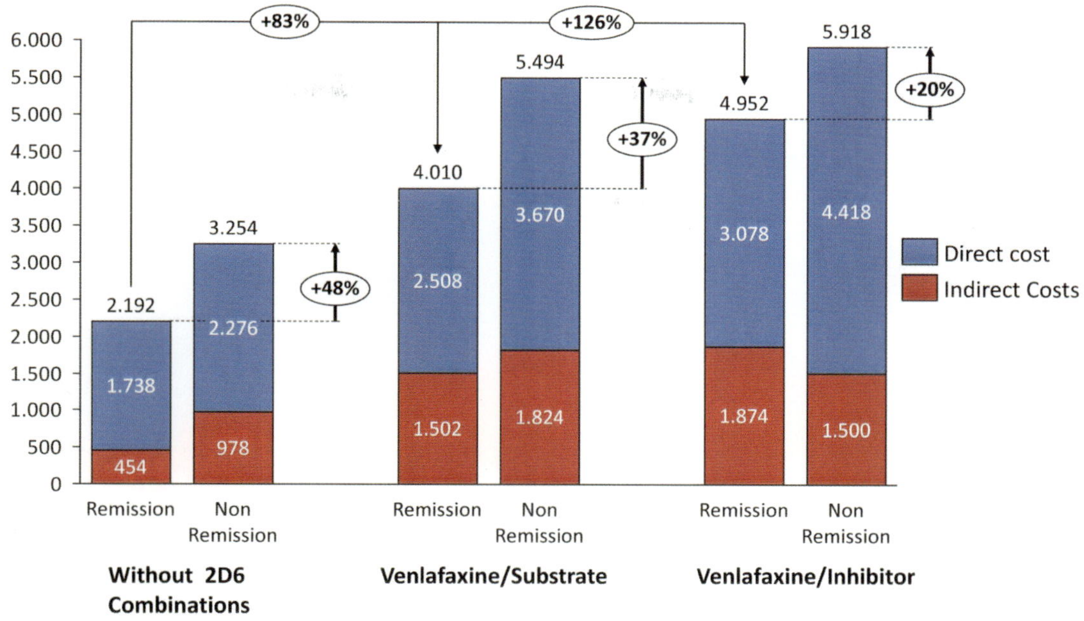

Figure 1. Distribution of healthcare and non-healthcare costs according to treatment response in study groups. Values expressed as means (in Euros).

24% of patients as a consequence of the administration of concomitant drugs, in particular CYP2D6 inhibitors or substrates [11].

The results of our study show that one in three patients with MDD treated with venlafaxine took a CYP2D6 substrate or inhibitor (23% venlafaxine-substrate and 10.3% venlafaxine-inhibitor), similar to the 27% found in the study by Preskorn [11]. In the present study, AD efficacy was greater, as shown both by the lower Hamilton scale scores and the higher percentage of patients with remission of symptoms, in patients in the no-combination group. In addition, there was a higher percentage of adverse events and higher healthcare and non-healthcare costs in patients in the venlafaxine-substrate and venlafaxine-inhibitor groups.

These findings suggest that, in patients with MDD, in whom medical and psychiatric comorbidity is fairly common and who may require various drug therapies, the pharmacokinetic properties of each medication should be taken into account to ensure that the response to and tolerability of AD treatment is not compromised.

Although this was not the objective of the study, the properties of a specific AD with respect to whether it is a CYP2D6 substrate or inhibitor may also affect the efficacy and safety of concomitant therapies. Many drugs are metabolised by CYP2D6, some of which are pro-drugs, metabolised by CYP2D6 into the active drug. These include tamoxifen, which is a selective modulator of the oestrogen receptor indicated for the treatment and prevention of breast cancer [28], which has been shown to reduce the risk of breast cancer by 50% [29]. Many antidepressants are more or less potent inhibitors of CYP2D6 and may affect the efficacy of tamoxifen by not permitting the active drug to be metabolised. A cohort study [26] of 2,430 patients found an increased risk of death related to breast cancer in women taking tamoxifen and concomitant paroxetine with a clear dose-response relationship and an association with the duration of overlap of the two treatments. Similarly, the efficacy of many opioids, such as tramadol, codeine and oxycodone is affected by the concomitant use of an AD that inhibits CYP2D6 [25,27].

Non-detection of polymorphic variations of genotype CYP2D6 that discriminate between slow, fast or intermediate metabolizers and accuracy of diagnosis are the two most important limitations of the study. In addition, there are the limitations inherent to studies using population-based data, such as under-reporting of diseases and possible variations among health professionals in the routine use of the different clinical screening scales. All limitations derived from the retrospective nature of this study are also applicable, primarily those related with quality of data.

Likewise, in the present study, the duration of the drug combinations in each study group was not controlled and, therefore, should be considered as a limitation. Because not all patients were concomitantly taking venlafaxine and substrates/ inhibitors during the whole follow-up period (12 months), we believe that this situation should be interpreted as another limitation of the study. Finally, the most severe cases of MDD and cases where the diagnosis was in doubt may not have been included, as these patients are normally treated at mental health centres.

A possible explanation for the overall results of the study, as well as a practical consequence, could therefore be that patients consuming substrates/inhibitors of CYP2D6 (in combination with venlafaxine) are less healthy, and are consequently expected to have greater use of health resources in the National Health System. Given these limitations, the results of this study show a clear relationship between reduced antidepressant efficacy of venlafaxine and the concomitant administration of CYP2D6 substrates or inhibitors in daily clinical practice. These findings suggest that, when deciding on an antidepressant therapy, the patient's other medication should be evaluated in order to avoid pharmacokinetic interactions that could reduce the efficacy of the antidepressant. Due to the high rate of comorbidity associated with MDD, which requires the use of concomitant medications, the ideal would be to have antidepressants with a simple metabolism that provided a more predictable antidepressant response, especially in patients with comorbidities and polypharmacy.

Author Contributions

Conceived and designed the experiments: ASM RNA PG BA. Performed the experiments: ASM. Analyzed the data: ASM. Contributed reagents/materials/analysis tools: ASM. Wrote the paper: ASM. Authorship and manuscript review: ASM PG BA MBT RNA. Final approval of manuscript: ASM PG BA MBT RNA.

References

1. Mathers CD, Loncar D (2006) Projections of global mortality and burden of disease from 2002 to 2030. PLoS Med 3: e442.
2. Haro JM, Palacín C, Vilagut G, Martínez M, Bernal M, et al. (2006) Prevalencia de los trastornos mentales y factores asociados: resultados del estudio ESEMeD-España. Med Clin (Barc) 126: 445–51.
3. Sicras-Mainar A, Blanca-Tamayo M, Gutiérrez-Nicuesa L, Salvatella-Pasant J, Navarro-Artieda R (2010) Impacto de la morbilidad, uso de recursos y costes en el mantenimiento de la remisión de la depresión mayor en España: estudio longitudinal de ámbito poblacional. Gac Sanit 24: 13–9.
4. Bellón JA, Moreno-Küstner B, Torres-González F, Montón-Franco C, GildeGómez-Barragán MJ, et al. (2008) Predicting the onset and persistence of episodes of depression in primary health care. The predictD-Spain study: methodology. BMC Public Health 25; 8: 256.
5. Keller MB (2003) Past, present and future directions for defining optimal treatment outcome in depression: remission and beyond. JAMA 289: 3152–60.
6. Clark K, Weir C (2012) A review of depression prevention in primary care. W V Med J 108: 64–8.
7. Preskorn SH (2010) Understanding outliers on the usual dose-response curve: Venlafaxine as a way to phenotype patients in terms of their CYP 2D6 status and why it matters. J Psychiatr Pract 16: 46–49.
8. Lobello KW, Preskorn SH, Guico-Pabia CJ, Jiang Q, Paul J, et al. (2010) Cytochrome P450 2D6 phenotype predicts antidepressant efficacy of venlafaxine: a secondary analysis of 4 studies in major depressive disorder. J Clin Psychiatry 71: 1482–7.
9. Sachse C, Brockmöller J, Bauer S, Roots I (1997) Cytochrome P450 2D6 variants in a Caucasian population: allele frequencies and phenotypic consequences. Am J Hum Genet 60: 284–95.
10. Zanger UM, Raimundo S, Eichelbaum M (2004) Cytochrome P450 2D6: overview and update on pharmacology, genetics, biochemistry. Naunyn Schmiedebergs Arch Pharmacol 369: 23–37.
11. Preskorn SH, Kane CP, Lobello K, Nichols AI, Fayyad R, et al. (2013) Cytochrome P450 2D6 phenoconversion is common in patients being treated for depression: implications for personalized medicine. J Clin Psychiatry 74: 614–21.
12. Otton SV, Ball SE, Cheung SW, Inaba T, Rudolph RL, et al. (1996) Venlafaxine oxidation in vitro is catalysed by CYP2D6. Br J Clin Pharmacol 41: 149–56.
13. Nichols AI, Lobello K, Guico-Pabia CJ, Paul J, Preskorn SH (2009) Venlafaxine metabolism as a marker of cytochrome P450 enzyme 2D6 metabolizer status. J Clin Psychopharmacol 29: 383–6.
14. Lamberts H, Wood M, Hofmans-Okkes IM (1993) The International Classification of Primary Care in the European Community. With a multi-language layer. Oxford: Oxford University Press.
15. American Psychiatric Association (2008) Diagnostic and Statistical Manual of Mental Disorders IV - Text Revision (DSM-IV-TR). Washington: American Psychiatric Association.
16. Conde V, Franch JL (1984) Escalas de evaluación comportamental para la cuantificación de la sintomatología psicopatológica en los trastornos angustiosos y depresivos. Departamento de psicología médica y de psiquiatría del Hospital Clínico de la Facultad de Medicina de Valladolid.
17. Wade AG, Despiégel N, Danchenko N, Saragoussi D, Verpillat P (2007) How does remission in major depressive disorder impact resource use in UK does: A General Practitioner Research Database (GPRD) based study. 23rd International Conference on Pharmacoepidemiology & Therapeutic Risk Management (ISPE) Québec City Canada, 19–22 August.
18. Shelton R (2006) Management of major depressive disorders following failure of antidepressant treatment. Prim Psychiatry 12: 73–82.
19. Charlson ME, Pompei P, Ales KL, Mackenzie CR (1987) A new method of classifying prognostic comorbidity in longitudinal studies: development and validation. J Chronic Dis 40: 373–83.
20. Weiner JP, Starfield BH, Steinwachs DM, Mumford LM (1991) Development and application of a population-oriented measure of ambulatory care case-mix. Med Care 29: 452–72.
21. Instituto Nacional de Estadística (2010) Encuesta de costes laborales del año 2010. Available: http://www.ine.es/infoine. Accessed: 2012 Jun.
22. Anonymous. (1991) Guidelines for ATC classification. Oslo: Nordic Collaborating Centre for Drug Statistics Methodology.
23. Preskorn SH, Nichols AI, Paul J, Patroneva AL, Helzner EC, et al. (2008) Effect of desvenlafaxine on the cytochrome P450 2D6 enzyme system. J Psychiatr Pract 14: 368–78.
24. Thompson SG, Barber JA (2000) How should cost data in pragmatic randomised trials be analysed? BMJ 320: 1197–200.
25. Poulsen L, Brøsen K, Arendt-Nielsen L, Gram LF, Elbaek K, et al. (1996) Codeine and morphine in extensive and poor metabolizers of sparteine: pharmacokinetics, analgesic effect and side effects. Eur J Clin Pharmacol 51: 289–95.
26. Kelly CM, Juurlink DN, Gomes T, Duong-Hua M, Pritchard KI, et al. (2010) Selective serotonin reuptake inhibitors and breast cancer mortality in women receiving tamoxifen: a population based cohort study. BMJ 8; 340.
27. Samer CF, Daali Y, Wagner M, Hopfgartner G, Eap CB, et al. (2010) The effects of CYP2D6 and CYP3A activities on the pharmacokinetics of immediate release oxycodone. Br J Pharmacol 160: 907–18.
28. Osborne CK (1998) Tamoxifen in the treatment of breast cancer. N Engl J Med 339: 1609–18.
29. Vogel VG, Costantino JP, Wickerham DL, Cronin WM, Cecchini RS, et al. (2006) National Surgical Adjuvant Breast and Bowel Project (NSABP). Effects of tamoxifen vs raloxifene on the risk of developing invasive breast cancer and other disease outcomes: the NSABP Study of Tamoxifen and Raloxifene (STAR) P-2 trial. JAMA 295: 2727–41.

2

Drinking Pattern, Abstention and Problem Drinking as Risk Factors for Depressive Symptoms: Evidence from Three Urban Eastern European Populations

Steven Bell[1]*, Annie Britton[1], Ruzena Kubinova[2], Sofia Malyutina[3,4], Andrzej Pajak[5], Yuri Nikitin[3], Martin Bobak[1]

1 Research Department of Epidemiology and Public Health, University College London, London, United Kingdom, **2** National Institute of Public Health, Prague, Czech Republic, **3** Institute of Internal and Preventive Medicine, Novosibirsk, Russia, **4** Novosibirsk State Medical University, Novosibirsk, Russia, **5** Institute of Public Health, Jagiellonian University, Krakow, Poland

Abstract

Purpose: To examine whether the frequency and amount of alcohol consumed in binge drinking sessions, total annual volume of alcohol consumed, problem drinking and abstaining from alcohol are associated with depressive symptoms in Eastern Europe.

Subjects and Methods: Cross-sectional data from a total of 24,381 participants from general population samples of the Czech Republic (N = 7,601), Russia (N = 6,908) and Poland (N = 9,872) aged 45–69 years in 2002–2005. Depressive symptoms were defined as ≥16 points on the Centre for Epidemiological Studies - Depression (CES-D) scale. Several alcohol related measures were derived using responses from the graduated frequency questionnaire. Binge drinking was defined at several sex-specific thresholds (ranging from 60+ to 140+ g of ethanol) and two frequencies (at least monthly or weekly). Total annual alcohol intake in grams was also extracted. Problem drinking was defined as ≥2 positive answers on the CAGE questionnaire.

Results: Problem drinking was consistently associated with approximately a 2-fold increase in odds of depressive symptoms across all countries and in both sexes. Abstaining from alcohol was typically associated with increased odds of depressive symptoms. Analyses separating lifelong abstainers and former drinkers in the Russian cohort revealed that this increased odds was driven by former drinkers. Amongst men, heavy frequent binge drinking was associated with increased odds of depressive symptoms in the Czech Republic and Poland. In women, heavy infrequent binge drinking was associated with increased odds of depressive symptoms in Russia and Poland. Only in Polish men was higher annual volume of alcohol intake associated with increased odds of depressive symptoms.

Conclusion: Abstaining from alcohol and problem drinking were associated with increased odds of depressive symptoms in these Eastern European populations. Annual volume of alcohol intake as well as frequency and amount of alcohol consumed in a binge drinking session were less consistently associated with depressive symptoms.

Editor: Antonio Verdejo García, University of Granada, Spain

Funding: SB was supported by a UK Economic and Social Research Council PhD Studentship. Both SB and AB are currently funded by the European Research Council (309337, PI: Britton, http://www.ucl.ac.uk/alcohol-lifecourse). The HAPIEE study was supported by grants from the Wellcome Trust (064947/Z, 081081/Z), the US National Institute of Aging (1R01 AG23522) and the MacArthur Foundation. The funders had no role in study design, data collection and analysis, decision to publish, or preparation of the manuscript.

Competing Interests: The authors have declared that no competing interests exist.

* Email: steven.bell@ucl.ac.uk

Introduction

Depression [1–3] and alcohol consumption [4] are widely acknowledged as important public health problems and there is ample evidence that the two are related [5,6]. The majority of research on the topic has focussed on the relationship between clinical disorders [7–9] with less attention drawn to the association between alcohol intake and depressive symptoms in the general (non-clinical) population [10,11]. Studies that have looked at the relationship between alcohol intake and depressive symptoms have produced conflicting findings [10–14].

Both the prevalence of depression [15,16] and alcohol consumption [4] are high in Eastern Europe compared to other regions. Little is known about the extent to which drinking patterns in this region, marked by heavy alcohol consumption and binge drinking [4,17], are linked with the high prevalence of depression. Examining the association between drinking pattern and depressive symptoms in populations with both high overall volume of alcohol intake combined with a pattern of heavy episodic drinking would allow for comparisons to be made to other drinking cultures whereby overall drinking volume is similar but drinking pattern is different (for example, Southern Europe [4]) or where drinking pattern is similar but overall volume of intake is lower (e.g. the Nordic regions [4]) to determine the extent to which drinking pattern plays a role in the development of depressive symptoms or whether it is mostly due to overall volume consumed.

Differentiating between different patterns of heavy drinking has been particularly encouraged in the context of Eastern Europe where a high prevalence of episodic heavy drinking exists [18–20]. Yet little research has specifically focussed on the effect of increasing dose of alcohol consumed per occasion *and* frequency of consuming these different doses of alcohol as risk factors for depression. It is probable that the biological effect of alcohol on the brain/body depends on cumulative dose, therefore examining the effect of different doses of consumption as well as the frequency of drinking makes intuitive sense. Others have, however, argued that it is problem drinking which is harmful to psychological health [21], but surprisingly few studies have examined the relationship between problem drinking and depression in Eastern Europe [22,23]. On the other spectrum of drinking, the extent to which non-drinking is associated with depression is also underexplored. The main uncertainty here relates to the degree to which the supposed beneficial psychological effects of moderate consumption [24,25] may be confounded by including former drinkers alongside lifelong abstainers in the non-drinking group [26,27].

Given the paucity of research on these important public health issues, the purpose of this study was to determine the extent to which binge drinking at different intensities (i.e. doses) and frequencies (e.g. on a monthly or weekly basis), annual drinking volume, problem drinking and abstention from alcohol are related to depressive symptoms in Eastern Europe.

Materials and Methods

Ethical statement

The University College London Hospital Research Ethics Committee Alpha approved the HAPIEE study. Ethical approval was also obtained from local research ethics committees at each HAPIEE site: National Institute of Public Health Ethics Committee (Prague, the Czech Republic), Jagellonian University Medical College Bioethics Committee (Krakow, Poland), and Institute of Internal and Preventive Medicine Ethics Committee (Novosibirsk, Russia). Participants provided written, informed consent.

The HAPIEE Study

Cross-sectional data from the baseline wave (2003–2005) of the Health, Alcohol and Psychosocial factors in Eastern Europe (HAPIEE) study [28] were used to explore the relationship between drinking pattern, problem drinking and abstaining from alcohol as risk factors for depressive symptoms. The study randomly recruited individuals aged between 45 to 69 years from electoral lists in Novosibirsk (Russia), and population registers in Krakow (Poland), Havirov/Karvina, Hradec Kralove, Jihlava, Kromeriz, Liberec and Usti nad Labem (Czech Republic). Questionnaires were identical across study sites and were translated to each language and back-translated to English to ensure comparability. The only difference between centres was the fact that the Polish questionnaire also included a filter question allowing those who reported not drinking[i] in the previous 12 months to skip the other questions in the alcohol section. A total of 28,947 subjects (overall response rate of 59%) were recruited. The analytic sample consisted of 24, 381 individuals after those with missing information on depressive symptom status (N = 3,274), alcohol consumption (N = 376) and covariates (N = 509) were excluded (categories not mutually exclusive). A multivariable logistic regression model revealed that those with missing data were more likely to have lower educational attainment and belong to the high deprivation group.

Assessment of dose and frequency of binge drinking

Data on drinking patterns come from the graduated frequency questionnaire [29,30]. The graduated frequency questionnaire asks participants how often in the previous 12 months they consumed more than *X* amount of alcohol with separate doses, equivalent to: ≥10 g, ≥40 g, ≥60 g, ≥100 g, ≥140 g and ≥ 180 g of pure ethanol (based on original local units defined as 0.5 litre of beer, 0.2 litre of wine and 0.05 litre of spirits, ranging from "10 and above" to "less than one" - 100 ml of beer, wine and spirit was assumed to contain 4 g, 10 g, or 36 g of ethanol, respectively). There were nine frequency responses, spanning from never to daily.

Given gender differences in alcohol consumption and metabolism [31], combined with low cell counts for certain response categories in women, separate binge drinking variables were derived for men and women. In men it was coded as follows: (1, reference category) always consuming between 1–59 g of alcohol per single drinking occasion, (2) consuming 60+ g on an occasional basis (defined as less than monthly), (3) 60–99 g in a single sitting at least monthly, (4) 100–139 g in a single sitting at least monthly, (5) 140+g in a single sitting at least monthly, (6) 60–99 g in a single sitting at least weekly, (7) 100–139 g in a single sitting at least weekly, (8) 140+g in a single sitting at least weekly and (9) past-year abstainers (those who reported no alcohol consumption in the previous 12 months on the graduated frequency questionnaire). For women, categories 4 and 5, and 7 and 8 were combined to form 100+g on an at least monthly or weekly basis respectively. We used frequency to determine the category drinkers belonged to in cases whereby participants reported exceeding one threshold on a monthly basis and another on a weekly basis (e.g. if a participant consumed 140+ g on a monthly basis and 60–99 g on a weekly basis then they would be classified as belonging to the 60–99 g on a weekly basis group). The rationale behind this decision is that frequency better reflects usual drinking habits than overall amount alone. Approximately 18 and 11% of men categorised as belonging to the 60–99 g in a single sitting on a weekly basis category drank 100 g or 140 g in a single occasion on a monthly basis, respectively. Around 19% of men belonging to the 100–139 g on a weekly basis category drank 140+ g in a single drinking episode on a monthly basis. Almost 13% of women belonging to the category of 60–99 g in a single sitting on a weekly basis drank 100+ g on one occasion monthly.

The purpose of deriving this variable was to compare each dose/frequency category (as well as abstention) with a non-binge drinking reference group always consuming between 1 and <59 g of alcohol per occasion; not simply, for example, looking at those who drank ≥100 grams in a single sitting on a monthly basis compared to those who did not consume this amount (a category which would then also include participants who were themselves binge drinkers albeit at a lower threshold). However, for the sake of completeness, we also estimated models examining the relationship between frequency of consuming 60+, 100+ and 140+g and depressive symptoms separately. For each dose of alcohol, frequency responses were as follows: (1) never, (2) 1–11 times per year, (3) 1–3 times per month, (4) weekly, and (5) past year abstainers. At doses of 100+ and 140+ g per occasion the category of never was divided into those always consuming between 1–59 g of alcohol per single drinking occasion (referent) and those who drank above 60 g but always less than *X* g per occasion. The estimates from these models can be found in *Information S1*.

Drinking volume

From the graduated frequency we also derived a measure of total volume of alcohol consumed in the previous year. We categorised consumption levels above 240 g (a threshold reflecting less than one drink per month) into sex-specific tertiles of consumption derived from the entire sample. These were 260–1740 g, 1750–6020 g and >6400 g for men, and 260–420 g, 430–1200 g and >1210 g for women. The final variable used in analyses consisted of the following categories: (1) abstainers, (2) ≤ 240 g per annum, (3) first tertile of consumption, (4) second tertile of consumption (reference category), and (5) third tertile of consumption.

Problem drinking

Problem drinking was assessed using the CAGE questionnaire [32,33]. CAGE is an acronym of the first four letters of the key words in each question: 1) "Have you ever felt you should Cut down on your drinking?", 2) "Have people ever Annoyed you by criticising your drinking?", 3) "Have you ever felt bad or Guilty about your drinking?", and 4) "Have you ever had a drink first thing in the morning to steady your nerves or get rid of a hangover (as an "Eye opener")?". Positive responses to two or more of the questions are commonly used as an indicator of problem drinking [34].

Former drinkers and lifelong abstainers

In the Russian cohort those who reported having not consumed alcohol in the past 12 months were asked whether they had previously consumed alcohol. These questions were used to stratify the abstainer group into former drinkers and life-long abstainers.

Assessment of depressive symptoms

Depressive symptoms were assessed using the 20-item Center for Epidemiologic Studies Depression (CES-D) scale [35]. The CES-D is a self-report questionnaire aimed to measure the presence of depressive symptoms in the past week (e.g. "I felt depressed" or "I was bothered by things that usually don't bother me"). Items are scored on a 4-point Likert scale, with response options relating to how frequent the participant experienced each of the 20 symptoms: (0) rarely or none of the time (less than 1 day); (1) some or a little of the time (1–2 days); (2) occasionally or a moderate amount of time (3–4 days); and (3) most or all of the time (5–7 days). Scores were combined to form an aggregate depression score on a scale of 0 to 60 and those with scores of 16 or above were considered to have depressive symptoms [36,37]. This threshold has been demonstrated to have acceptable specificity and sensitivity in comparison to clinical interview based measures of depressive disorder [38,39].

Covariates

The following covariates were used in analyses: age, marital status (married/cohabiting [reference category], single, divorced/separated and widowed) [40,41], educational attainment (university, secondary/vocational [reference category], primary or less) [42,43], material deprivation level score [44,45] which was based on three questions concerning how often the participants' household did not have enough money to buy food or clothes, or to pay bills such as housing, heating and electricity, with the possible answers "never", "rarely", "sometimes", "often" or "all the time", coded as 0–4. These items were summed and then categorised into three groups: low (reference category; scores of 0–1), intermediate (scores of 2–8) and high (scores of 9–12). Smoking status (never smoked [reference category], current smoker, ex-smoker) was also controlled for [40,46].

Statistical Analysis

Logistic regression was used to estimate odds ratios (ORs) and associated 95% confidence intervals (CIs) for depressive symptoms by binge drinking dose/frequency, annual volume of alcohol intake as well as problem drinking. Separate models were fitted for each drinking measure as including all drinking components in the same model would likely represent over-adjustment [47] and therefore bias the effect estimates (estimates from models including all drinking variables simultaneously are made available for interested readers in *Information S2*).

To compare the consistency of associations across countries, we tested for interactions between drinking variables and cohort; we found p-values <0.01 in all interaction tests. Models were further stratified by gender (frequency/dose variables differed by sex). Within all centres, we present two models: model 1 was adjusted for age only, and model 2 was adjusted for all covariates.

All models were fitted using Stata 13.1 [48]. An alpha level of 0.05 was considered statistically significant for all analyses.

Results

Sample composition

Table 1 outlines descriptive statistics by country and gender. Briefly, among men, problem drinking was more common in Russia followed by Poland and the Czech Republic. Binge drinking in general was also more common in Russian men with almost 30% of respondents reporting binge drinking on a weekly basis compared to approximately 18% of Czech Republic men and 7% of Polish men. Men from the Czech Republic and Russia consumed a higher volume of alcohol annually than those from Poland. A greater proportion of Polish men abstained from alcohol in the previous year, followed by Russia and the Czech Republic. Depressive symptoms were also more common in Polish men.

Among women, abstaining rates were high in Poland doubling the rate of both Russia and the Czech Republic. Problem drinking was highest for women from the Czech Republic followed by those from Russia and Poland. A greater proportion of those from the Czech Republic and Russia engaged in binge drinking on a monthly or weekly basis, although the behaviour was not common in any country (especially heavy binge drinking). Women from the Czech Republic had a higher annual intake of alcohol than women from Russia and Poland. Depressive symptoms were more common amongst women; almost a quarter of women from the Czech Republic and, 34 and 33% of women from Russia and Poland were identified as having depressive symptoms.

Regression estimates

For men (Table 2), in the Czech Republic significant increased odds of depressive symptoms were observed for those drinking 140+g on a weekly basis (OR 1.92, CI 1.16–3.17) in comparison to those always drinking <60 g in a single sitting. In Poland, binge drinking on a weekly basis was associated with increased odds of depressive symptoms irrespective of the amount consumed in a single session (however upon adjustment for confounding factors the effects were attenuated). Russian men who consumed between 100 to 139 g of ethanol in a single sitting on a monthly basis had lower odds of depressive symptoms (OR 0.53, CI 0.31–0.89) than those who always drank <60 g in a single sitting and this reduced odds was maintained after adjustment for confounding factors (OR 0.47, CI 0.28–0.81). Men who abstained from alcohol in the previous 12 months also had higher odds of depressive symptoms

Table 1. Descriptive information by country and sex.

	Czech				Russia				Poland			
	Men		Women		Men		Women		Men		Women	
	N	%	N	%	N	%	N	%	N	%	N	%
Depressive symptoms												
No	3052	86.2	3092	76.2	2636	85.0	2526	66.4	3789	79.3	3412	67.0
Yes	489	13.8	968	23.8	465	15.0	1281	33.6	988	20.7	1683	33.0
Drinking session dose/frequency												
Abstainer	227	6.4	738	18.2	418	13.5	620	16.3	1090	22.8	2439	47.9
Always <60 g in a single sitting	887	25.1	2091	51.5	444	14.3	2451	64.4	1511	31.6	2069	40.6
60+g occasionally	1091	30.8	837	20.6	579	18.7	464	12.2	1215	25.4	443	8.7
60–99 g monthly	450	12.7	226	5.6	358	11.5	173	4.5	361	7.6	87	1.7
100–139 g† monthly	159	4.5	78	1.9	205	6.6	32	0.8	131	2.7	26	0.5
140+g monthly	107	3.0	--	--	170	5.5	--	--	152	3.2	--	--
60–99 g weekly	399	11.3	56	1.4	462	14.9	53	1.4	186	3.9	23	0.5
100–139 g† weekly	121	3.4	34	0.8	259	8.4	14	0.4	62	1.3	8	0.2
140+g weekly	100	2.8	--	--	206	6.6	--	--	69	1.4	--	--
Annual drinking volume												
Abstainer	227	6.4	738	18.2	418	13.5	620	16.3	1090	22.8	2439	47.9
<=240 g	389	11.0	1165	28.7	137	4.4	1274	33.5	565	11.8	1185	23.3
1st tertile	753	21.3	388	9.6	757	24.4	933	24.5	1315	27.5	423	8.3
2nd tertile	888	25.1	669	16.5	820	26.4	581	15.3	1140	23.9	589	11.6
3rd tertile	1284	36.3	1100	27.1	969	31.3	399	10.5	667	14.0	458	9.00
CAGE score												
<2	2940	90.0	3193	97.3	2066	77.0	3126	98.1	3198	88.2	2556	98.3
2+	326	10.0	88	2.7	617	23.0	61	1.9	430	11.8	45	1.7
Age (mean, SD)	3541	58.4 (7.2)	4060	57.7 (7.1)	3101	58.1 (7.0)	3807	57.9 (7.1)	4777	57.9 (7.0)	5095	57.5 (7.0)
Marital status												
Married/cohabiting	2976	84.0	2776	68.4	2743	88.5	2308	60.6	4139	86.6	3399	66.7
Single	105	3.0	98	2.4	70	2.3	172	4.5	197	4.1	357	7.0
Divorced/separated	347	9.8	615	15.1	166	5.4	549	14.4	261	5.5	465	9.1
Widowed	113	3.2	571	14.1	122	3.9	778	20.4	180	3.8	874	17.2
Educational attainment												
Primary or less	205	5.8	725	17.9	182	5.9	227	6.0	464	9.7	718	14.1
Secondary/vocational	2667	75.3	2900	71.4	1870	60.3	2524	66.3	2920	61.1	3025	59.4
University	669	18.9	435	10.7	1049	33.8	1056	27.7	1393	29.2	1352	26.5
Smoking status												

Table 1. Cont.

	Czech				Russia				Poland			
	Men		Women		Men		Women		Men		Women	
	N	%	N	%	N	%	N	%	N	%	N	%
Never	1121	31.7	2214	54.5	759	24.5	3225	84.7	1325	27.7	2602	51.1
Current	1055	29.8	962	23.7	1505	48.5	392	10.3	1717	35.9	1442	28.3
Former	1365	38.6	884	21.8	837	27.0	190	5.0	1735	36.3	1051	20.6
Material deprivation												
Low	2247	66.3	2396	59.0	1462	47.2	961	25.2	2854	59.7	2544	49.9
Intermediate	1140	32.2	1580	38.9	1493	48.2	2498	65.6	1680	35.2	2203	43.2
High	54	1.5	84	2.1	146	4.7	348	9.1	243	5.09	348	6.8

†The figures presented for the category of 100–139 g in a single sitting for women also contain those drinking 140+ g; see methods section. Some percentage totals may exceed 100 due to rounding.

in the Czech Republic (adjusted OR 1.55, CI 1.05–2.28) as well as Poland (adjusted OR 1.59, CI 1.31–1.94). In terms of annual volume of alcohol consumed, those who abstained from alcohol had consistently higher odds of depressive symptoms than those in the second tertile of consumption (after full adjustment this effect was attenuated and became non-significant in the Czech Republic but the overall OR continued to indicate increased odds). In Russia and Poland, those drinking ≤240 g of alcohol annually had increased odds of depressive symptoms when compared to those in the second tertile of consumption, as did those belonging to the first tertile of consumption in Russia (adjusted OR 1.39, CI 1.04, 1.87). Only in Poland was there an increased risk in the third tertile of annual alcohol consumption (adjusted OR 1.42, CI 1.11, 1.81)

For women (Table 3), those who abstained from alcohol in the previous 12 months had increased odds of depressive symptoms when compared to those always drinking <60 g in a single sitting in the Czech Republic (adjusted OR 1.30, CI 1.07–1.59) and Poland (adjusted OR 1.35, CI 1.18, 1.54). In the Czech Republic, women consuming 100 g+ on a weekly basis had increased odds of depressive symptoms (OR 2.45, CI 1.23–4.90) however this was attenuated after controlling for confounding factors (OR 1.93, CI 0.94–3.96). In both Russia (adjusted OR 3.31, CI 1.52–6.55) and Poland (adjusted OR 2.84, CI 1.26–6.41) women consuming 100+ g on a monthly basis had increased odds of depressive symptoms in comparison to those who always drank <60 g in a single sitting. When looking at differences in the odds of depressive symptoms by total volume of alcohol consumed in the previous year, abstainers in all countries had higher odds than those in the second tertile of alcohol intake. In Russia, those with an intake of ≤240 g had higher odds of depressive symptoms (adjusted OR 1.31, CI 1.05–1.64).

Problem drinking was consistently associated with increased odds of depressive symptoms across all countries in both men (Table 2) and women (Table 3).

When stratifying the abstainer group into former drinkers and life-long abstainers (Table 4) in the Russian cohort, neither abstainer category had increased odds of depressive symptoms compared to those always drinking <60 g in a single sitting for men, while for women, former drinkers had increased odds (adjusted OR 1.37, CI 1.09–1.72) but not lifelong abstainers. Former drinkers had higher odds of depressive symptoms in all models relating to annual alcohol intake in comparison to those in the second tertile of consumption (adjusted ORs of 1.55, CI 1.10, 2.17 and 1.64, CI 1.23, 2.17 for men and women respectively).

Discussion

Summary of findings

In this large population based study in Eastern Europe, we found that problem drinking was consistently associated with an increased prevalence of depressive symptoms in all populations and both sexes. With binge drinking, the results were slightly less consistent. In men, frequent heavy binge drinking (140+ g in a sitting at least once a week) was associated with increased odds of depressive symptoms in the Czech Republic and Poland. Interestingly, Russian men who drank 100–139 g of alcohol in a single sitting on a monthly basis had lower odds of depressive symptoms than those always drinking less than 60 g in a single sitting. Among women, there was a tendency for those who engaged in heavy binge drinking (100+g in a single sitting) to have higher odds of depressive symptoms but the odds ratios were not statistically significant in the case of at least weekly binge drinking.

Table 2. Odds ratios (95% confidence intervals) for depressive symptoms by binge drinking dose/frequency, annual drinking volume and problem drinking by country in men.

	Czech (N = 3541)		Russia (N = 3101)		Poland (N = 4777)	
	Age adjusted	Fully adjusted‡	Age adjusted	Fully adjusted	Age adjusted	Fully adjusted
Binge drinking dose/frequency						
Abstainer	1.73** [1.19,2.51]	1.55* [1.05,2.28]	1.12 [0.79,1.59]	1.03 [0.71,1.48]	1.67*** [1.38,2.01]	1.59*** [1.31,1.94]
Always <60 g in a single sitting	1.00 (ref.)	1.00 (ref.)	1.00 (ref.)	1.00 (ref.)	1.00 (ref.)	1.00 (ref.)
60+g occasionally	0.88 [0.68,1.16]	0.98 [0.74,1.28]	0.77 [0.55,1.08]	0.77 [0.55,1.10]	0.88 [0.72,1.08]	0.88 [0.72,1.08]
60–99 g monthly	0.92 [0.66,1.30]	1.01 [0.71,1.44]	0.86 [0.59,1.25]	0.81 [0.55,1.21]	0.98 [0.73,1.31]	0.92 [0.68,1.25]
100–139 g monthly	0.91 [0.55,1.51]	1.01 [0.60,1.69]	0.53* [0.31,0.89]	0.47** [0.28,0.81]	1.06 [0.68,1.67]	0.97 [0.61,1.55]
140+g monthly	1.30 [0.76,2.23]	1.18 [0.68,2.05]	1.18 [0.75,1.87]	1.02 [0.63,1.66]	0.78 [0.50,1.24]	0.67 [0.42,1.07]
60–99 g weekly	0.84 [0.59,1.21]	0.83 [0.57,1.21]	0.66* [0.45,0.97]	0.68 [0.46,1.00]	1.44* [1.01,2.06]	1.38 [0.95,2.01]
100–139 g weekly	0.92 [0.52,1.62]	0.89 [0.50,1.59]	0.78 [0.51,1.21]	0.77 [0.49,1.21]	2.36** [1.38,4.04]	1.71 [0.96,3.04]
140+g weekly	1.92* [1.16,3.17]	1.67 [1.00,2.81]	0.98 [0.62,1.53]	0.83 [0.52,1.32]	1.93* [1.14,3.26]	1.53 [0.88,2.65]
Annual drinking volume						
Abstainer	1.72** [1.18,2.50]	1.43 [0.97,2.11]	1.64** [1.18,2.26]	1.55** [1.11,2.17]	1.89*** [1.53,2.32]	1.88*** [1.52,2.34]
≤240 g	1.08 [0.76,1.52]	0.99 [0.70,1.41]	1.68* [1.05,2.69]	1.61 [0.99,2.63]	1.25 [0.96,1.62]	1.32* [1.01,1.72]
1st tertile	0.97 [0.73,1.28]	0.97 [0.73,1.30]	1.36* [1.02,1.81]	1.39* [1.04,1.87]	1.04 [0.84,1.28]	1.08 [0.87,1.34]
2nd tertile	1.00 (ref.)	1.00 (ref.)	1.00 (ref.)	1.00 (ref.)	1.00 (ref.)	1.00 (ref.)
3rd tertile	0.87 [0.68,1.12]	0.83 [0.64,1.07]	1.18 [0.90,1.56]	1.17 [0.88,1.55]	1.48** [1.17,1.88]	1.42** [1.11,1.81]
Problem drinking†						
No	1.00 (ref.)	1.00 (ref.)	1.00 (ref.)	1.00 (ref.)	1.00 (ref.)	1.00 (ref.)
Yes	2.18*** [1.65,2.89]	2.09*** [1.56,2.78]	1.82*** [1.44,2.31]	1.66*** [1.29,2.13]	3.17*** [2.55,3.94]	2.76*** [2.20,3.48]

*** $p<0.001$;
** $p<0.01$;
* $p<0.05$.
†Models concerning problem drinking (CAGE score 2+) are restricted to those who consumed alcohol in the previous 12 months (Czech N = 3266, Russia N = 2683, Poland N = 3828).
‡Full adjustment = age, marital status, educational attainment, material deprivation level and smoking status.

Abstaining from alcohol was also associated with increased odds of depressive symptoms in comparison to moderate drinking except in Russia; however, compared to the second tertile of annual alcohol consumption, abstainers had consistently higher odds of depressive symptoms. Analyses attempting to disentangle lifelong non-drinkers from former drinkers typically revealed significantly increased odds of depressive symptoms in former drinkers.

Interpretation and comparison to other work

These findings corroborate previous studies in Central and Eastern Europe which have found binge drinking to be associated with increased rates of depressive symptoms [22], including earlier analyses of the HAPIEE data [15]. However, the models used previously [15] differ substantially from those used here. The previous analyses used a relatively low dose of alcohol (<20 g, including abstainers) as the reference category (in comparison to the referent group used in this study, i.e. always consuming <60 g in a single sitting and excluding abstainers) and they used the mean dose of alcohol in a single drinking session as the main exposure (using a maximum dose of ≥80 g). While the previous analyses found increased odds of depressive symptoms in binge drinkers, the previous definition did not take into account the frequency of binge drinking or the graded increase in the amount of alcohol consumed in a binge drinking session (i.e. different doses above 60 g). When the intensity and frequency of binge drinking are accounted for, as in our analyses, it appears that both elements are important in terms of the association with depressive symptoms.

An unexpected finding was that Russian men who consumed 100–139 g in a single sitting at least monthly had lower odds of depressive symptoms than those who always consumed less than 60 g in a drinking occasion. A possible explanation for this finding is that those who drank heavily did so with friends and therefore social participation served as a protective factor against depression, whilst also increasing the opportunity to drink at hazardous levels [49,50]. However, given that this result was not replicated in the Czech Republic or Polish cohorts (or in women) appropriate caution should be applied in the interpretation this this finding.

To our knowledge only one other study has examined abstaining from alcohol as a risk factor for poor mental health in Eastern Europe, focussing on Russian men [51]. Our findings are generally consistent with that study in that we found abstaining was not associated with greater odds of depressive symptoms in Russia when looking at drinking pattern (effect estimates indicated poorer mental health for abstaining Russians in both studies but these effects did not reach statistical significance) but in analyses of the association between annual drinking volume and depressive symptoms, Russians who abstained from alcohol actually had significantly increased odds of depression.

Table 3. Odds ratios (95% confidence intervals) for depressive symptoms by binge drinking dose/frequency, annual drinking volume and problem drinking by country in women.

	Czech (N = 4060)		Russia (N = 3807)		Poland (N = 5095)	
	Age adjusted	Fully adjusted‡	Age adjusted	Fully adjusted	Age adjusted	Fully adjusted
Binge drinking dose/frequency						
Abstainer	1.48*** [1.22,1.79]	1.30** [1.07,1.59]	1.19 [0.99,1.44]	1.14 [0.94,1.37]	1.43*** [1.25,1.62]	1.35*** [1.18,1.54]
Always <60 g in a single sitting	1.00 (ref.)	1.00 (ref.)	1.00 (ref.)	1.00 (ref.)	1.00 (ref.)	1.00 (ref.)
60+g occasionally	1.06 [0.88,1.29]	1.10 [0.90,1.35]	0.91 [0.73,1.13]	0.85 [0.68,1.07]	1.24 [1.00,1.55]	1.17 [0.93,1.47]
60–99 g monthly	0.80 [0.56,1.14]	0.81 [0.57,1.17]	1.02 [0.73,1.43]	1.01 [0.72,1.41]	0.99 [0.62,1.59]	0.90 [0.54,1.48]
100+g monthly	1.46 [0.89,2.41]	1.38 [0.82,2.32]	3.31** [1.62,6.77]	3.16** [1.52,6.55]	2.85** [1.31,6.19]	2.84* [1.26,6.41]
60–99 g weekly	1.06 [0.56,1.99]	1.09 [0.57,2.08]	1.22 [0.69,2.16]	1.26 [0.71,2.25]	0.86 [0.34,2.20]	0.81 [0.31,2.13]
100+g weekly	2.45* [1.23,4.90]	1.93 [0.94,3.96]	1.30 [0.43,3.90]	0.96 [0.31,2.97]	1.47 [0.35,6.17]	1.53 [0.34,6.86]
Annual drinking volume						
Abstainer	1.52*** [1.19,1.95]	1.32* [1.02,1.70]	1.39** [1.09,1.78]	1.37* [1.06,1.76]	1.56*** [1.28,1.91]	1.48*** [1.19,1.83]
≤240 g annually	1.14 [0.90,1.43]	1.11 [0.88,1.41]	1.31* [1.06,1.63]	1.31* [1.05,1.64]	1.22 [0.98,1.52]	1.18 [0.94,1.49]
1st tertile	1.05 [0.78,1.42]	0.97 [0.71,1.32]	1.04 [0.83,1.30]	1.10 [0.87,1.38]	1.01 [0.76,1.34]	1.00 [0.74,1.33]
2nd tertile	1.00 (ref.)	1.00 (ref.)	1.00 (ref.)	1.00 (ref.)	1.00 (ref.)	1.00 (ref.)
3rd tertile	0.98 [0.78,1.24]	1.00 [0.79,1.27]	1.25 [0.95,1.64]	1.28 [0.96,1.69]	1.29 [0.99,1.68]	1.30 [0.99,1.72]
Problem drinking†						
No	1.00 (ref.)	1.00 (ref.)	1.00 (ref.)	1.00 (ref.)	1.00 (ref.)	1.00 (ref.)
Yes	2.36*** [1.52,3.66]	2.28*** [1.45,3.59]	2.51*** [1.51,4.18]	2.38** [1.41,4.03]	3.89*** [2.12,7.16]	3.37*** [1.77,6.42]

*** p<0.001;
** p<0.01;
* p<0.05.
†Models concerning problem drinking (CAGE score 2+) are restricted to those who consumed alcohol in the previous 12 months (Czech N = 3541, Russia N = 3101, Poland N = 4777).
‡Full adjustment = age, marital status, educational attainment, material deprivation level and smoking status.

In our data, problem drinkers had consistently increased odds of depressive symptoms. This finding is in line with previous findings on the topic of depression and alcohol consumption in Eastern Europe [22,23]. In studies elsewhere, problem drinking has been demonstrated to increase the risk of prevalent [9,22,52–56] and incident [6–8,57] depression independent of the amount of alcohol a person consumes or the manner in which that they consume it [21,58].

Table 4. Odds ratios (95% confidence intervals) for former drinkers and lifelong abstainers on depressive symptoms in the Russian HAPIEE cohort.

	Men			Women		
	N	Age adjusted	Fully adjusted‡	N	Age adjusted	Fully adjusted
Binge drinking dose/frequency						
Always <60 g in a single sitting	–	1.00 [1.00,1.00]	1.00 [1.00,1.00]	–	1.00 [1.00,1.00]	1.00 [1.00,1.00]
Former drinker	388	1.12 [0.78,1.59]	1.02 [0.71,1.48]	369	1.41** [1.13,1.77]	1.37** [1.09,1.72]
Lifelong abstainer	30	1.17 [0.46,2.98]	1.07 [0.41,2.80]	251	0.92 [0.70,1.22]	0.86 [0.65,1.14]
Annual drinking volume						
2nd tertile	–	1.00 [1.00,1.00]	1.00 [1.00,1.00]	–	1.00 [1.00,1.00]	1.00 [1.00,1.00]
Former drinker	388	1.63** [1.17, 2.27]	1.55** [1.10, 2.17]	369	1.65*** [1.25, 2.18]	1.64*** [1.23, 2.17]
Lifelong abstainer	30	1.72 [0.69, 4.33]	1.63 [0.63, 4.23]	251	1.07 [0.78, 1.48]	1.03 [0.74, 1.43]

*** p<0.001;
** p<0.01;
* p<0.05.
‡Full adjustment = age, marital status, educational attainment, material deprivation level and smoking status.

Strengths and weaknesses

Specific strengths of this analysis include the large sample size of each country – providing relatively good statistical power (with certain exceptions outlined below). Furthermore, standardised internationally validated tools were used to collect information on individual drinking episodes and depressive symptoms. Data from the graduated frequency questionnaire were then used to create a variable which took into account both dose and frequency of binge drinking and derive total annual alcohol intake.

There are, however, also several shortcomings. First, these analyses are based on cross-sectional data. It is plausible that the relationship would differ over time and examining the association over multiple occasions may provide additional aetiological insights into the possibly bi-directional relationship between alcohol consumption and depressive symptoms [5,59,60] (that is, depressive symptoms may cause people to drink in binges, and drinking in binges may exacerbate depressive symptoms). Therefore further work using longitudinal data is warranted.

Another limitation is that in some of our statistical models, abstainers had to be grouped into a single aggregate category of past year non-drinkers, although the reasons for present/recent non-drinking are likely to be heterogeneous. Many other investigators have pointed out the weaknesses of using an aggregate group of abstainers [26,27,61] as a comparison group for moderate (and other) drinkers. There are valid concerns that moderate drinking may inadvertently be attributed as having beneficial effects compared to non-drinking when the reality may be that this difference is due to residual confounding [62] or failure to distinguish former drinkers and occasional drinkers from the lifelong abstaining group [27,63]. In our study we were able to stratify the abstainer group into former drinkers and lifelong abstainers in Russia (Table 4). We found that there were increased odds of depressive symptoms amongst former drinkers, supporting the argument that the increased odds of depressive symptoms among abstainers may largely be driven by former drinkers as previously reported elsewhere [64].

A third limitation is that the frequency of consuming <60 g in a single sitting was not taken into account. The reference group used in these analyses may therefore contain a number of occasional or, conversely, frequent drinkers which may bias the relationship observed [27]. However, additional analyses did not detect a significant association between depressive symptoms and drinking frequency in this group (with the exception of Russian women, where those drinking very infrequently (only 1–5 times per year) had increased odds of depression; data not presented). It is also possible that the reference group contains some individuals who have reduced their alcohol consumption over time due to ill-health [65,66]. There was no information available to account for this possibility at baseline, and interpretation of the above findings should be made with this in mind.

Fourth, there may also be concerns about the small number of female binge drinkers identified in the study, especially categories relating to heavy and frequent binge drinking. The odds ratios for female drinkers have wide confidence intervals and should be interpreted with appropriate caution.

A fifth limitation relates to both alcohol and depressive symptom measures being based on self-reported data. Self-report measures of alcohol consumption have been consistently demonstrated to provide inaccurate estimates of consumption [67,68] and self-report measures of depressive symptoms are not (necessarily) equivalent to clinical diagnoses [69].

Sixth, participants were aged between 45 and 69 years of age. It is plausible that the same relationship might not be present in younger or older populations. Studies examining the relationship between alcohol use disorders and major depression earlier in the life-course also find a consistent relationship between problematic drinking and depression [7] suggesting that the association between these two measures might be consistent across the life-course. However, drinking pattern is known to fluctuate over time [70] and hazardous drinking declines with age [71] – this may explain why we do not see a consistent picture with respect to the association between binge drinking or annual volume of alcohol consumed and depressive symptoms in our sample. Analyses focussed on life-course patterns of alcohol intake in relation to depressive symptomology may provide important additional information, such as whether there are periods in the life-course whereby binge drinking is most commonly linked with depressive symptoms or if the relationship between drinking pattern and depressive symptoms is best explained by accumulated exposure of life-time drinking. Such hypotheses strengthen the argument that longitudinal work on this topic is warranted.

Finally, the rates of abstention in Poland were higher than in other populations in HAPIEE and than what we would expect from population level surveys [4]. Almost 35% of the Polish sample reported being non-drinkers at baseline. The reason for such a high rate is believed to be related to the Polish questionnaire containing a filter question which allowed for participants to skip the alcohol related questions if they indicated being non-drinkers in the last 12 months. However, the associations of abstention with depressive symptoms in Polish subjects were similar to Czech participants, as would be expected from the geographical and cultural closeness of these two populations. This suggests that the filter questions did not introduce a major bias.

Conclusions

Our findings indicate that dose of alcohol consumed in a binge drinking session and the frequency of doing so may contribute to the burden of depression in Eastern Europe but problem drinking was the alcohol variable consistently associated with increased odds of depressive symptoms in all countries, indicating that it is likely to be a useful predictor of depression in Eastern Europe. It is possible that the increased odds of depressive symptoms observed amongst non-drinkers is driven by former drinkers. Future work will however need to investigate whether this relationship holds when predicting depressive symptoms prospectively using a longitudinal design.

Supporting Information

Information S1 Estimates from models relating the frequency of drinking >60, 100 and 140 g in the past year to depressive symptoms.

Information S2 Estimates from models whereby binge drinking dose/frequency, annual drinking volume and problem drinking are simultaneously included in the same model.

Acknowledgments

We would like to thank all individuals participating in the HAPIEE study as well as all members of the HAPIEE study team.

Author Contributions

Conceived and designed the experiments: SB AB MB RK SM AP YN. Performed the experiments: SB AB MB RK SM AP YN. Analyzed the data: SB. Wrote the paper: SB. Revised the manuscript critically for important intellectual content and approved the final draft: AB RK SM AP YN MB.

References

1. Becker AE, Kleinman A (2013) Mental Health and the Global Agenda. N Engl J Med 369: 66–73. doi:10.1056/NEJMra1110827
2. Mathers CD, Loncar D (2006) Projections of Global Mortality and Burden of Disease from 2002 to 2030. PLoS Med 3: e442. doi:10.1371/journal.pmed.0030442
3. Patel V, Jenkins R, Lund C, the PLoS Medicine Editors (2012) Putting Evidence into Practice: The PLoS Medicine Series on Global Mental Health Practice. PLoS Med 9: e1001226. doi:10.1371/journal.pmed.1001226
4. World Health Organisation (2012) Alcohol in the European Union. Consumption, harm and policy approaches. Copenhagen, Denmark: World Health Organisation Regional Office for Europe. Available: http://www.euro.who.int/__data/assets/pdf_file/0003/160680/e96457.pdf. Accessed 25 April 2012.
5. Mueser KT, Drake RE, Wallach MA (1998) Dual diagnosis: A review of etiological theories. Addict Behav 23: 717–734. doi:10.1016/S0306-4603(98)00073-2
6. Boden JM, Fergusson DM (2011) Alcohol and depression. Addiction 106: 906–914. doi:10.1111/j.1360-0443.2010.03351.x
7. Fergusson DM, Boden JM, Horwood LJ (2009) Tests of Causal Links Between Alcohol Abuse or Dependence and Major Depression. Arch Gen Psychiatry 66: 260–266. doi:10.1001/archgenpsychiatry.2008.543
8. Boschloo L, van den Brink W, Penninx BWJH, Wall MM, Hasin DS (2012) Alcohol-use disorder severity predicts first-incidence of depressive disorders. Psychol Med 42: 695–703. doi:10.1017/S0033291711001681
9. Grant BF, Harford TC (1995) Comorbidity between DSM-IV alcohol use disorders and major depression: results of a national survey. Drug Alcohol Depend 39: 197–206. doi:10.1016/0376-8716(95)01160-4
10. Haynes JC, Farrell M, Singleton N, Meltzer H, Araya R, et al. (2005) Alcohol consumption as a risk factor for anxiety and depression: Results from the longitudinal follow-up of the National Psychiatric Morbidity Survey. Br J Psychiatry 187: 544–551. doi:10.1192/bjp.187.6.544
11. Paljärvi T, Koskenvuo M, Poikolainen K, Kauhanen J, Sillanmäki L, et al. (2009) Binge drinking and depressive symptoms: a 5-year population-based cohort study. Addiction 104: 1168–1178. doi:10.1111/j.1360-0443.2009.02577.x
12. Wang J, Patten SB (2001) Alcohol consumption and major depression: findings from a follow-up study. Can J Psychiatry 46: 632–638.
13. Wang J, Patten SB (2002) Prospective study of frequent heavy alcohol use and the risk of major depression in the Canadian general population. Depress Anxiety 15: 42–45. doi:10.1002/da.1084
14. Graham K, Massak A, Demers A, Rehm J (2007) Does the Association Between Alcohol Consumption and Depression Depend on How They Are Measured? Alcohol Clin Exp Res 31: 78–88. doi:10.1111/j.1530-0277.2006.00274.x
15. Bobak M, Pikhart H, Pajak A, Kubinova R, Malyutina S, et al. (2006) Depressive symptoms in urban population samples in Russia, Poland and the Czech Republic. Br J Psychiatry 188: 359–365. doi:10.1192/bjp.188.4.359
16. Ferrari AJ, Charlson FJ, Norman RE, Patten SB, Freedman G, et al. (2013) Burden of Depressive Disorders by Country, Sex, Age, and Year: Findings from the Global Burden of Disease Study 2010. PLoS Med 10: e1001547. doi:10.1371/journal.pmed.1001547
17. Popova S, Rehm J, Patra J, Zatonski W (2007) Comparing alcohol consumption in central and eastern Europe to other European countries. Alcohol Alcohol 42: 465–473. doi:10.1093/alcalc/agl124
18. Room R (2005) Commentary: Pattern of drinking and the Russian heart. Int J Epidemiol 34: 788–790. doi:10.1093/ije/dyi117
19. Bobak M, Room R, Pikhart H, Kubinova R, Malyutina S, et al. (2004) Contribution of drinking patterns to differences in rates of alcohol related problems between three urban populations. J Epidemiol Community Health 58: 238–242. doi:10.1136/jech.2003.011825
20. Leon DA, Shkolnikov VM, McKee M (2009) Alcohol and Russian mortality: a continuing crisis. Addiction 104: 1630–1636. doi:10.1111/j.1360-0443.2009.02655.x
21. Bulloch A, Lavorato D, Williams J, Patten S (2012) Alcohol Consumption and Major Depression In The General Population: The Critical Importance of Dependence. Depress Anxiety 29: 1058–1064. doi:10.1002/da.22001
22. Zhan W, Shaboltas A, Skochilov R, Kozlov A, Krasnoselskikh T (2012) Gender Differences in the Relationship between Alcohol Use and Depressive Symptoms in St. Petersburg, Russia. J Addict Res Ther 3. doi:10.4172/2155-6105.1000124
23. Averina M, Nilssen O, Brenn T, Brox J, Arkhipovsky V, et al. (2005) Social and lifestyle determinants of depression, anxiety, sleeping disorders and self-evaluated quality of life in Russia. Soc Psychiatry Psychiatr Epidemiol 40: 511–518. doi:10.1007/s00127-005-0918-x
24. Peele S, Brodsky A (2000) Exploring psychological benefits associated with moderate alcohol use: a necessary corrective to assessments of drinking outcomes? Drug Alcohol Depend 60: 221–247. doi:10.1016/S0376-8716(00)00112-5
25. Baum-Baicker C (1985) The psychological benefits of moderate alcohol consumption: A review of the literature. Drug Alcohol Depend 15: 305–322. doi:10.1016/0376-8716(85)90008-0
26. Fillmore KM, Stockwell T, Chikritzhs T, Bostrom A, Kerr W (2007) Moderate Alcohol Use and Reduced Mortality Risk: Systematic Error in Prospective Studies and New Hypotheses. Ann Epidemiol 17: S16–S23.
27. Stockwell T, Greer A, Fillmore K, Chikritzhs T, Zeisser C (2012) How good is the science? BMJ 344: e2276.
28. Peasey A, Bobak M, Kubinova R, Malyutina S, Pajak A, et al. (2006) Determinants of cardiovascular disease and other non-communicable diseases in Central and Eastern Europe: Rationale and design of the HAPIEE study. BMC Public Health 6: 255. doi:10.1186/1471-2458-6-255
29. Rehm J (1998) Measuring Quantity, Frequency, and Volume of Drinking. Alcohol Clin Exp Res 22: 4s–14s. doi:10.1111/j.1530-0277.1998.tb04368.x
30. Greenfield TK (2000) Ways of measuring drinking patterns and the difference they make: experience with graduated frequencies. J Subst Abuse 12: 33–49. doi:10.1016/S0899-3289(00)00039-0
31. Bell S, Britton A (2011) Alcohol and men's health. Trends Urol Mens Health 2: 9–12. doi:10.1002/tre.206
32. Mayfield D, McLeod G, Hall P (1974) The CAGE questionnaire: validation of a new alcoholism screening instrument. Am J Psychiatry 131: 1121–1123.
33. Ewing JA (1984) Detecting Alcoholism: The CAGE Questionnaire. JAMA J Am Med Assoc 252: 1905–1907. doi:10.1001/jama.1984.03350140051025
34. Fiellin DA, Reid MC, O'Connor PG (2000) Screening for alcohol problems in primary care: a systematic review. Arch Intern Med 160: 1977–1989. doi:10.1001/archinte.160.13.1977
35. Radloff LS (1977) The CES-D Scale. Appl Psychol Meas 1: 385–401. doi:10.1177/014662167700100306
36. Beekman ATF, Deeg DJ., van Tilburg T, Smit JH, Hooijer C, et al. (1995) Major and minor depression in later life: a study of prevalence and risk factors. J Affect Disord 36: 65–75. doi:10.1016/0165-0327(95)00061-5
37. Ferketich AK, Schwartzbaum JA, Frid DJ, Moeschberger ML (2000) Depression as an Antecedent to Heart Disease Among Women and Men in the NHANES I Study. Arch Intern Med 160: 1261–1268. doi:10.1001/archinte.160.9.1261
38. Breslau N (1985) Depressive symptoms, major depression, and generalized anxiety: A comparison of self-reports on CES-D and results from diagnostic interviews. Psychiatry Res 15: 219–229. doi:10.1016/0165-1781(85)90079-4
39. Beekman AT, Deeg D, Van Limbeek J, Braam A, De Vries M, et al. (1997) Criterion validity of the Center for Epidemiologic Studies Depression scale (CES-D): results from a community-based sample of older subjects in The Netherlands. Psychol Med 27: 231–236.
40. Merrick EL, Horgan CM, Hodgkin D, Garnick DW, Houghton SF, et al. (2008) Unhealthy Drinking Patterns in Older Adults: Prevalence and Associated Characteristics. J Am Geriatr Soc 56: 214–223. doi:10.1111/j.1532-5415.2007.01539.x
41. Van de Velde S, Bracke P, Levecque K (2010) Gender differences in depression in 23 European countries. Cross-national variation in the gender gap in depression. Soc Sci Med 71: 305–313. doi:10.1016/j.socscimed.2010.03.035
42. Bjelland I, Krokstad S, Mykletun A, Dahl AA, Tell GS, et al. (2008) Does a higher educational level protect against anxiety and depression? The HUNT study. Soc Sci Med 66: 1334–1345. doi:10.1016/j.socscimed.2007.12.019
43. Grittner U, Kuntsche S, Gmel G, Bloomfield K (2013) Alcohol consumption and social inequality at the individual and country levels—results from an international study. Eur J Public Health 23: 332–339. doi:10.1093/eurpub/cks044
44. Bobak M, Mckee M, Rose R, Marmot M (1999) Alcohol consumption in a national sample of the Russian population. Addiction 94: 857–866. doi:10.1046/j.1360-0443.1999.9468579.x
45. Pikhartova J, Chandola T, Kubinova R, Bobak M, Nicholson A, et al. (2009) Neighbourhood socioeconomic indicators and depressive symptoms in the Czech Republic: a population based study. Int J Public Health 54: 283–293. doi:10.1007/s00038-009-8029-1
46. Boden JM, Fergusson DM, Horwood LJ (2010) Cigarette smoking and depression: tests of causal linkages using a longitudinal birth cohort. Br J Psychiatry 196: 440–446. doi:10.1192/bjp.bp.109.065912
47. Schisterman EF, Cole SR, Platt RW (2009) Overadjustment Bias and Unnecessary Adjustment in Epidemiologic Studies. Epidemiology 20: 488–495. doi:10.1097/EDE.0b013e3181a819a1
48. StataCorp (2013) Stata Statistical Software: Release 13. College Station, TX: StataCorp LP.
49. Bobrova N, West R, Malyutina D, Malyutina S, Bobak M (2010) Gender Differences in Drinking Practices in Middle Aged and Older Russians. Alcohol Alcohol 45: 573–580. doi:10.1093/alcalc/agq069
50. Peirce RS, Frone MR, Russell M, Cooper ML, Mudar P (2000) A longitudinal model of social contact, social support, depression, and alcohol use. Health Psychol 19: 28–38. doi:10.1037/0278-6133.19.1.28
51. Dissing AS, Gil A, Keenan K, McCambridge J, McKee M, et al. (2013) Alcohol consumption and self-reported (SF12) physical and mental health among working-aged men in a typical Russian city: a cross-sectional study. Addiction 108: 1905–1914. doi:10.1111/add.12257
52. Swendsen JD, Merikangas KR, Canino GJ, Kessler RC, Rubio-Stipec M, et al. (1998) The comorbidity of alcoholism with anxiety and depressive disorders in four geographic communities. Compr Psychiatry 39: 176–184. doi:10.1016/S0010-440X(98)90058-X
53. Burns L, Teesson M (2002) Alcohol use disorders comorbid with anxiety, depression and drug use disorders: Findings from the Australian National Survey

of Mental Health and Well Being. Drug Alcohol Depend 68: 299–307. doi:10.1016/S0376-8716(02)00220-X
54. Smith GW, Shevlin M (2008) Patterns of Alcohol Consumption and Related Behaviour in Great Britain: A Latent Class Analysis of the Alcohol Use Disorder Identification Test (AUDIT). Alcohol Alcohol 43: 590–594. doi:10.1093/alcalc/agn041
55. Bolton JM, Robinson J, Sareen J (2009) Self-medication of mood disorders with alcohol and drugs in the National Epidemiologic Survey on Alcohol and Related Conditions. J Affect Disord 115: 367–375. doi:10.1016/j.jad.2008.10.003
56. Boschloo L, Vogelzangs N, van den Brink W, Smit JH, Veltman DJ, et al. (2012) Alcohol use disorders and the course of depressive and anxiety disorders. Br J Psychiatry 200: 476–484. doi:10.1192/bjp.bp.111.097550
57. Flensborg-Madsen T, Mortensen EL, Knop J, Becker U, Sher L, et al. (2009) Comorbidity and temporal ordering of alcohol use disorders and other psychiatric disorders: results from a Danish register-based study. Compr Psychiatry 50: 307–314. doi:10.1016/j.comppsych.2008.09.003
58. Boschloo L, Vogelzangs N, van den Brink W, Smit JH, Veltman DJ, et al. (2012) Authors' reply. Br J Psychiatry 201: 326–327. doi:10.1192/bjp.201.4.326a
59. Meyer RE (1986) Psychopathology and addictive disorders. New York, USA: Guildford Press. 362 p.
60. Bell S, Britton A (2014) An exploration of the dynamic longitudinal relationship between mental health and alcohol consumption: a prospective cohort study. BMC Med 12: 91. doi:10.1186/1741-7015-12-91
61. Kerr WC, Ye Y (2010) Relationship of Life-Course Drinking Patterns to Diabetes, Heart Problems, and Hypertension Among Those 40 and Older in the 2005 U.S. National Alcohol Survey. J Stud Alcohol Drugs 71: 515–525.
62. Naimi TS, Brown DW, Brewer RD, Giles WH, Mensah G, et al. (2005) Cardiovascular risk factors and confounders among nondrinking and moderate-drinking U.S. adults. Am J Prev Med 28: 369–373. doi:10.1016/j.amepre.2005.01.011
63. Caldwell TM, Rodgers B, Power C, Clark C, Gamble SA (2006) Drinking histories of self-identified lifetime abstainers and occasional drinkers: findings from the 1958 British Birth cohort study. Alcohol Alcohol 41: 650–654. doi:10.1093/alcalc/agl088
64. Lucas N, Windsor TD, Caldwell TM, Rodgers B (2010) Psychological Distress in Non-Drinkers: Associations with Previous Heavy Drinking and Current Social Relationships. Alcohol Alcohol 45: 95–102. doi:10.1093/alcalc/agp080
65. Shaper AG, Wannamethee G, Walker M (1988) Alcohol and mortality in British men: explaining the U-shaped curve. The Lancet 332: 1267–1273.
66. Hu Y, Pikhart H, Malyutina S, Pajak A, Kubinova R, et al. (2014) Alcohol consumption and physical functioning among middle-aged and older adults in Central and Eastern Europe: Results from the HAPIEE study. Age Ageing: Advance Access. doi:10.1093/ageing/afu083
67. Chikirzhs T, Fillmore K, Stockwell T (2009) A healthy dose of scepticism: Four good reasons to think again about protective effects of alcohol on coronary heart disease. Drug Alcohol Rev 28: 441–444. doi:10.1111/j.1465-3362.2009.00052.x
68. Laatikainen T, Alho H, Vartiainen E, Jousilahti P, Sillanaukee P, et al. (2002) Self-reported alcohol consumption and association to carbohydrate-deficient transferrin and gamma-glutamyltransferase in a random sample of the general population in the Republic of Karelia, Russia and in North Karelia, Finland. Alcohol Alcohol 37: 282–288. doi:10.1093/alcalc/37.3.282
69. Myers JK, Weissman MM (1980) Use of a self-report symptom scale to detect depression in a community sample. Am J Psychiatry 137: 1081–1084.
70. Fillmore KM (1987) Prevalence, Incidence and Chronicity of Drinking Patterns and Problems Among Men as a Function of Age: a longitudinal and cohort analysis. Br J Addict 82: 77–83. doi:10.1111/j.1360-0443.1987.tb01440.x
71. O'Malley PM (2004) Maturing out of problematic alcohol use. Alcohol Res Health 28: 202–204.

3

Genetic Prediction of Antidepressant Drug Response and Nonresponse in Korean Patients

Shinn-Won Lim[1], Hong-Hee Won[1], Hyeran Kim[2], Woojae Myung[2], Seonwoo Kim[3], Ka-Kyung Kim[4], Bernard J. Carroll[5], Jong-Won Kim[4]*, Doh Kwan Kim[2]*

1 Center for Clinical Research, Samsung Biomedical Research Institute, Seoul, Korea, **2** Department of Psychiatry, Samsung Medical Center, Sungkyunkwan University School of Medicine, Seoul, Korea, **3** Biostatistics Unit, Samsung Biomedical Research Institute, Seoul, Korea, **4** Department of Laboratory Medicine and Genetics, Samsung Medical Center, Sungkyunkwan University School of Medicine, Seoul, Korea, **5** Pacific Behavioral Research Foundation, Carmel, California, United States of America

Abstract

Genetic polymorphism contributes to variation in response to drug treatment of depression. We conducted three independent 6-week treatment studies in outpatients with major depressive disorder (MDD) to develop a pharmacogenomic model predicting response and nonresponse. We screened candidate genomic markers for association with response to selective serotonin reuptake inhibitors (SSRIs). No patients had received any antidepressant drug treatment in the current episode of depression. Outcome evaluation was blinded to drug and genotype data. The prediction model derived from a development sample of 239 completer cases treated with SSRIs comprised haplotypes and polymorphisms related to serotonin synthesis, serotonin transport, glutamate receptors, and GABA synthesis. The model was evaluated prospectively for prediction of outcome in a validation sample of 176 new SSRI-treated completer cases. The model gave a prediction in 60% of these cases. Predictive values were 85% for predicted responders and 86% for predicted nonresponders, compared to prior probabilities of 66% for observed response and 34% for observed nonresponse in those cases (both $P<0.001$). Convergent cross-validation was obtained through failure of the model to predict outcomes in a third independent sample of 189 completer cases who received non-SSRI antidepressants. We suggest proof of principle for genetic guidance to use or avoid SSRIs in a majority of Korean depressed patients.

Editor: Judith Homberg, Radboud University, Netherlands

Funding: This study was supported by grants from National Research Foundation of Korea funded by the Korea government (MEST, R0A 2007-000-20129-0, to D.K.K.), the Korean Health Technology R&D Project, Ministry of Health & Welfare, Republic of Korea (A110339, to D.K.K.), and the Brain Research Program through the National Research Foundation of Korea, funded by the Ministry of Science, ICT, and Future Planning (NRF-2013M3C7A1073000, to J.W.K.). The funders had no role in study design, data collection and analysis, decision to publish, or preparation of the manuscript.

Competing Interests: Hyeran Kim and Woojae Myung are affiliated to Samsung Medical Center. Samsung Medical Center is a public utility foundation which is administratively separate from the Samsung Corporation.

* Email: paulkim@skku.edu (DKK); kimjw@skku.edu (J-WK)

These authors contributed equally to this work.

Introduction

Response rates in drug treatment of major depression are variable and often less than 50% in "real world" studies [1], and there are no biomarkers to direct choice of antidepressant drug class. Genetic markers hold promise for improving this record [2–4].

Many studies have focused on a few genes related to the primary actions of the drugs. Genetic polymorphism in the serotonin transporter (5-hydroxytryptamine transporter, 5-HTT), has been linked to antidepressant response to selective serotonin reuptake inhibitors (SSRIs) [5–7], although not in all studies [8]. Among the factors affecting functional response to antidepressant drugs are multiple secondary neurobiological mechanisms, environmental factors, ethnicity, and drug class. Based on our earlier reports [5,9], we adopted an expanded survey of candidate genes using single nucleotide polymorphism (SNP) microarray methods. Candidate genes were selected for the primary targets and secondary mechanisms affected by antidepressant drugs. We used a candidate gene strategy rather than an exploratory genome wide association study (GWAS) which requires much larger sample sizes [10].

Here we report on a 3-stage study (Figure 1) of multiple candidate genes for predicting response and nonresponse to SSRIs in depressed patients. After identifying a predictive model for SSRI response in the derivation sample, we subjected the model to validation testing in the second, independent, sample of patients, who also received SSRI treatment. The cross-validation sample, also independent, was treated with non-SSRI drugs. This third sample served 3 purposes – as a partial solution to the absence of a placebo-treated group; to evaluate whether the predictive SSRI model generalized to another class of antidepressant drug; and for exploration of gene markers of response to non-SSRI agents. We hypothesized that the predictive model for SSRI response would predict response to SSRI treatment in the validation sample, whilst it would not predict response to non-SSRI drugs in the cross-validation sample. These predictions are consistent with other reports of drug class differences [9,11].

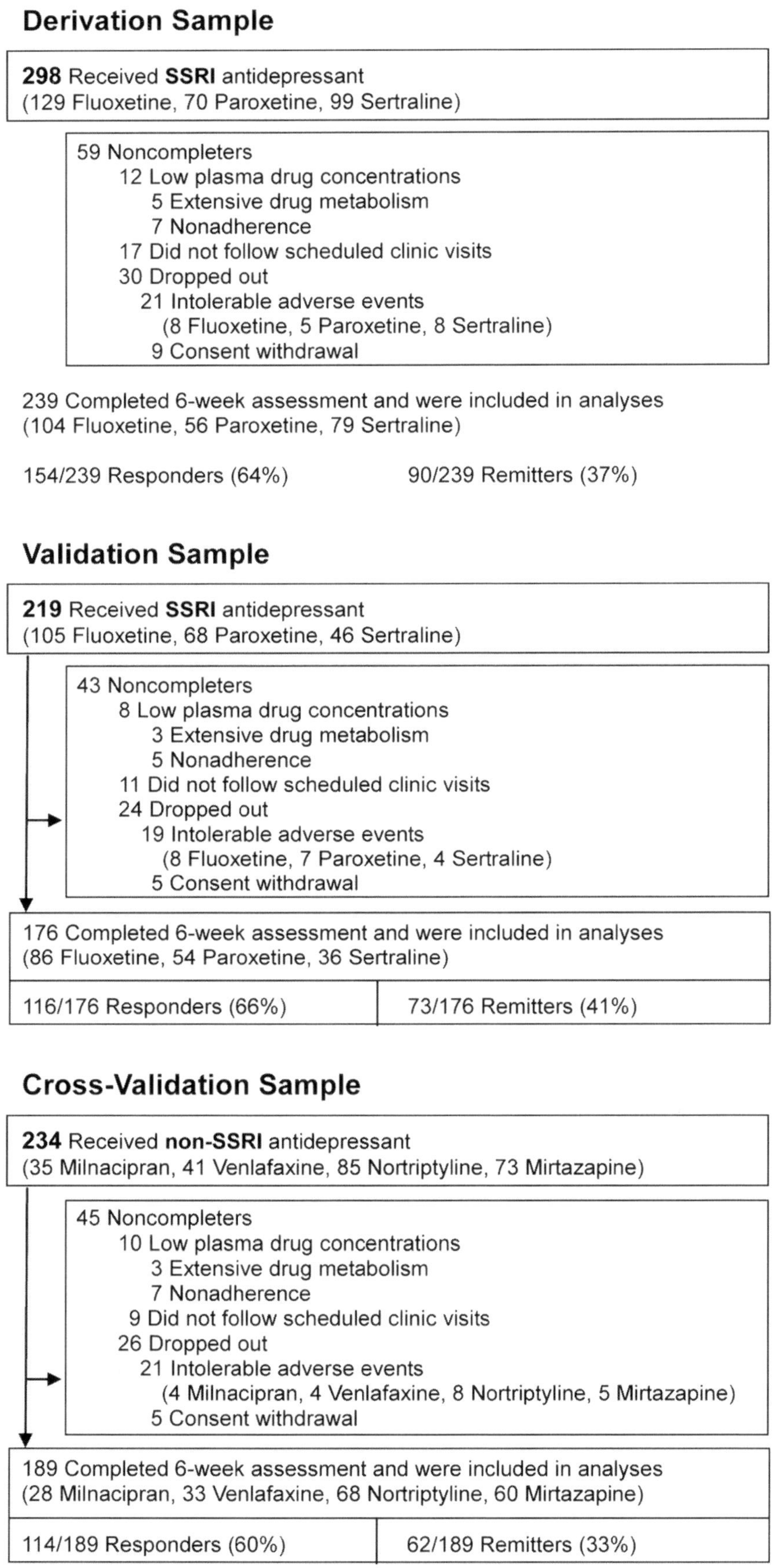

Figure 1. Enrollment, attrition, drug treatments, and outcomes of patients in all samples.

Methods

Participants

We studied 3 independent cohorts totaling 751 Korean adult outpatients with major depression. These samples were completely separate from our previous reports [5,9]. The first (derivation) sample (N = 298) received SSRI drugs. The second (validation) sample (N = 219) also received SSRI drugs. The third (cross-validation) sample (N = 234) received non-SSRI drugs. No patients had received any antidepressant drug treatment during the current episode of depression. The study was conducted in a naturalistic clinical setting rather than in a placebo-controlled clinical trial [12,13]. The protocol was approved by the ethics review board of Samsung Medical Center, Seoul, Korea. Signed informed consent was obtained from all participants. The study is registered (NCT00817375) in ClinicalTrials.gov.

The assessment and quality control procedures have been fully described previously [5,9]. A total 782 participants were recruited from patients seeking care for depression at a university hospital from October 1997 through July 2007. Thirty-one cases were excluded: 6 patients did not have a significant other to obtain collateral diagnostic information, 4 patients had significant medical conditions, 7 patients had a concomitant Axis I psychiatric disorder, and 16 patients did not have a minimum 17-item HAM-D score of 15. Two cases met 2 of these exclusion criteria. Thus, a total of 751 Korean outpatients with MDD were enrolled. All were clinically referred and all were of unrelated Korean ancestry. Figure 1 displays retention and attrition data for the 3 independent clinical samples. As this is a discovery project, outcome analyses included only subjects who completed 6 weeks of treatment with adequate blood levels (Figure 1). Extensive drug metabolizers were distinguished from nonadherent cases by clinical review after a low blood level was detected. Overall, 604 patients (80.4%) completed the protocol.

Enrolled patients met the *Diagnostic and Statistical Manual of Mental Disorders, Fourth Edition* (DSM-IV) criteria for MDD without psychotic features. The diagnosis was based on an initial clinical interview, followed by a structured research interview, the Samsung Psychiatric Evaluation Schedule (SPES). The affective disorder section of the SPES uses the Korean version of the *Structured Clinical Interview for the Diagnostic and Statistical Manual of Mental Disorders, Fourth Edition*. The SPES provides additional information including cognitive screening, comorbid psychiatric diagnoses, psychosocial variables (age, sex, age of onset, duration of current episode, episode number), family history and initial Hamilton Depression Rating Scale (HAM-D) [14] severity score. These diagnostic interviews involved the patient and at least one family member. The final diagnosis was made after review of ongoing clinical observations, medical records, past histories, and the DSM-IV criteria, by a board-certified psychiatrist. Inclusion criteria were 18 years of age or older, the existence of a current nonpsychotic unipolar major depressive episode as verified by DSM-IV criteria, a minimum 17-item HAM-D score of 15, and ability to provide informed consent. To be included in these discovery analyses, patients also were required to adhere to prescribed medication and to have an adequate plasma antidepressant drug level measured at 6 weeks. Exclusion criteria were pregnancy, significant medical conditions, abnormal baseline laboratory values, unstable psychiatric features (e.g., suicide attempt), histories of alcohol or drug dependence, seizure disorder, neurological illness including significant cognitive impairment, or concomitant Axis I psychiatric disorder. Patients with MDD who met DSM-IV criteria for the specifier '*Severe With Psychotic Features*' were excluded because they would normally receive concurrent antipsychotic medication. As stated above, no patients had received antidepressant drug treatment in the current episode before enrolment in this study. In addition, no patient had received non-antidepressant psychotropic medication within 2 weeks of the study. We also verified that no patients had received fluoxetine, which has a long half-life, for any reason within the preceding 4 weeks.

Procedures

Patients received monotherapy for 6 weeks with one of three commonly used SSRI drugs or one of four non-SSRI antidepressants, by clinician's choice (Figure 1). In this naturalistic study, choice of drug was driven by the preference of the physician, with consideration of anticipated side effects in at-risk individuals [15]. Dose titration was completed within two weeks. Trough plasma samples were drawn at the end of week 6 for plasma drug concentrations. Lorazepam 0.5–1 mg was allowed at bedtime for insomnia. Patients were seen by a psychiatrist, who monitored their adverse events by the Udvalg for Kliniske Undersogelser (UKU) scale [16] at weeks 0, 1, 2, 4, and 6. The 17-item Hamilton scale for depression (HAM-D) [14] was administered by a single trained rater every two weeks. The rater and genotyper were blinded to the hypotheses and to drug assignment. HAM-D and genotype data were not disclosed to the psychiatrist, and the rater was blinded to the genotype data. To maintain the blindness, a trained research coordinator managed the data and schedules. At six weeks, response was defined according to standard conventions [4] as $\geq 50\%$ decrease in the HAM-D score, and remission as a HAM-D score ≤ 7.

The protocol completion rates were 80% (derivation sample), 80% (validation sample), and 81% (cross-validation sample) (Figure 1). For comparison, protocol completion rates in controlled clinical trials of antidepressant drugs typically are 70–75% [17]. As shown in Figure 1, dropouts occurred for the usual clinical and administrative reasons, and we excluded cases with evidence of nonadherence or extensive drug metabolism inferred from the finding of low plasma drug concentrations at week 6. The clinical characteristics of non-completers did not differ significantly from completers in any cohort (data not shown). The data reported in the Results apply to the 604 completer cases: 239 in the derivation cohort; 176 in the validation SSRI cohort; and 189 in the cross-validation non-SSRI cohort (Figure 1).

Candidate genes and selection of SNP markers

We focused on candidate genes of neurotransmitter metabolic enzymes, transporters and receptors (Table S1). We selected 79 candidate genes, based on their likely importance for immediate or delayed mechanisms of antidepressant action. We combined knowledge-based and function-based tagging selection approaches (Figure S1). We selected 155 SNPs through a literature survey on the significant SNPs related to antidepressant response, and 1657 SNPs by tagging based on potential functional importance (Table S2).

After screening for availability of Golden Gate Bead Array analysis (Illumina, Inc. San Diego, CA), 1502 SNPs were genotyped. 67 SNPs with a call rate of less than 95% and 35 SNPs with a minor allele frequency less than 5% were excluded. Finally, 1400 SNPs were prepared.

To enable comparison with SNP data using different SNP genotyping platforms, we imputed genotypes for untyped SNPs using the IMPUTE software [18].

Table 1. Characteristics of patients in derivation sample, validation sample, and cross-validation sample.

Characteristics	Derivation Sample			Validation Sample				Cross-Validation Sample			
	SSRI Treated Group			SSRI Treated Group			P^{+}	Non-SSRI Treated Group			P^{++}
	Responder	Nonresponder	*P*	Responder	Nonresponder	*P*		Responder	Nonresponder	*P*	
Response Rate (%)[a]	154/239 (64.4%)			116/176 (65.9%)			1.00	114/189 (60.3%)			0.84
Remission Rate (%)[a]	90/239 (37.7%)			73/176 (41.5%)			0.96	62/189 (32.8%)			0.62
Gender, Female (%)[a]	180/239 (75.3%)			136/176 (77.3%)			1.00	137/189 (72.5%)			1.00
	119/154 (66.1%)	61/85 (71.8%)	0.35	91/116 (78.5%)	45/60 (75.0%)	0.70		83/114 (72.8%)	54/75 (72.0%)	1.00	
Age, Mean±SD (Range), Year[b]	59.8±13.7 (19–86)			62.3±12.7 (24–87)			0.11	58.7±13.3 (22–82)			0.82
	59.1±14.0 (19–86)	61.1±13.2 (24–85)	0.35	62.0±12.3 (27–87)	62.7±13.4 (24–83)	0.47		58.7±13.0 (22–82)	59.4±13.9 (25–82)	0.21	
Family History of Depression (%)[a]	46/239 (19.3%)			34/176 (19.3%)			1.00	39/189 (20.6%)			1.00
	33/154 (21.4%)	13/85 (15.3%)	0.30	23/116 (19.8%)	11/60 (18.3%)	1.00		23/114 (20.2%)	16/75 (21.3%)	0.86	
Duration of Index Episode, Mean±SD (Range), Month[b]	9.6±14.1 (1–92)			8.8±13.2 (1–92)			1.00	10.8±15.9 (1–120)			0.82
	9.1±15.3 (1–92)	10.5±11.4 (1–71)	0.04	8.2±12.1 (1–63)	10.0±15.2 (1–92)	0.36		11.1±18.7 (1–120)	10.4±10.5 (1–37)	0.13	
No. of Episodes, Mean±SD (Range)[b]	2.2±1.8 (1–16)			2.3±2.0 (1–16)			1.00	2.2±2.1 (1–19)			1.00
	2.2±2.0 (1–16)	2.1±1.2 (1–6)	0.31	2.3±2.2 (1–16)	2.2±1.8 (1–12)	0.86		2.1±1.8 (1–11)	2.4±2.4 (1–19)	0.20	
Age at First Episode, Mean±SD (Range), Year[b]	53.0±15.1 (16–82)			55.6±14.5 (15–82)			0.18	51.2±15.0 (15–77)			0.56
	52.4±15.7 (16–81)	54.3±13.9 (19–82)	0.47	55.4±14.4 (20–81)	56.0±15.0 (15–82)	0.66		51.5±14.4 (15–77)	50.9±15.9 (15–75)	0.90	
HAM-D Baseline, Mean±SD (Range)[b]	20.9±4.8 (15–40)			19.2±3.4 (15–32)				21.5±5.1 (15–40)			
	20.8±5.3 (15–40)	21.0±4.0 (15–31)	0.45[c]	19.1±3.2 (15–29)	19.4±3.7 (15–32)	1.00		21.4±5.1 (15–40)	21.6±5.2 (15–36)	1.00[c]	
HAM-D After, Mean±SD (Range)[b]	10.2±5.6 (0–26)			9.5±5.3 (0–30)				11.7±6.5 (1–35)			
	7.0±3.1 (0–15)	16.0±4.3 (9–26)	<0.01[c]	6.5±2.8 (0–14)	15.3±4.0 (9–30)	<0.01		7.4±3.1 (1–17)	18.1±4.6 (10–35)	<0.01[c]	

Abbreviations: SSRI, selective serotonin reuptake inhibitor; HAM-D, Hamilton depression rating score.
[a]Fisher's exact test.
[b]Mann-Whitney test.
[c]Corrected by Bonferroni's correction for multiple testing.
[+]Comparison between derivation sample and validation sample.
[++]Comparison between derivation sample and cross-validation sample.

Statistical analysis

We performed tests of five genetic modes (dominant, recessive, genotype, allele, and additive) for each SNP with the use of Fisher's exact test and the Cochran-Armitage test [19]. The mode most strongly associated with response was considered the best-fitting genetic mode for each SNP. These significance levels were calculated and corrected with the false discovery rate (FDR) control [20].

Haplotype blocks were defined in the derivation sample by confidence intervals using Haploview [21,22]. Associations between haplotype blocks and response were tested using Fisher's exact test with the FDR control. Multivariable analyses for SNPs and for haplotype blocks found to be significant in univariable analyses were performed using multiple logistic regression and the Generalized Estimating Equations method [23], respectively.

Prediction models for response and nonresponse were constructed using multiple logistic regression. We constructed two types of prediction model. First, only polymorphic markers were considered (polymorphism model, section 4 of Text S2). Second, in addition to SNPs and VNTR markers, haplotypes were included and considered in the model (HAP-SNP model). Before constructing a combined haplotype-SNP (HAP-SNP) model, haplotypes were re-defined as a pair of two haplotypes (for example, *TPH2* H3-A is defined as a pair of two haplotypes (GCATGG and GCATGG) because the haplotypes are clustered data. We used the operational criteria of probability>0.8 for predicting response (better than the optimal response rate expected with combined drug and cognitive behavioral therapy in common psychiatric disorders such as depression and anxiety) [24,25], and response probability <0.3 for predicting nonresponse (lower than conservative estimates of the expected response rate with placebo in controlled clinical trials for depression [26]). This approach stratified each sample as predicted responders, predicted nonresponders, and indeterminate cases (no prediction). Excluding the indeterminate cases, we calculated overall accuracy, positive predictive value (PPV), negative predictive value (NPV), sensitivity and specificity, and areas under the receiver operating curve (AUC). The significance of the change from prior probabilities in the absence of genotyping to posterior probabilities from the prediction model was tested by the Chi square Goodness of Fit method. The PPVs and NPVs between the derivation set and the validation set were compared by Fisher's exact test.

The study was powered for the outcomes of observed response and nonresponse (see Text S1, section 4). All p values were reported as two-sided, and *P* values <0.05 were considered statistically significant. Analyses were performed with the use of the SAS software, version 9.13.

Detailed methods of function-based tagging selection of SNP markers, genotyping, power analysis and quantification of plasma drug levels are described in Text S1 (Supplementary Method).

Results

Clinical characteristics

Demographic variables, response and remission rates, severity ratings, and salient clinical variables of the three samples are shown in Table 1. HAM-D scores indicated moderate to severe depression. Observed response rates exceeded 60% in all groups. Responders and nonresponders did not differ at baseline on any variable, except for duration of episode in the derivation sample. Choice of SSRI drug did not influence outcomes overall (response rate to fluoxetine, paroxetine and sertraline: 65.4%, 64.3% and 63.3%, see Table S3) or in relation to any genotype (Table S3). Plasma drug levels in responders and nonresponders were not significantly different (Table S4).

Significant polymorphic markers for SSRI response

In the derivation sample, ten of 1400 candidate SNPs showed significant associations ($P<0.05$) with response after FDR correction (Table 2). These resided in four genes: four in *TPH2*, two in *GRIK2*, two in *GAD1*, and two in *SLC6A4*. The *TPH2* gene was most strongly associated with SSRI response. The rs4760815 in intron 6 of *TPH2* showed the strongest association ($P = 1.26\times10^{-5}$), and rs11179027, rs17110532 and rs17110747 in *TPH2* were also significantly associated ($P = 1.57\times10^{-5}$, 8.86×10^{-5} and 1.94×10^{-4}).

The second strongest associations with response to SSRIs were found in rs543196 and rs572487 in intron 2 of *GRIK2* ($P = 4.84\times10^{-5}$ and 1.36×10^{-4}). Another strong association was found in *GAD1*, where rs3828275 in intron 3 and rs12185692 located ~2.5 kb upstream of this gene showed strong association ($P = 6.89\times10^{-5}$ and 2.33×10^{-4}).

Two SNPs, rs2066713 and rs2020942, in the serotonin transporter gene (*SLC6A4*) also showed strong association with SSRI response ($P = 1.26\times10^{-4}$ and 2.96×10^{-4}). Previously, we reported that 44 bp insertion/deletion polymorphisms in the promoter region (*5-HTTLPR*) and variable number of tandem repeat (VNTR) *s/l* polymorphisms in intron 2 (*STin2*) of *SLC6A4* were associated with response to SSRIs [5,9]. We also genotyped these two VNTRs, and they once again showed significant associations with response to SSRIs ($P<0.01$) (Table 2).

Haplotype analysis for SSRI response

We further analyzed the four major genes (*TPH2*, *GRIK2*, *GAD1* and *SLC6A4*) which have multiple significant SNPs by examining linkage disequilibrium (LD) structures and haplotypes. Six haplotype blocks in those genes except *GAD1* were significantly associated with SSRI response (FDR corrected $P<0.05$). Among five haplotype blocks observed in *TPH2*, the third (H3), fourth (H4) and fifth (H5) blocks were significantly associated with response ($P<0.01$) (Figure 2A). When we examined haplotypes and LD structure separately for the responders and nonresponders to SSRI drugs, LD was stronger and haplotype blocks were longer in the responders than the nonresponders (Figure S2).

Among 16 haplotype blocks constructed from 78 SNPs of *GRIK2*, the eighth ($P = 9.6\times10^{-4}$) and ninth ($P = 9.6\times10^{-4}$) haplotype blocks were significantly associated with SSRI response (Figure 2B). Only one haplotype block from 12 SNPs of *SLC6A4* was significantly associated ($P = 1.3\times10^{-2}$) (Figure 2C). However, two haplotype blocks from ten SNPs of *GAD1* were not significantly associated with response to SSRI drugs (Figure 2D).

Prediction model for SSRI response

Using the stated operational criteria for predicting observed response and nonresponse to SSRIs (see Method; statistical analysis), the two prediction models demonstrated similar predictive performance. The HAP-SNP model made predictions for 54% of cases (129/239), compared with 46% (110/239) of patients using the polymorphism model. For this reason, we report on the HAP-SNP model as the optimal prediction model for response to SSRI treatment in this study. Genotypic combinations of the HAP-SNP model are presented in Table 3.

Moreover, we examined the effect of duration of episode, which differed between responders and nonresponders (Table 1), in the modeling but found that this clinical feature did not contribute significantly.

Table 2. The SNPs most strongly associated with SSRI response ($P < 0.05$ after FDR correction) and the strongly associated polymorphisms in *SLC6A4* from our previous study [9].

Gene	Chromosome	Position[a]	SNP	Responsive Allele	RAF in Responders	RAF in Nonresponders	MAF	*P* Value[b]	*P* Value by Bonferroni's Correction	*P* Value by Controlling FDR	Genetic Mode	Heterozygote Odds Ratio (95% CI)	Homozygote Odds Ratio (95% CI)
TPH2	12	70658496	rs4760815	T	0.60	0.41	0.50	1.26×10^{-5}	0.02	0.02	Dominant	3.77 (3.55–4.00)	4.39 (2.08–9.29)
TPH2	12	70663579	rs11179027	C	0.55	0.34	0.44	1.57×10^{-5}	0.02	0.02	Allele	2.69 (1.45–4.99)	4.77 (2.17–10.49)
GRIK2	6	102158042	rs543196	C	0.65	0.46	0.44	4.84×10^{-5}	0.07	0.02	Additive	1.69 (0.83–3.45)	5.02 (2.18–11.53)
GAD1	2	171390986	rs3828275	G	0.72	0.64	0.31	6.89×10^{-5}	0.10	0.02	Genotype	0.31 (0.17–0.55)	1.24 (0.43–3.62)
TPH2	12	70650935	rs17110532	C	0.42	0.24	0.33	8.86×10^{-5}	0.12	0.02	Allele	2.02 (1.14–3.59)	5.36 (1.93–14.87)
SLC6A4	17	25575791	rs2066713	C	0.96	0.86	0.07	1.26×10^{-4}	0.18	0.03	Recessive	0.48 (0.03–8.42)	2.27 (0.14–36.87)
GRIK2	6	102157181	rs572487	G	0.59	0.41	0.48	1.36×10^{-4}	0.19	0.03	Additive	1.65 (1.54–1.77)	4.76 (2.09–10.86)
TPH2	12	70712221	rs17110747	A	0.31	0.16	0.25	1.94×10^{-4}	0.27	0.03	Allele	2.53 (1.37–4.69)	3.88 (1.25–11.99)
GAD1	2	171379072	rs12185692	C	0.71	0.65	0.31	2.33×10^{-4}	0.33	0.04	Genotype	0.35 (0.20–0.62)	1.57 (0.49–5.03)
SLC6A4	17	25571040	rs2020942	G	0.95	0.85	0.09	2.96×10^{-4}	0.42	0.04	Additive	1.27 (1.21–1.34)	4.56 (0.41–51.22)

Gene	Chromosome	VNTR	*P* Value[b]	*P* Value by Bonferroni's Correction	*P* Value by Controlling FDR	Genetic Mode	Odds Ratio (95% CI)
SLC6A4	17	*5-HTT* VNTR in promoter (*5-HTTLPR*)	6.00×10^{-3}	NA	NA	*ss* vs. *sl*+*ll*	2.18 (1.27–3.75)
SLC6A4	17	*5-HTT* VNTR in intron 2 (*STin2*)	2.00×10^{-4}	NA	NA	*ll* vs. *sl*+*ss*	3.86 (1.90–7.84)

Abbreviations: SNP, single-nucleotide polymorphism; SSRI, selective serotonin reuptake inhibitor; RAF, responsive allele frequency; FDR, false discovery rate; VNTR, variable number of tandem repeat; MAF, minor allele frequency; NA, not applicable.

[a]Genomic position (NCBI Build 36).

[b]Fisher's exact test.

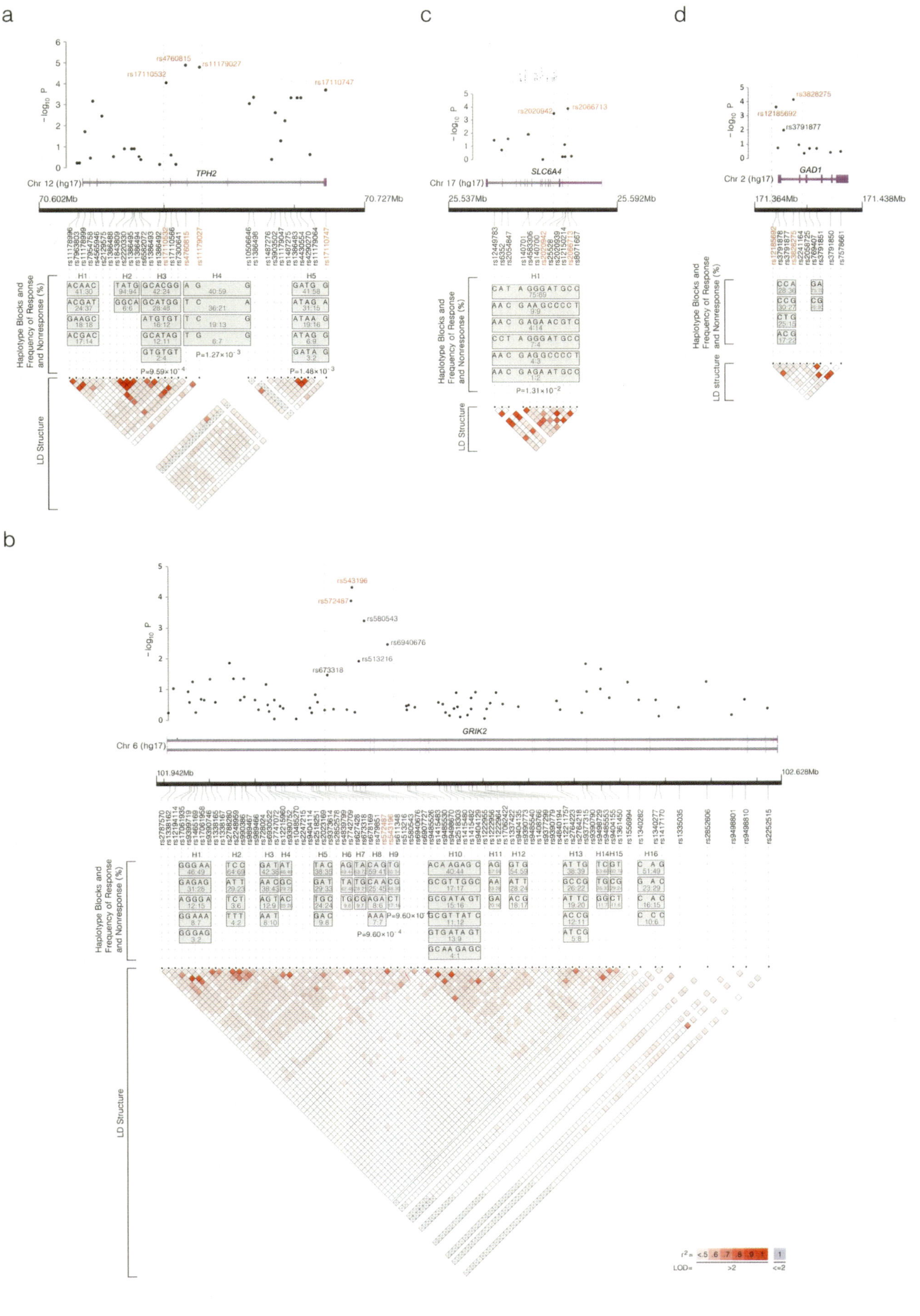
a
c
d
rs4760815
rs11179027
rs17110532
rs17110747
TPH2
Chr 12 (hg17)
70.602Mb
70.727Mb
P=9.59×10⁻⁴
P=1.27×10⁻³
P=1.48×10⁻³
rs2020942
rs2066713
SLC6A4
Chr 17 (hg17)
25.537Mb
25.592Mb
P=1.31×10⁻²
rs3828275
rs12185692
rs3791877
GAD1
Chr 2 (hg17)
171.364Mb
171.438Mb
b
rs543196
rs572487
rs580543
rs6940676
rs513216
rs673318
GRIK2
Chr 6 (hg17)
101.942Mb
102.628Mb
P=9.60×10⁻⁴
−log10 P
Haplotype Blocks and Frequency of Response and Nonresponse (%)
LD Structure
r² = <.5 .6 .7 .8 .9 1 1
LOD= >2 <=2

Figure 2. Linkage disequilibrium (LD) and haplotype structure of (a) *TPH2*, (b) *GRIK2*, (c) *SLC6A4*, and (d) *GAD1*. The LD structure in the lower panel is based on the measure of r^2. Dark red indicates strong LD between two markers with high r^2 and a logarithm of odds (LOD) score of greater than 2.0. Haplotype frequencies of responders and nonresponders are also shown in each box in order (responders: nonresponders). The figure was prepared with LocusView2.0 (http://www.broad.mit.edu/mpg/locusview). Significant SNPs inscribed in red are plotted with their association analysis p values (as $-\log_{10}$ values) in the upper panel. Haplotype blocks and estimated haplotypes for each block are presented in the middle panel. (a) Among 30 SNPs screened in *TPH2*, four SNPs (colored red), rs17110532, rs4760815, rs11179027 and rs17110747, were significantly associated (see Table 2). The third (H3), fourth (H4) and fifth haplotype (H5) blocks were significantly associated with drug response ($P<0.05$ after FDR correction). (b) Among 78 SNPs in *GRIK2*, two SNPs (colored red), rs543196 and rs572487, were significantly associated. Four SNPs, rs580543, rs6940676, rs513216, and rs673318, adjacent to the peak SNPs also showed high associations. The eighth (H8) and ninth (H9) blocks were significantly associated with response ($P<0.05$ after FDR correction). (c) Among 12 SNPs in *SLC6A4*, two SNPs (colored red), rs2066713 and rs2020942, were significantly associated with response. The first haplotype (H1) block was significantly associated with response ($P<0.05$ after FDR correction). (d) Among ten SNPs in *GAD1*, two SNPs (colored red), rs3828275 and rs12185691, were significantly associated (see Table 2). No haplotype blocks were significantly associated with response.
doi:10.1371/journal.pone.0107098.g002

The HAP-SNP model contained polymorphic markers and haplotype blocks: *TPH2* (H3) ($P<0.001$), *SLC6A4* (H1) ($P<0.001$), rs543196 of *GRIK2* ($P<0.001$), rs3828275 of *GAD1* ($P=0.01$), and *5-HTTLPR* of *SLC6A4* ($P=0.04$), and showed an AUC of 0.82, which is considered an overall good performance [27]. The model predicted outcome for 54% of completer cases (129/239) in the derivation sample, with 90 predicted responders (>80% predicted probability of response) and 39 predicted nonresponders (<30% predicted probability of response) (Figure 3A). The observed outcomes in these 129 cases were 85 responders and 44 nonresponders (observed response rate 66%). For these 129 cases, 79 of 85 observed responders were correctly predicted (sensitivity 93%; 95% confidence interval [CI] 88%–98%), as were 33 of 44 observed nonresponders (specificity 75%; [62%–88%]). The positive predictive value (PPV) was 88% (79/90; [81%–95%]) and the negative predictive value (NPV) was 85% (33/39; [74%–96%]). The overall accuracy of prediction was 112 of 129 predicted cases (87%; [81%–93%]). The prior probabilities of observed response (66%) and nonresponse (34%) in the absence of genotyping increased to posterior probabilities of 88% and 85%, respectively ($P<0.001$ in each case). For the remaining 110 cases with predicted probability of response between 30% and 80%, posterior probabilities did not differ significantly from prior probabilities of response or nonresponse.

Validation of prediction model

In the validation sample of 176 new completer cases treated with SSRI drugs, the distributions of clinical characteristics and genetic markers did not differ from the derivation sample (Table 1, Table S5). Seven of the top 10 SNPs that showed the strongest association with SSRI treatment response in the derivation sample were significantly associated in the validation sample (Table S6). In this validation cohort, the prior probabilities were 66% for response (116 of 176) and 34% for nonresponse (60 of 176) (Table 1). The HAP-SNP model made predictions for 60% (106/176) of these patients, with 84 predicted responders and 22 predicted nonresponders (Figure 3B). The observed outcomes in these 106 predicted cases were 74 responders and 32 nonresponders (Figure 3B). The overall accuracy of prediction was 85% (90/106; [78%–92%]). Sensitivity and specificity were 96% (71/74; [91%–100%]) and 59% (19/32; [42%–76%]), respectively. This specificity result was not significantly lower than in the derivation sample ($P=0.21$). Among these 106 cases, the prior probabilities of observed response (70%) and nonresponse (30%) in the absence of genotyping increased to posterior probabilities of 85% (PPV; 71/84; [77%–92%]) and 86% (NPV; 19/22; [72%–100%]), respectively ($P<0.001$ in each case). These PPV and NPV results did not significantly differ from the corresponding values (PPV = 88%, NPV = 85%) in the derivation sample (Fisher's exact test, $P=0.66$, $P=1.00$, respectively). Of note, the model predicted 59% (19 of 32) of observed nonresponders in the validation sample with 86% accuracy (Figure 3B).

Cross-validation of prediction model

In the third phase of this study we tested whether the HAP-SNP model that predicted response to SSRIs also predicted outcomes in patients treated with non-SSRI antidepressants. In an independent sample of 189 protocol completers (Figure 1), we compared response and nonresponse predicted for SSRIs by the HAP-SNP model with observed response and observed nonresponse to non-SSRI antidepressants. The distributions of clinical characteristics and genetic markers did not differ from the derivation sample in this cross-validation sample (Table 1, Table S5). The observed response rate was 60% (114/189). The genetic associations with observed response to SSRI drugs were not replicated for observed response to non-SSRI agents (Table S7). Figure S3 shows a lack of correlation between the association analysis P values of groups receiving SSRIs and non-SSRIs (Pearson $r=0.02$). No SNP markers in the non-SSRI group reached a significant level of association with response after FDR correction.

Consistent with these gene association differences, the observed responses to non-SSRI drugs differed significantly from the predictions made by the HAP-SNP model that predicted response to SSRIs. The model made predictions for 84 (44%) of the 189 cases in the cross validation sample (61 predicted responders (73%) and 23 predicted nonresponders (27%)). There were 43 observed responders (70.5%) among the 61 predicted responders (PPV), and 11 observed nonresponders (47.8%) among the 23 predicted nonresponders (NPV). These values were significantly different from the corresponding PPV and NPV values in the derivation sample. (Fisher's exact test, $P=0.01$, $P<0.01$, respectively). Within this group of 84 cases, the observed outcomes were 55 responders (65%) and 29 nonresponders (35%). These are the prior probabilities of response and nonresponse among predicted cases, not significantly different from the full cohort of 189 cases (60% and 40%, respectively).

Text S2 provides additional descriptions of secondary analyses (Supplementary Results), which describes (1) comparisons of the three cohorts in respect of genotypes, clinical characteristics, and plasma drug levels in relation to response status; (2) SNP associations with the secondary outcome of remission; (3) a test of the top 10 SNPs in the response prediction model for possible associations with the diagnosis of major depression – with no significant association being found; (4) details of the polymorphism prediction model that was replaced by the HAP-SNP model; (5) secondary conditional probability analyses in the cross-validation cohort, demonstrating a double dissociation of observed versus expected outcomes: cases predicted by the HAP-SNP model to do poorly with SSRI treatment actually had significantly better observed outcomes with non-SSRI treatment, while cases

Table 3. Genotypic combinations of haplotype-SNP (HAP-SNP) prediction model.

	TPH2 (H3)*	SLC6A4 (H1)[†]	rs543196	rs3828275	5-HTTLPR	
Predicted responder	H3-B	H1-A	CC	AA	ss	>80% (n = 90)
	H3-B	H1-A	CC	GG	ss	
	H3-B	H1-A	CC	AA	sl+ll	
	H3-B	H1-A	TC	AA	ss	
	H3-B	H1-A	CC	GG	sl+ll	
	H3-B	H1-A	TC	GG	ss	
	H3-B	H1-A	CC	AG	ss	
	H3-B	H1-A	TC	AA	sl+ll	
Predicted Nonresponder	H3-B	H1-B	TT	GG	ss	<30% (n = 39)
	H3-B	H1-B	TC	AG	ss	
	H3-A	H1-A	TT	AA	ss	
	H3-A	H1-B	CC	AA	ss	
	H3-A	H1-A	TC	GG	sl+ll	
	H3-A	H1-A	CC	AG	sl+ll	
	H3-B	H1-B	TT	AA	sl+ll	
	H3-A	H1-A	TT	GG	ss	
	H3-A	H1-A	TC	AG	ss	
	H3-A	H1-B	CC	GG	ss	
	H3-B	H1-B	TT	GG	sl+ll	
	H3-B	H1-B	TC	AG	sl+ll	
	H3-A	H1-A	TT	AA	sl+ll	
	H3-B	H1-B	TT	AG	ss	
	H3-A	H1-B	CC	AA	sl+ll	
	H3-A	H1-B	TC	AA	ss	
	H3-A	H1-A	TT	GG	sl+ll	
	H3-A	H1-A	TC	AG	sl+ll	
	H3-A	H1-B	CC	GG	sl+ll	
	H3-A	H1-A	TT	AG	ss	
	H3-A	H1-B	TC	GG	ss	
	H3-A	H1-B	CC	AG	ss	
	H3-B	H1-B	TT	AG	sl+ll	
	H3-A	H1-B	TC	AA	sl+ll	
	H3-A	H1-B	TT	AA	ss	
	H3-A	H1-A	TT	AG	sl+ll	
	H3-A	H1-B	TC	AA	sl+ll	
	H3-A	H1-B	CC	AG	sl+ll	
	H3-A	H1-B	TT	GG	ss	
	H3-A	H1-B	TC	AG	ss	
	H3-A	H1-B	TT	AA	sl+ll	
	H3-A	H1-B	TT	GG	sl+ll	
	H3-A	H1-B	TC	AG	sl+ll	
	H3-A	H1-B	TT	AG	ss	
	H3-A	H1-B	TT	AG	sl+ll	

Abbreviations: SNP, single-nucleotide polymorphism; *5-HTTLPR,* serotonin-transporter-linked polymorphic region.
*H3-A is defined as a pair of two haplotypes (GCATGG and GCATGG), and H3-B as the other cases.
[†]H1-A is defined as any pairs constituting of the CATAGGGATGCC, CATAGGGACGCC, CATAGGAACGTC, CCTAGGGATGCC, AATAGGGATGCC, AACGAGGCCCCT, AACGAGAATGCC and AACGAAGCCCCT haplotypes, and H1-B as any pairs including at least one haplotype among the AACGAGAACGTC, CATAGGGCCCCC and CATGAGGATGCC haplotypes.

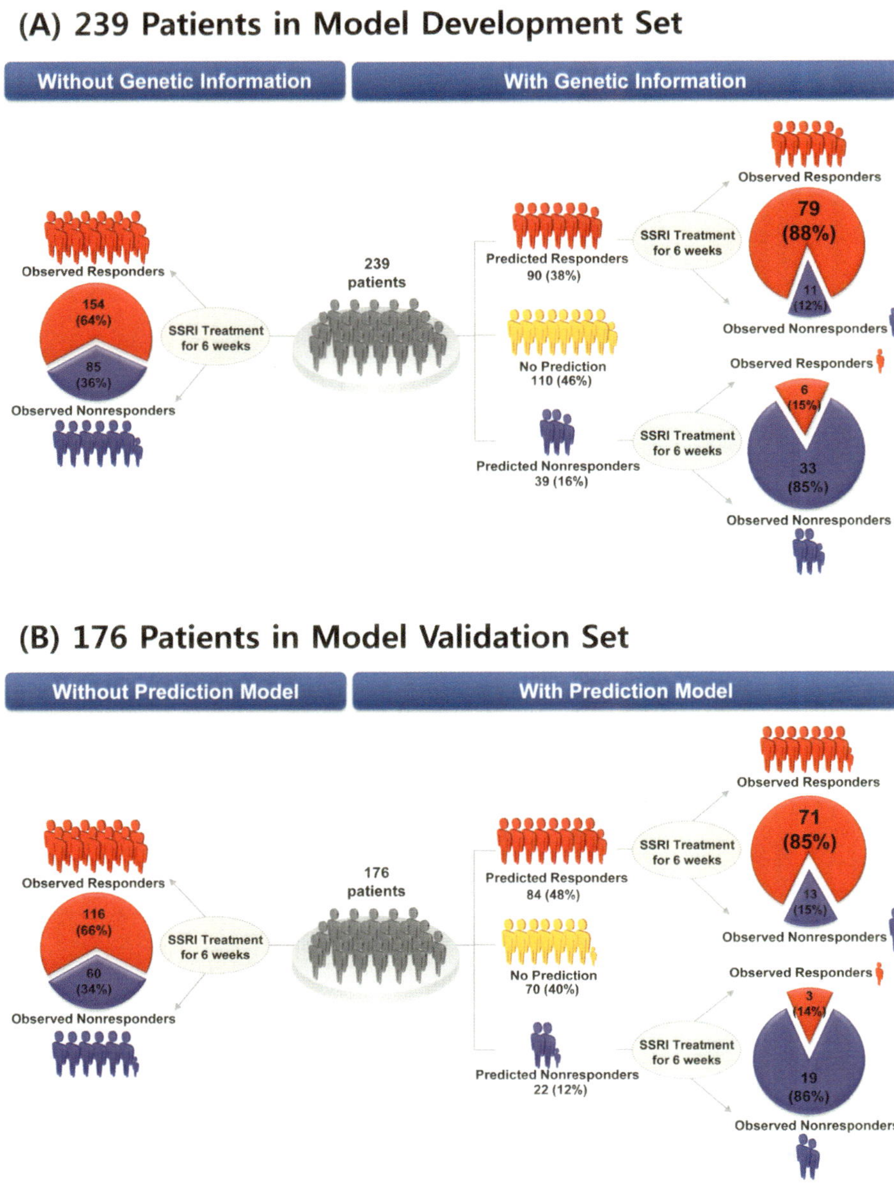

Figure 3. Clinical performance of selective serotonin reuptake inhibitor (SSRI) response prediction model using genetic information. Results of genetic prediction of response or nonresponse to SSRIs (a) in initial derivation sample (n = 239) and (b) validation sample (n = 176) of completer patients with major depression.

predicted by the HAP-SNP model to do well with SSRI treatment actually had significantly worse observed outcomes with non-SSRI drugs.

Discussion

The markers associated with response to SSRI drugs comprised ten SNPs from the *TPH2*, *SLC6A4*, *GRIK2*, and *GAD1* genes and six haplotypes from the *TPH2*, *SLC6A4*, and *GRIK2* genes (Table 2 and Figure 2). Thus, SSRI response was associated with polymorphisms in serotonin, glutamate, and GABA related genes. *TPH2* showed the most significant association with SSRI response. *TPH2* encodes the rate-limiting enzyme of brain serotonin production [28].

Comparison with previous studies

Our finding of association between *TPH2* and SSRI response is consistent with prior evidence from studies in an animal model and human post mortem neurochemistry [29,30]. We found associations of SSRI response with 4 SNPs in *TPH2* (rs4760815, rs11179027, rs17110532, and rs17110747). A previous small study found that three SNPs in *TPH2*, rs1843809 and rs1386492 of intron 5, and rs1487276 of intron 8, were associated with drug response after 12 weeks of SSRI treatment (Figure S4) [31]. However, there was no significant association between those three SNPs and SSRI response in the present study.

Another study performed in a European population investigated nine SNPs in the *TPH2* gene, and found two SNPs, rs10879346 and rs1487278, were significantly related to antidepressant response [32]. Additionally, rs2171363 was significant in a

Chinese population [33]. We imputed these three SNPs using genotype data, because they were not genotyped in our study. The imputed SNPs showed significant associations with SSRI response (Figure S4). These results from imputed data increase the possibility that the predictive markers suggested in our data will be replicable in other populations.

Our previous studies indicated that two VNTRs in the 2nd intron (*STin2*) and promoter (*5-HTTLPR*) of *SLC6A4* are associated with SSRI response [5,9]. In this study, we examined the two VNTRs and 12 SNPs in the *SLC6A4* gene, and found both VNTRs and two SNPs were significantly associated with SSRI response (Table 2). The two SNPs, rs2066713 and rs2020942, were located in intron 1 and intron 3, respectively. A previous study reported that these two SNPs have no association with SSRI response at 12 weeks in an ethnically mixed population [31], but another U.S. study reported that rs2066713 showed a trend towards association with SSRI response [34]. Three polymorphisms significantly associated with SSRI response, rs2066713 of intron 1, VNTR of intron 2, and rs2020942 of intron 3, were tightly linked (Table S8). When we constructed a haplotype from 12 SNPs of the *SLC6A4* gene, the haplotype was significantly associated with SSRI response (Figure 2C). It was also reported in a Caucasian population that a haplotype constructed from 21 SNPs of the *SLC6A4* gene was significant [31]. Thus, our results here and previously [5,9] are consistent with much previous work and with a previous meta-analysis [35] which concluded that the *SLC6A4* gene is an informative genetic marker for SSRI response. Moreover, a recent meta-analysis study [36] that examined Caucasian and Asian populations separately confirmed the importance of ethnicity for interpreting pharmacogenetic studies [37]. This is in contrast to an earlier meta-analysis [38] that disregarded ethnicity and found no overall association of *5-HTTLPR* genotype and responsiveness. Porcelli and colleagues reported in Caucasians that *5-HTTLPR* may be a predictor of antidepressant response, while in Asians it is not. These inconsistencies in the evidence for an association between *5-HTTLPR* and antidepressant response in Asian populations may result also from the established genetic variability within broad Asian ethnic groups. For instance, the genotype distribution of *5-HTTLPR* in Han Chinese is closer to the Caucasian profile than to the Japanese or Korean profile [37].

We did not confirm the claim that the serotonin receptor gene *HTR2A* is associated with SSRI response [8]. We found no association for any of the 28 markers in the *HTR2A* gene in our population (rs7997012, FDR corrected $P = 0.47$). In addition, the original report [8] has not been consistently replicated [12,39].

We found that both glutamate (*GRIK2*) and GABA (*GAD1*) related genes are associated with SSRI response. Both these abundant neurotransmitters are implicated in mood circuitry. Our result with *GRIK2* might be related to a report claiming *GRIK4* is associated with response to the SSRI citalopram [40]. We found that two SNPs in intron 1 of the *GRIK2* gene (rs543196 and rs572487) and two haplotypes including each SNP were significantly associated with SSRI response, and several neighboring SNPs showed a trend towards association (Table 2 and Figure 2B). The *GRIK2* gene encodes glutamate receptors, which respond to glutamate for excitatory transmission in mood circuits. There are abnormalities in glutamatergic neurotransmission in depressed patients [41], and the glutamate system is influenced by SSRIs [42,43].

We know of no previous reports that GABA (*GAD1*) related genes are associated with SSRI response. *GAD1* is the key enzyme of the GABA neurotransmitter system. We found that two SNPs in the *GAD1* gene (rs3828275 of intron3 and rs12185692 of 5′-untranslated region) were significantly associated with SSRI response (Table 2). Abnormalities in GABA neurotransmission have been noted in depression [44]. Overall, the genetic profile of our HAP-SNP model for prediction of response to SSRIs is consistent with drug actions involving the neuromodulator serotonin, followed by effects on the mood circuits that employ glutamate and GABA [45].

Study limitation and strength

A recent meta-analysis identified no individual SNP associations with a genome-wide significance for response to SSRI drugs in depression. That null result includes our own findings [46]. One candidate reason for this apparent non-confirmation may be the ethnic distinctiveness of our population. It is previously reported that response to the SSRI citalopram in African American depressed patients was poorer than in Caucasian Americans and it was suggested that this variance in response may be explained by an allelic frequency difference in rs7997012 of *HTR2A* between the two population samples [8]. Three recent genome-wide association studies [12,13,47] failed to identify gene associations with response to antidepressant drugs in depression. These failures underscore the heterogeneity of the clinical depression phenotype, and the complex gene-environment nature of the disorder. In addition, these large, multi-site studies risk incurring methodological problems such as heterogeneity of case material, ethnic heterogeneity, measurement error, and variable recruitment practices [48,49]. By comparison, strengths of our study design include single site performance by an experienced research team, strictly blinded quality control, ethnic homogeneity, inclusion of only clinically referred cases, clinical diagnoses by experienced psychiatrists in advance of confirmatory research diagnostic interviews [50], outcome assessments in person rather than by telephone, and verification of adequate antidepressant blood levels. We also required that all cases were unexposed to antidepressant drugs in the current episode of depression before enrolment in this study. By these means, heterogeneity and confounding of the case material were controlled, and we succeeded in identifying and validating significant genetic predictors of response with manageable sample sizes.

The prediction model examined *observed* response and nonresponse: without a placebo control group we have no basis to predict specific drug response. The gain of information from the predictive model is substantial, especially in the prediction of nonresponse. For the 16% of completer cases (39/239) that our HAP-SNP model predicts will be nonresponders in the derivation sample (Figure 3A), the relative risk of observed nonresponse is 3.3 in comparison to all other cases, and 6.9 in comparison to the cases whom the model predicts will be responders. In the validation sample, these relative risks are 3.2 and 5.6, respectively (Figure 3B). For comparison, the relative risk of a poor outcome is 1.5 in the 27% of patients receiving clopidogrel who have loss of function polymorphisms in *CYP2C19* [51].

The genetic determinants of observed response to SSRI drugs (Table 2) were not associated with response to non-SSRI antidepressant drugs (Table S7). Thus, these results are consistent with the previous reports [9,11] that pharmacologically different antidepressants are associated with different genetic determinants of response. A further, indirect, inference is that the significant markers for observed response to SSRI drugs may be unrelated to nonspecific response factors ("placebo effect") in our patients. However, we should mention that previous antidepressant treatment history in prior episodes of depression might have influenced the clinicians' choice of non-SSRI treatment in the cross-validation sample. We cannot positively rule out this possible confound in this naturalistic study, even though the cross-validation sample closely resembled the SSRI-treated samples on relevant clinical variables (Table 1).

The convergent data from the validation and cross-validation samples suggest that for approximately half the total cases who adhere to treatment, a gene-based recommendation of SSRI or non-SSRI agent as first-line treatment may be possible with 85% confidence, and that this represents a significant improvement over base rates of response and nonresponse in the absence of genotype information for those cases.

The ethnic homogeneity of our sample may be viewed as either a strength or a limitation, and our prediction model needs to be evaluated in other populations. However, the predictive markers suggested in the European [32] and Chinese studies [33] were replicable in our population from imputed data of *TPH2* (Figure S4). Moreover, the ethnic homogeneity of our sample with the appropriate power may overcome the problems of population stratification which can occur in ethnically mixed populations [8]. Additionally, we could not detect any evidence of population stratification between responders and nonresponders in the 1400 genetic markers of our subjects by the Structure 2.2 software [52] and by quantile-quantile plots of the association results (Figure S5 and Figure S6).

Our prediction model does not include clinical variables. Duration of depressive episode was the only clinical or demographic variable that differed between responders and nonresponders, and only in the derivation sample (Table 1). This clinical variable was eliminated when it was found to be nonsignificant in the logistic regression analyses. Thus, while clinical features are somewhat related to antidepressant response, they may not be independently predictive after correction for genomic factors [32].

Implications

Our HAP-SNP model appears to achieve the goal of gene-based selection of drug class in just over 50% of adherent cases. Though it remains an objective, we do not yet know whether it is realistic to expect significantly better predictive power than 50% in such a complex and heterogeneous disorder as DSM-IV defined major depression. Nevertheless, this extent of genetic prediction is potentially cost-effective [53]. In particular, 59% of the anticipated nonresponders could be identified without the expense and delay associated with a failed trial of SSRIs. In order to evaluate the applicability of genetic predictors in clinical practice, Intent-to-Treat (ITT) analyses and cost analyses will be required. However, ITT is not the appropriate framework for discovery purposes such as this study. Moreover, all potential biomarkers for prediction of antidepressant response in practice settings are destined to be subject to the attrition that we observed (at least 20%), if not much more [54]. While our results need to be confirmed in other populations, and will doubtless be refined with further experience, to the best of our knowledge, no genetic models possessing comparable power have been proposed and validated for the prediction of antidepressant drug class response.

Web Resources

dbSNP: http://www.ncbi.nlm.nih.gov/projects/SNP

FESD: http://sysbio.kribb.re.kr:8080/fesd

HapMap: http://hapmap.org

Tagger: http://www.broad.mit.edu/mpg/tagger

Supporting Information

Figure S1 Selection of 1502 candidate SNPs from 79 candidate genes.

Figure S2 Difference in linkage disequilibrium (LD) structure of TPH2 between responders and nonresponders. The LD structure is based on the measure of r^2. LD was stronger among responders than among nonresponders. The region including three different haplotype blocks, H2, H3, and a part of H4 in the nonresponder group was observed as a single long haplotype, H2 (12 SNPs) in the responder group.

Figure S3 Association analysis of SSRI and non-SSRI treated groups. Association analysis p values (as $-\log_{10}$ values) of 1400 polymorphic markers were plotted. No correlation of p values between SSRI treated and non-SSRI treated groups was observed. (A) Association analysis p values between antidepressant response and single-nucleotide polymorphisms (SNPs) in the SSRI treated group are sorted in descending order. The plot of the p values of the SSRI treated group is distributed by continuous curve form and that of the non-SSRI treated group by scattered form. (B) The distribution of high $-\log_{10}$ p values on each axis demonstrates that distinct SNPs were associated with response to each class of antidepressant drug.

Figure S4 Comparison of association analysis results for *TPH2* with previous studies. Red filled diamonds indicate genotyped SNPs in this study and red blank diamonds imputed SNPs. Blue filled triangles, blue blank triangles, and dark green crosses indicate association results studied in Tzvetkov et al. 2008, Peters et al. 2004, and Tsai et al. 2009, respectively. The same SNPs between studies are linked by dotted lines. The significant SNPs, rs10879346 and rs1487278, in Tzvetkov et al. 2008 study and rs2171363 in Tsai et al. 2009 study were replicated in our imputation study, suggesting that associations in the current study might be replicable in other populations (See Discussion of Manuscript).

Figure S5 Population structure in the derivation sample of SSRI treated patients. Population structure was estimated from 10 000 iterated simulations using the Structure 2.2 software. Red and green circles indicate responders and nonresponders, respectively. We set the number (K) of possible sub-populations as three (cluster 1, cluster 2 and others). If there was population stratification, individual circles would be grouped near one of the clusters according to their overall genetic similarity. We did not observe any clear pattern of clustering between responders and nonresponders. No evidence of population stratification between two groups was observed in our sample.

Figure S6 Quantile-quantile (QQ) plots for association tests of 1400 SNPs. For each of five genetic modes of (A) genotype, (B) additive, (C) allele, (D) dominant, and (E) recessive, QQ plots of the results of association with selective serotonin reuptake inhibitor (SSRI) response are shown in blue. No overall departures of the observed p values from the expected p values were observed in the QQ plots. Median value of $-\log_{10} P$ values ranged from 0.24 to 0.34 according to the genetic mode.

Table S1 Candidate genes and 1502 selected SNPs.

Table S2 Summary of selected SNPs according to SNP selection method.

Table S3 Associations of significant SNP markers with response for individual SSRI drugs in derivation sample.

Table S4 Plasma levels of antidepressants for responders and nonresponders.

Table S5 Distribution of genotypes of the SNPs most strongly associated with response to SSRIs in derivation sample, in validation sample, and in cross-validation sample.

Table S6 Association analysis results in validation samples of top 10 SNPs significantly associated with SSRI response in derivation samples.

Table S7 SNPs most strongly associated with response to non-SSRI drugs.

Table S8 Linkage disequilibrium (LD) between predictive markers.

Text S1 Supplementary Methods: 1. Function-based tagging selection of single-nucleotide polymorphism markers; 2. Genotyping, 3. Plasma drug levels; 4. Power analysis.

Text S2 Supplementary Results: 1. Characteristics of study subjects; 2. SNPs most strongly associated with remission in SSRI treated group; 3. Association with depression diagnosis for top 10 SNPs significantly associated with SSRI response; 4. Polymorphism prediction model for SSRI treatment; 5. Cross validation results with HAP-SNP prediction model.

Acknowledgments

We thank Sang-En Lee and Heejin Bae from Medical Information and Medical Service of Samsung Medical Center for their assistance in drawing Figure 3 and text editing. And we thank Jong Min Woo from Inje University for his advice on the likely cost-effectiveness of genetic screening in depression. We also thank William H. Wilson from Duke University Medical Center for advice on statistical analyses.

Author Contributions

Conceived and designed the experiments: DKK SL HW WM HK SK JK BJC. Performed the experiments: SL HW JK. Analyzed the data: HW SK BJC. Contributed reagents/materials/analysis tools: SL KK. Wrote the paper: DKK JK SL HW WM SK BJC.

References

1. Trivedi MH, Rush AJ, Wisniewski SR, Nierenberg AA, Warden D, et al. (2006) Evaluation of outcomes with citalopram for depression using measurement-based care in STAR*D: implications for clinical practice. Am J Psychiatry 163: 28–40.
2. Laje G, Perlis RH, Rush AJ, McMahon FJ (2009) Pharmacogenetics studies in STAR*D: strengths, limitations, and results. Psychiatr Serv 60: 1446–1457.
3. Licinio J, Wong ML (2010) Pharmacogenomics of antidepressants: what is next? Mol Psychiatry 15: 445.
4. Kato M, Serretti A (2010) Review and meta-analysis of antidepressant pharmacogenetic findings in major depressive disorder. Mol Psychiatry 15: 473–500.
5. Kim DK, Lim SW, Lee S, Sohn SE, Kim S, et al. (2000) Serotonin transporter gene polymorphism and antidepressant response. Neuroreport 11: 215–219.
6. Pollock BG, Ferrell RE, Mulsant BH, Mazumdar S, Miller M, et al. (2000) Allelic variation in the serotonin transporter promoter affects onset of paroxetine treatment response in late-life depression. Neuropsychopharmacology 23: 587–590.
7. Smeraldi E, Zanardi R, Benedetti F, Di Bella D, Perez J, et al. (1998) Polymorphism within the promoter of the serotonin transporter gene and antidepressant efficacy of fluvoxamine. Mol Psychiatry 3: 508–511.
8. McMahon FJ, Buervenich S, Charney D, Lipsky R, Rush AJ, et al. (2006) Variation in the gene encoding the serotonin 2A receptor is associated with outcome of antidepressant treatment. Am J Hum Genet 78: 804–814.
9. Kim H, Lim SW, Kim S, Kim JW, Chang YH, et al. (2006) Monoamine transporter gene polymorphisms and antidepressant response in Koreans with late-life depression. JAMA 296: 1609–1618.
10. McMahon FJ (2010) Pioneering first steps and cautious conclusions. Biol Psychiatry 67: 99–100.
11. Perlis RH, Fijal B, Dharia S, Heinloth AN, Houston JP (2010) Failure to replicate genetic associations with antidepressant treatment response in duloxetine-treated patients. Biol Psychiatry 67: 1110–1113.
12. Ising M, Lucae S, Binder EB, Bettecken T, Uhr M, et al. (2009) A genomewide association study points to multiple loci that predict antidepressant drug treatment outcome in depression. Arch Gen Psychiatry 66: 966–975.
13. Garriock HA, Kraft JB, Shyn SI, Peters EJ, Yokoyama JS, et al. (2010) A genomewide association study of citalopram response in major depressive disorder. Biol Psychiatry 67: 133–138.
14. Hamilton M (1967) Development of a rating scale for primary depressive illness. Br J Soc Clin Psychol 6: 278–296.
15. Karasu TB, Gelenberg A, Merriam A, Wang P (2000) Treatment of patients with major depressive disorder. In: McIntyre JS, Charles SC, editors.American Psychiatric Association Practice Guidelines for the Treatment of Psychiatric Disorders Compendium 2000. 2nd ed.Arlington, Virginia: American Psychiatric Association. pp. 413–495.
16. Lingjaerde O, Ahlfors UG, Bech P, Dencker SJ, Elgen K (1987) The UKU side effect rating scale. A new comprehensive rating scale for psychotropic drugs and a cross-sectional study of side effects in neuroleptic-treated patients. Acta Psychiatr Scand Suppl 334: 1–100.
17. Cipriani A, Furukawa TA, Salanti G, Geddes JR, Higgins JP, et al. (2009) Comparative efficacy and acceptability of 12 new-generation antidepressants: a multiple-treatments meta-analysis. Lancet 373: 746–758.
18. Marchini J, Howie B, Myers S, McVean G, Donnelly P (2007) A new multipoint method for genome-wide association studies by imputation of genotypes. Nat Genet 39: 906–913.
19. Armitage P (1955) Tests for linear trends in proportions and frequencies. Biometrics 11: 375–386.
20. Storey JD, Tibshirani R (2003) Statistical significance for genomewide studies. Proc Natl Acad Sci U S A 100: 9440–9445.
21. Barrett JC, Fry B, Maller J, Daly MJ (2005) Haploview: analysis and visualization of LD and haplotype maps. Bioinformatics 21: 263–265.
22. Gabriel SB, Schaffner SF, Nguyen H, Moore JM, Roy J, et al. (2002) The structure of haplotype blocks in the human genome. Science 296: 2225–2229.
23. Liang KY, Zeger SL (1986) Longitudinal data analysis using generalized linear models. Biometrika 73: 13–22.
24. Keller MB, McCullough JP, Klein DN, Arnow B, Dunner DL, et al. (2000) A comparison of nefazodone, the cognitive behavioral-analysis system of psychotherapy, and their combination for the treatment of chronic depression. N Engl J Med 342: 1462–1470.
25. Walkup JT, Albano AM, Piacentini J, Birmaher B, Compton SN, et al. (2008) Cognitive behavioral therapy, sertraline, or a combination in childhood anxiety. N Engl J Med 359: 2753–2766.
26. Walsh BT, Seidman SN, Sysko R, Gould M (2002) Placebo response in studies of major depression: variable, substantial, and growing. JAMA 287: 1840–1847.
27. Wigton RS, Connor JL, Centor RM (1986) Transportability of a decision rule for the diagnosis of streptococcal pharyngitis. Arch Intern Med 146: 81–83.
28. Zhang X, Beaulieu JM, Sotnikova TD, Gainetdinov RR, Caron MG (2004) Tryptophan hydroxylase-2 controls brain serotonin synthesis. Science 305: 217.
29. Shishkina GT, Kalinina TS, Dygalo NN (2007) Up-regulation of tryptophan hydroxylase-2 mRNA in the rat brain by chronic fluoxetine treatment correlates with its antidepressant effect. Neuroscience 150: 404–412.
30. Lim JE, Pinsonneault J, Sadee W, Saffen D (2007) Tryptophan hydroxylase 2 (TPH2) haplotypes predict levels of TPH2 mRNA expression in human pons. Mol Psychiatry 12: 491–501.
31. Peters EJ, Slager SL, McGrath PJ, Knowles JA, Hamilton SP (2004) Investigation of serotonin-related genes in antidepressant response. Mol Psychiatry 9: 879–889.
32. Tzvetkov MV, Brockmoller J, Roots I, Kirchheiner J (2008) Common genetic variations in human brain-specific tryptophan hydroxylase-2 and response to antidepressant treatment. Pharmacogenet Genomics 18: 495–506.
33. Tsai SJ, Hong CJ, Liou YJ, Yu YW, Chen TJ, et al. (2009) Tryptophan hydroxylase 2 gene is associated with major depression and antidepressant treatment response. Prog Neuropsychopharmacol Biol Psychiatry 33: 637–641.
34. Kraft JB, Peters EJ, Slager SL, Jenkins GD, Reinalda MS, et al. (2007) Analysis of association between the serotonin transporter and antidepressant response in a large clinical sample. Biol Psychiatry 61: 734–742.
35. Serretti A, Kato M, De Ronchi D, Kinoshita T (2007) Meta-analysis of serotonin transporter gene promoter polymorphism (5-HTTLPR) association with

selective serotonin reuptake inhibitor efficacy in depressed patients. Mol Psychiatry 12: 247–257.
36. Porcelli S, Fabbri C, Serretti A (2012) Meta-analysis of serotonin transporter gene promoter polymorphism (5-HTTLPR) association with antidepressant efficacy. Eur Neuropsychopharmacol 22: 239–258.
37. Myung W, Lim SW, Kim S, Kim H, Chung JW, et al. (2013) Serotonin transporter genotype and function in relation to antidepressant response in Koreans. Psychopharmacology (Berl) 225: 283–290.
38. Taylor MJ, Sen S, Bhagwagar Z (2010) Antidepressant response and the serotonin transporter gene-linked polymorphic region. Biol Psychiatry 68: 536–543.
39. Peters EJ, Slager SL, Jenkins GD, Reinalda MS, Garriock HA, et al. (2009) Resequencing of serotonin-related genes and association of tagging SNPs to citalopram response. Pharmacogenet Genomics 19: 1–10.
40. Paddock S, Laje G, Charney D, Rush AJ, Wilson AF, et al. (2007) Association of GRIK4 with outcome of antidepressant treatment in the STAR*D cohort. Am J Psychiatry 164: 1181–1188.
41. Rosenberg DR, Mirza Y, Russell A, Tang J, Smith JM, et al. (2004) Reduced anterior cingulate glutamatergic concentrations in childhood OCD and major depression versus healthy controls. J Am Acad Child Adolesc Psychiatry 43: 1146–1153.
42. Barbon A, Popoli M, La Via L, Moraschi S, Vallini I, et al. (2006) Regulation of editing and expression of glutamate alpha-amino-propionic-acid (AMPA)/kainate receptors by antidepressant drugs. Biol Psychiatry 59: 713–720.
43. Martinez-Turrillas R, Frechilla D, Del Rio J (2002) Chronic antidepressant treatment increases the membrane expression of AMPA receptors in rat hippocampus. Neuropharmacology 43: 1230–1237.
44. Kalueff AV, Nutt DJ (2007) Role of GABA in anxiety and depression. Depress Anxiety 24: 495–517.
45. Price JL, Drevets WC (2010) Neurocircuitry of mood disorders. Neuropsychopharmacology 35: 192–216.
46. GENDEP Investigators, MARS Investigators, STAR*D Investigators (2013) Common genetic variation and antidepressant efficacy in major depressive disorder: a meta-analysis of three genome-wide pharmacogenetic studies. Am J Psychiatry 170: 207–217.
47. Tansey KE, Guipponi M, Perroud N, Bondolfi G, Domenici E, et al. (2012) Genetic predictors of response to serotonergic and noradrenergic antidepressants in major depressive disorder: a genome-wide analysis of individual-level data and a meta-analysis. PLoS Med 9: e1001326.
48. Demitrack MA, Faries D, Herrera JM, DeBrota D, Potter WZ (1998) The problem of measurement error in multisite clinical trials. Psychopharmacol Bull 34: 19–24.
49. Kraemer HC, Glick ID, Klein DF (2009) Clinical trials design lessons from the CATIE study. Am J Psychiatry 166: 1222–1228.
50. Carroll BJ (1984) Problems with diagnostic criteria for depression. J Clin Psychiatry 45: 14–18.
51. Mega JL, Close SL, Wiviott SD, Shen L, Hockett RD, et al. (2009) Cytochrome p-450 polymorphisms and response to clopidogrel. N Engl J Med 360: 354–362.
52. Pritchard JK, Stephens M, Donnelly P (2000) Inference of population structure using multilocus genotype data. Genetics 155: 945–959.
53. Braithwaite RS, Meltzer DO, King JT, Jr., Leslie D, Roberts MS (2008) What does the value of modern medicine say about the $50,000 per quality-adjusted life-year decision rule? Med Care 46: 349–356.
54. Lawrenson RA, Tyrer F, Newson RB, Farmer RD (2000) The treatment of depression in UK general practice: selective serotonin reuptake inhibitors and tricyclic antidepressants compared. J Affect Disord 59: 149–157.

Associations between Depression and Diabetes in the Community: Do Symptom Dimensions Matter? Results from the Gutenberg Health Study

Jörg Wiltink[1]*, Matthias Michal[1], Philipp S. Wild[2,3,4], Astrid Schneider[5], Jochem König[5], Maria Blettner[5], Thomas Münzel[3], Andreas Schulz[3], Matthias Weber[6], Christian Fottner[6], Norbert Pfeiffer[7], Karl Lackner[8], Manfred E. Beutel[1]

1 Department of Psychosomatic Medicine and Psychotherapy, University Medical Center of the Johannes Gutenberg-University Mainz, Mainz, Germany, **2** Center for Thrombosis and Hemostasis, University Medical Center of the Johannes Gutenberg-University Mainz, Mainz, Germany, **3** Department of Medicine 2, University Medical Center of the Johannes Gutenberg-University Mainz, Mainz, Germany, **4** German Center for Cardiovascular Research (DZHK), partner site RhineMain, Mainz, Mainz, Germany, **5** Institute of Medical Biostatistics, Epidemiology and Informatics, University Medical Center of the Johannes Gutenberg-University Mainz, Mainz, Germany, **6** Department of Medicine 1, University Medical Center of the Johannes Gutenberg-University Mainz, Mainz, Germany, **7** Department of Ophthalmology, University Medical Center of the Johannes Gutenberg-University Mainz, Mainz, Germany, **8** Institute of Clinical Chemistry and Laboratory Medicine, University Medical Center of the Johannes Gutenberg-University Mainz, Mainz, Germany,

Abstract

Objectives: While a bidirectional relationship between diabetes and depression has been established, there is little knowledge if the associations are due to somatic-affective or cognitive-affective dimensions of depression.

Research Design and Methods: In a population-based, representative survey of 15.010 participants we therefore studied the associations of the two dimensions of depression with diabetes and health care utilization among depressed and diabetic participants. Depression was assessed by the Patient Health Questionnaire PHQ-9.

Results: We found a linear and consistent association between the intensity of depression and the presence of diabetes increasing from 6.9% in no or minimal depression to 7.6% in mild, 9% in moderate and 10.5% in severe depression. There was a strong positive association between somatic-affective symptoms but not with cognitive-affective symptoms and diabetes. Depression and diabetes were both independently related to somatic health care utilisation.

Conclusions: Diabetes and depression are associated, and the association is primarily driven by the somatic-affective component of depression. The main limitation of our study pertains to the cross-sectional data acquisition. Further longitudinal work on the relationship of obesity and diabetes should differentiate the somatic and the cognitive symptoms of depression.

Editor: Robert Stewart, Institute of Psychiatry, United Kingdom

Funding: This work/the Gutenberg Health Study is funded through the government of Rhineland-Palatinate ('Stiftung Rheinland Pfalz für Innovation', contract number AZ 961-386261/733), the research programs 'Wissen schafft Zukunft' and 'Schwerpunkt Vaskuläre Prävention' of the Johannes Gutenberg-University of Mainz and its contract with Boehringer Ingelheim and PHILIPS Medical Systems including an unrestricted grant for the Gutenberg Health Study. Philipp S. Wild is funded by the Federal Ministry of Education and Research (BMBF 01EO1003). The funders had no role in study design, data collection and analysis, decision to publish, or preparation of the manuscript.

Competing Interests: All authors declare that they have no competing interest relevant to the subject matter of the manuscript that have occurred over the last two years, or that are expected in the foreseeable future.

* Email: joerg.wiltink@unimedizin-mainz.de

Introduction

With an increasing prevalence diabetes has become a significant public health burden (e.g. [1]). About 10 percent of diabetes patients also suffer from clinically significant depressive symptoms, and between 25 and 30 percent reported subclinical depressive symptoms (e.g. [2–4]).

There is evidence from longitudinal studies that depressive symptoms contribute to the incidence of diabetes in addition to obesity or antidepressant drug use (e.g. [5]). A recent meta-analysis based on 23 studies with more than 400.000 participants and a mean follow-up of 8.3 years by Rotella & Mannucci [6] found that the yearly incidence of diabetes was higher in the initially depressed compared to the nondepressed participants (0.72 vs. 0.47%).

Several meta-analyses on longitudinal data have indicated a bidirectional relationship between diabetes and depression, however, evidence for the direction that diabetes causes depression is somewhat weaker (e.g. [7,8]; for overview: [9,10]). Comorbid depression is consistently related to diabetes complications (diabetic retinopathy, nephropathy, neuropathy, macrovascular complications, and sexual dysfunction) [11] and also to treatment nonadherence [12]. Insulin-dependent diabetes patients have to cope with specific problems as difficulties with the integration of treatment into daily live, self-responsibility, dietary restrictions, or fear of complications, all contributing to depression and reducing medication adherence and therefore impair regulation of blood glucose leading to diabetes complications in later life. In addition, adverse health behavior (e.g. smoking, physical inactivity) associated with depression may compound diabetic complications [13].

Most studies focused on depressive symptoms in general as indicated e.g. by the PHQ sum score [14] or diagnostic interviews. For different somatic conditions (e.g. cardiovascular disease, obesity) only the somatic-affective symptoms were associated with poor medical outcome [15–18]. Studies differentiating cognitive-affective and somatic-affective depressive symptoms in diabetes are rare (e.g. [19,20]). To our knowledge, no study to date has investigated the associations of somatic-affective and cognitive-affective symptoms to diabetes in a large population based study.

In our cross-sectional population based sample we sought to answer the following issues:

1) Are intensity and symptomatology of depression associated to diabetes?
2) How are depression and diabetes associated to the utilization of mental and somatic health care?

We expected an increased prevalence of depressive symptoms among diabetic participants. We also expected a closer relationship between diabetes and somatic-affective depressive symptoms rather than cognitive-affective depressive symptoms. We further expected more frequent health care utilization and psychopharmacological treatments in the participants suffering from both diabetes and depressive symptoms.

Materials and Methods

Procedure and study sample

We investigated cross-sectional data of N = 15.010 participants enrolled in the Gutenberg Health Study (GHS) from 2007 to 2012. The GHS is a population-based, prospective, observational single-center cohort study in the Rhine-Main-Region in western Mid-Germany. The GHS has been approved by the local ethics committee and by the local and federal data safety commissioners. The primary aim of the study is to evaluate and improve cardiovascular risk stratification. The sample was drawn randomly from the local registry in the city of Mainz and the district of Mainz-Bingen. The sample was stratified 1:1 for gender and residence and in equal strata for decades of age. Inclusion criteria were age 35 to 74 years and written informed consent. Persons with insufficient knowledge of German language, or those who reported that they were not able to visit the study center on their own (due to their physical and/or mental condition) were excluded. The response rate (defined as the recruitment efficacy proportion, i.e. the number of persons with participation in or appointment for the baseline examination divided by the sum of number of persons with participation in or appointment for the baseline examination plus those with refusal and those who were not contactable) was 60.3% for the first 5.000 participants. Due to the ongoing recruitment of the GHS, which is conducted in waves, a final statement concerning the response rate cannot be made at this time. The design and the rationale of the Gutenberg Health Study (GHS) have been described in detail elsewhere [21].

Materials and Assessment

The 5-hour baseline-examination in the study center comprised evaluation of prevalent classical cardiovascular risk factors and clinical variables, a computer-assisted personal interview, laboratory examinations from a venous blood sample, blood pressure and anthropometric measurements. In general, all examinations were performed according to standard operating procedures (SOPs) by certified medical technical assistants.

Primary outcome measures

Depression. Depression was measured by the Patient Health Questionnaire (PHQ-9); caseness was defined by a score ≥10 with a sensitivity of 81% and a specificity of 82% for depressive disorder (14). Depressive symptoms were classified as "minimal" (score 5 to 9), "mild" (score 10 to 14), "moderately severe" (score 15 to 19) and "severe" (score >20) [22]. The somatic-affective and cognitive-affective dimensions of depression were defined according to prior studies [23–25]. Four PHQ-9 items related to problems with sleep, fatigability, appetite, and psychomotor agitation/retardation were classified as somatic-affective symptoms, whereas 5 items, related to lack of interest, depressed mood, negative feelings about self, concentration problems and suicidal ideation, were classified as cognitive-affective symptoms of depression [16,18]. While we were aware, that dimensions of depression (cognitive-affective and somatic-affective) in the community might differ from those in cardiovascular settings, we used the same dimensions for comparison purposes and due to their high face validity and comparability.

Diabetes. *Diabetes* was defined in individuals with a definite diagnosis of diabetes by a physician or a blood glucose level of ≥ 126 mg/dl in the baseline examination after an overnight fast of at least 8 hours or a blood glucose level of ≥200 mg/dl in the baseline examination after a fasting period <8 hours.

Health care utilization. We determined two variables indicating health care utilization regarding mainly somatic or mainly mental problems. We assessed whether subjects had *consulted somatic physicians* (general practitioner or medical specialists) and whether they had *consulted psychotherapists/psychiatrists* during the last 4 weeks.

Potential confounders. In addition to age and sex we predefined a comprehensive set of confounders with a potential relation to diabetes and/or depression.

Life style factors. *The socioeconomic status* (SES) was defined according to Lampert's and Kroll's Scores of SES range from 3 to 27 while 3 indicates the lowest SES and 27 the highest SES [26].

Anxiety. *Generalized anxiety* was assessed with the two screening items of the short form of the GAD-7 (Generalized Anxiety Disorder [GAD] – 7 Scale) [27,28]. A sum score of 3 and more (range 0–6) out of these two items indicates generalized anxiety with good sensitivity (86%) and specificity (83%) [28]. *Panic disorder* was screened with the brief PHQ panic module. Caseness was defined if at least two of the first four PHQ panic questions are answered with "yes" [29].The German version of the Mini-Social Phobia Inventory (Mini-Spin) [30] was used to detect *social anxiety*. Utilizing a cut-off score of 6 (range 0–12), the Mini-Spin is supposed to separate between individuals with generalized social anxiety disorder and controls with good sensitivity (89%) and specificity (90%) [30,31]. Suffering from *any anxiety* was defined by reaching the cut-off in at least one of the three above mentioned scales [31].

Somatic conditions. *Hypertension* was diagnosed, if antihypertensive drugs were taken, or a mean systolic blood pressure of ≥140 mmHg in the 2nd and 3rd standardized measurement after 8 and 11 minutes of rest or a mean diastolic blood pressure of ≥ 90 mmHg in the 2nd and 3rd standardized measurement after 8 and 11 minutes of rest. *Obesity* was defined as a Body-Mass-Index (BMI) ≥30 kg/m^2. *Dyslipidemia* was defined as a definite diagnosis of dyslipidemia by a physician or an LDL/HDL-ratio of >3.5. The presence of further somatic conditions was assessed within a structured interview: "Has a physician ever diagnosed: constriction of your coronary heart vessels (*coronary heart disease*, CHD), *atrial fibrillation*, *cancer*, *myocardial infarction*, or *stroke*?"

Psychotropic medication. The following *psychotropic medications* potentially affecting mood and/or metabolism were chosen as confounders: non-selective monoamine reuptake inhibitors, selective serotonin reuptake inhibitor, other antidepressants, antipsychotics, anxiolytics, hypnotics/sedatives, antiepileptics, opioids.

Statistical analysis

Statistical analysis was done by IBM SPSS Statistics 20 (IBM, Chicago, IL).

Data are presented as numbers/percentage, mean (and 1.96-fold standard deviation) or median (and 1st, 3rd quartile) as appropriate.

To determine prevalence rates of diabetes stratified by severity of depressive symptoms we weighted our data by age and gender based on the population in the region of Mainz/Mainz-Bingen.

Odds ratios of single items differentiating the diabetic and non-diabetic populations were computed by ordinal logistic regression analyses (cumulative logit) of the PHQ-9 items on diabetes status. The models were adjusted by age, sex and SES.

To analyse the relationship between depression and diabetes, we computed separate linear regression models with depression (PHQ-9 sum score) as the dependent variable. Model 1 was without adjustment; in model 2 we adjusted for age, gender and socioeconomic status (SES) as potential confounders of depression and diabetes. Depressive symptoms were additionally evaluated with two separate analyses: a) using somatic-affective symptoms of depression (PHQ somatic-affective sum score) and b) using cognitive-affective symptoms (PHQ cognitive-affective sum score) as dependent variables. For these analyses we additionally adjusted (model 3) for cognitive-affective symptoms (dependent variable: somatic affective symptoms) and for somatic-affective symptoms (dependent variable: cognitive affective symptoms). Dependent variables were transformed in order to optimize the regression model: ln(PHQ-9 sumscore +5), ln(somatic-affective sum score +5), ln(cognitive-affective sum score +2), where ln denotes the natural logarithm.

To determine relations between depression (caseness: PHQ sum score <10 vs. PHQ sum score >= 10), diabetes and health care utilization we used logistic regression models with the dichotomous variables a) *consultation of somatic physicians* and b) *consultation of psychotherapists/psychiatrists* as the dependent variables and diabetes, depression and their interaction term (diabetes × depression) as independent variables. Models were adjusted for age, gender, socioeconomic status (SES), any anxiety and somatic conditions. In order to reduce total number of predictors we performed a variable selection for somatic conditions (obesity, hypertension, dyslipidemia, atrial fibrillation, CHD, myocardial infarction, stroke, cancer). Only those somatic conditions significantly related to health care utilization (logistic regression model with backward enter procedure) were entered into our regression. For the visualization of the results of these logistic regression models we computed model based estimates of marginal population means for each of the four groups defined by presence or absence of diabetes and depression.

All p-values correspond to 2-tailed tests.

Results

Sample characteristics

Table 1 shows the sociodemographic characteristics (age, sex, SES), depressive symptoms, anxiety, psychotropic medication, somatic conditions and health care utilization stratified for severity of depressive symptoms (no/minimal to moderately severe/severe).

The mean age of the participants was 55.0 years (range 35–74 years). 7428 were male (50.4%), and 7303 participants were female (49.6%). The majority of the participants reported a low level of education (less than 10th grade). About 1/3 had completed high school.

Prevalence of diabetes (weighted by age and gender) in the group of participants with no or only minimal depressive symptoms was 5.8%, mild depression 6.4%, moderate 7.5% and moderately severe/severe depression 9.1%. There was a considerable proportion of participants with an untreated or undetected (unaware) diabetes (no or only minimal depressive symptoms 0.6%, mild depression 0.4%, moderate depression 0.4% and moderately severe/severe 0.3%). Unawareness among diabetics decreased with increasing depression: no or only minimal depressive symptoms 10.2%, mild depression 6.9%, moderate depression 5.1% and moderately severe/severe 3.4%.

Associations between depression and diabetes

In our linear regression model, diabetes was significantly positively related to depressive symptoms after controlling for age, gender, socioeconomic status (SES). Using only the somatic-affective symptoms of depression as dependent variable and additionally controlling for the cognitive-affective symptoms, the same picture emerged. Cognitive-affective symptoms of depression were unrelated to diabetes. See table 2.

Figure 1 shows depressive symptoms for the diabetic and non-diabetic population.

Diabetics scored higher than non-diabetics in the following three items: "Feeling tired or having little energy" (item 4; OR 1.31), "Poor appetite or overeating" (item 5; OR 1.49), and "Moving or speaking so slowly that other people could have noticed. Or the opposite being so fidgety or restless that you have been moving around a lot more than usual" (item 8; OR 1.26). The three items all belong to the somatic-affective symptoms of depression.

Relation between depression, diabetes and health care utilization

We analysed the relationship between depression (dichotomous; cut-off >= 10), diabetes and health care utilization with logistic regression models.

After controlling for age, gender, SES, substantial symptoms of anxiety, and somatic conditions only depression was significantly related to consultations of psychotherapists/psychiatrists (OR 15.2 [95%CI 9.4, 24.7; p<.001]), diabetes was not (OR 0.70 [95%CI 0.16, 2.98; p = .62]), and neither was the interaction between depression and diabetes (p = .58).

Again, after controlling for the aforementioned variables (age, gender, SES, anxiety, and somatic conditions) depression (OR

Table 1. Sample characteristics stratified for severity of depressive symptoms (N = 14.731).

	PHQ score			
	0-4-5	**5–9**	**10–14**	**15–27**
Number	**9566**	**4032**	**856**	**277**
Sex, female	45.3%	56.6%	59.9%	61.4%
Age, in years; mean (SD)	55.3 (11.2)	54.5 (11.0)	53.2 (10.3)	51.6 (9.8)
SES, (3-21), median (1st, 3rd quartile)	13 (10/17)	12 (9/16)	11 (9/15)	11 (8/14)
Depressive symptoms				
Somatic-affective, median (1st/3rd quartile)	1 (1/2)	4 (3/4)	6 (5/7)	9 (7/10)
Cognitive-affective, median (1st,/3rd quartile)	0 (0/1)	3 (2/4)	5 (4/6)	9 (8/10)
Any Anxiety	3.4%	18.5%	55.2%	86.1%
Psychopharmacological treatment	4.8%	12.3%	24.0%	41.5%
Somatic conditions				
Diabetes	6.9%	7.6%	9.0%	10.5%
Diabetes untreated/unaware	0.7%	0.4%	0.5%	0.4%
Obesity (BMI> = 30)	23.2%	27.2%	30.5%	38.8%
Hypertension	50.1%	48.7%	47.3%	49.6%
Dyslipidemia	28.6%	29.9%	34.2%	35.4%
Atrial fibrillation	2.6%	2.9%	2.4%	3.3%
CHD	4%	4.7%	5.5%	5.8%
Myocardial infarction	2.6%	3.5%	3.0%	3.3%
Stroke	1.6%	2.0%	3.1%	1.8%
Cancer	8.5%	10.2%	10.2%	7.2%
> three somatic conditions	3.0%	4.0%	5.1%	5.7%
Health care utilization (last 4 weeks)				
Consulted somatic physicians	39.4%	47.1%	57.9%	64.6%
Consulted psychotherapists/psychiatrists	0.2%	0.4%	2.1%	9%

1.73 [95%CI 1.48, 2.01; p<.001]) and diabetes (OR 2.00 [95%CI 1.72, 2.33; p<.001]) were significantly related to consultations of somatic physicians, the interaction between depression and diabetes (p = .42) was not.

Results of the logistic regression models (least square means of frequency of health care utilization stratified by depression and diabetes) can be found in Table 3.

Discussion and Conclusions

The principal findings of this paper are a) a strong association between diabetes and depression; b) this was primarily due to somatic-affective rather than cognitive-affective symptoms and c) depression and diabetes were both independently related to somatic health care utilisation.

We found a linear and consistent association of the intensity of depression with the presence of diabetes increasing from 6.9% in no or minimal depression to 7.6% in mild, 9% in moderate and 10.5% in severe depression; i.e. the prevalence of diabetes in severe vs. no depression was elevated substantially (1.5 fold). This finding corresponds to the findings of earlier population based studies (e.g. [2,4]).

When controlling for comorbid somatic and mental (anxiety) conditions, we found a strong positive association of diabetes with

Table 2. Linear regression analyses of diabetes and depression (N = 14631–14639).

	Depressive symptoms (PHQ)	Somatic-affective symptoms	Cognitive-affective symptoms
	B (95% CI)	**B (95% CI)**	**B (95% CI)**
Model 1	0.037 (−0.025, 0.100)	0.079 (0.016, 0.141)	−0.016 (−0.078, 0.046)
Model 2	0.108 (0.045, 0.170)	0.138 (0.075, 0.201)	0.048 (−0.015, 0.112)
Model 3	..	0.110 (0.059, 0.161)	−0.032 (−0.083, 0.019)

Model 1: without adjustment; Model 2: adjusted for age, gender and socioeconomic status (SES); Model 3: additionally adjusted for cognitive-affective symptoms (dependent variable: somatic affective symptoms) and for somatic-affective symptoms (dependent variable: cognitive affective symptoms).

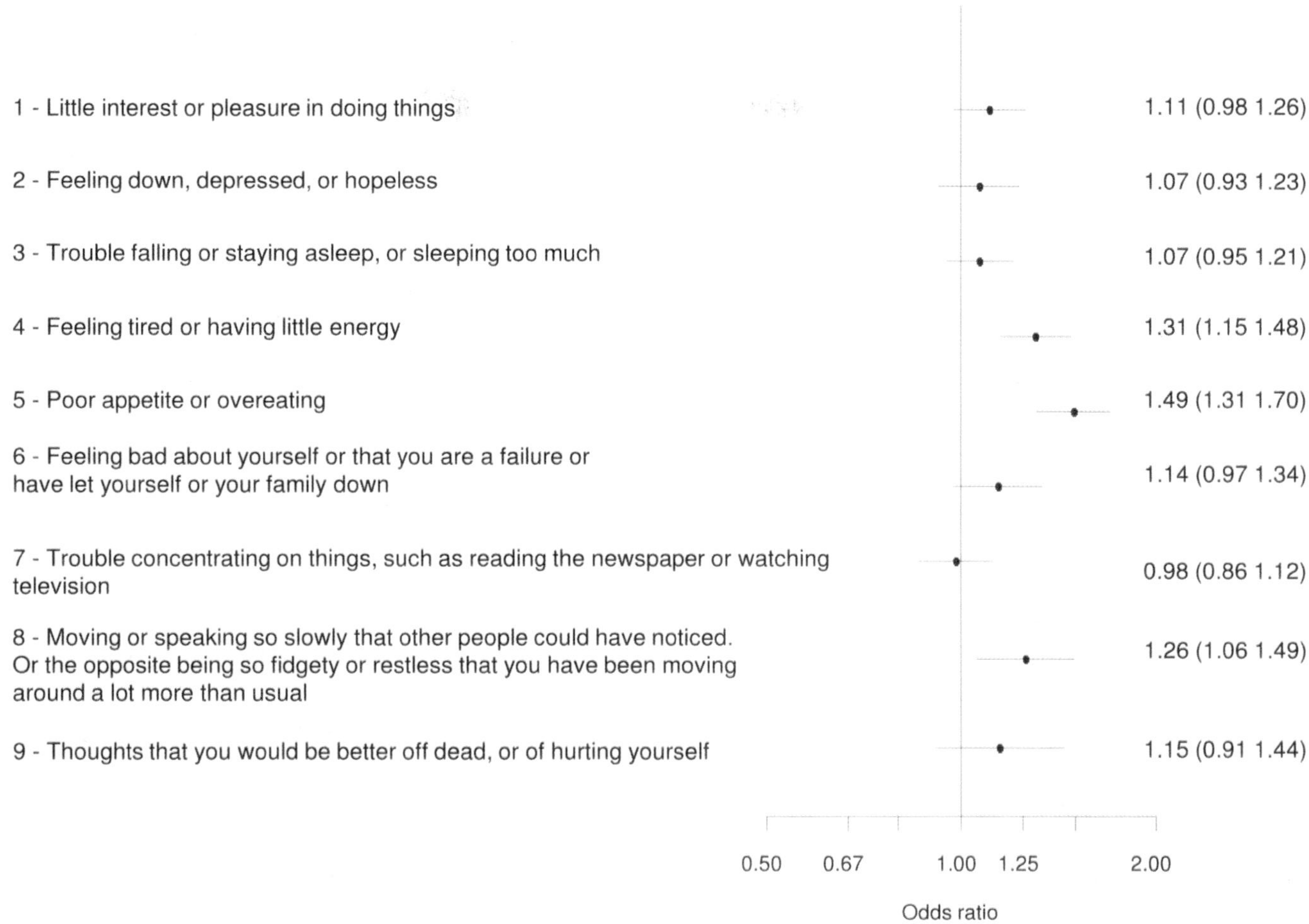

Figure 1. Depressive Symptoms (PHQ): Comparison between the diabetic and non-diabetic population. Ordinal logistic regression analyses (cumulative logit) of PHQ-9 items on diabetes status, models adjusted by age, sex and SES. Odds ratio above 1 indicate a trend towards a higher item response in diabetics. ORs and 95%CI are presented.

somatic-affective symptoms, but no association with cognitive-affective symptoms. Our findings narrow down the association of depression and diabetes to the somatic-affective dimension. These associations are likely to work both ways: Somatic-affective depressive symptoms are associated with metabolic risk factors for diabetes (obesity, dyslipidemia), which we have demonstrated in a previous paper [16]. Also, metabolic changes in diabetics and the associated inflammation may induce somatic-affective depression (e.g. Sleep disorder, fatigue, increased or decreased appetite, psychomotor changes).

Somatic and mental health care utilization also increased with depression: The majority of severely depressed (64.6% vs. 39.4% no depression) had consulted a physician in the past 4 weeks, and 9% (vs. 0.2%) had consulted a psychiatrist or a psychotherapist. Depressive symptoms were mostly treated pharmacologically, and depression was also associated with psychotherapeutic health care, but to a lesser degree. Taking comorbid conditions into account and controlling for other somatic diseases and anxiety, somatic health care utilization was predicted independently both by depression and by diabetes, i.e. both depressed and diabetic

Table 3. Health care utilization stratified by diabetes and depression (adjusted proportions).

	Consultation of psychotherapists/psychiatrists	Consultation of somatic physicians
	% (95%CI)	% (95%CI)
Depression/Diabetes		
Yes/yes	1.07 (0.25, 4.50)	88.4 (82.1, 92.7)
Yes/no	2.40 (1.41, 4.04)	79.9 (75.9, 83.4)
No/yes	0.14 (0.02, 0.99)	82.1 (78.3, 85.3)
No/no	0.30 (0.17, 0.51)	69.9 (65.4, 74.0)

participants had a high somatic health care utilization. However, the lack of an interaction implies that depressive diabetics do not receive more intensive medical treatment than non-depressive diabetics, although it has been demonstrated that depression increased complications and mortality in diabetics [11,32]. This may indicate an under-supply in those critical patients. As the success of collaborative health care projects suggests [33,34], depressed patients with comorbid somatic disorders may need more communication between somatic and mental health practitioners.

The main limitation of our study pertains to the cross-sectional data acquisition. Therefore, causal inferences are not possible. Due to the fact that people with less severe complaints are more likely to take part in a community study selection bias might have occurred towards oversampling those with the less severe depressive symptoms. Therefore, our results might not be generalizable to persons with major depressive disorders. Also, we relied on data of validated questionnaires, however, we could not use expert clinical ratings of depression.

The strengths are a) the well characterized, representative sample of participants living in the Rhine-Main region in Germany b) the inclusion of younger participants starting at the age of 35 years and b) the relatively large sample size.

Further, prospective work on the relationship of obesity and diabetes should also a) differentiate the somatic and the cognitive symptoms of depression in elucidating the mechanisms relating depression and diabetes (e.g. genetics, pro-inflammatory cytokines) including moderators (e.g. change in antidepressive or antidiabetic medication, psychotherapy) and b) target effective interventions to prevent and reduce depression in diabetes patients.

Author Contributions

Conceived and designed the experiments: JW MM MB. Analyzed the data: A. Schneider JK JW MM MEB. Contributed to the writing of the manuscript: JW MM MEB PSW A. Schneider JK MB TM A. Schulz MW CF NP KL.

References

1. Moulton AD, Albright AL, Gregg EW, Goodman RA (2013) Law, public health, and the diabetes epidemic. Am J Prev Med 45:486–493.
2. Ali S, Stone MA, Peters JL, Davies MJ, Khunti K (2006) The prevalence of co-morbid depression in adults with Type 2 diabetes: a systematic review and meta-analysis. Diabet Med 23:1165–1173.
3. Anderson RJ, Freedland KE, Clouse RE, Lustman PJ (2001) The prevalence of comorbid depression in adults with diabetes: a meta-analysis. Diabetes Care 24:1069–1078.
4. Hermanns N, Kulzer B, Krichbaum M, Kubiak T, Haak T (2005) Affective and anxiety disorders in a German sample of diabetic patients: prevalence, comorbidity and risk factors. Diabet Med 22:293–300.
5. Knol MJ, Twisk JW, Beekman AT, Heine RJ, Snoek FJ, et al. (2006) Depression as a risk factor for the onset of type 2 diabetes mellitus. A meta-analysis. Diabetologia 49:837–845.
6. Rotella F, Mannucci E (2013) Depression as a risk factor for diabetes: a meta-analysis of longitudinal studies. J Clin Psychiatry 74:31–37.
7. Mezuk B, Eaton WW, Albrecht S, Golden SH (2008) Depression and type 2 diabetes over the lifespan: a meta-analysis. Diabetes Care 31:2383–2390.
8. Pan A, Keum N, Okereke OI, Sun Q, Kivimaki M, et al. (2012) Bidirectional association between depression and metabolic syndrome: a systematic review and meta-analysis of epidemiological studies. Diabetes Care 35:1171–1180.
9. Renn BN, Feliciano L, Segal DL (2011) The bidirectional relationship of depression and diabetes: a systematic review. Clin Psychol Rev 31:1239–1246.
10. Wagner G, Icks A, Albers B, Abholz HH (2012) [Type 2 diabetes mellitus and depressive symptoms: what is the cause of what? A systematic literature review]. Dtsch Med Wochenschr 137:523–528.
11. de Groot M, Anderson R, Freedland KE, Clouse RE, Lustman PJ (2001) Association of depression and diabetes complications: a meta-analysis. Psychosom Med 63:619–630.
12. Gonzalez JS, Peyrot M, McCarl LA, Collins EM, Serpa L, et al. (2008) Depression and diabetes treatment nonadherence: a meta-analysis. Diabetes Care 31:2398–2403.
13. Michal M, Wiltink J, Reiner I, Kirschner Y, Wild PS, et al. (2013) Association of mental distress with smoking status in the community: Results from the Gutenberg Health Study. J Affect Disord 146:355–360.
14. Löwe B, Gräfe K, Zipfel S, Witte S, Loerch B, et al. (2004) Diagnosing ICD-10 depressive episodes: superior criterion validity of the Patient Health Questionnaire. *Psychother Psychosom* 73:386–390.
15. Kuper H, Nicholson A, Kivimaki M, Aitsi-Selmi A, Cavalleri G, et al. (2009) Evaluating the causal relevance of diverse risk markers: horizontal systematic review. *BMJ* 339:b4265.
16. Michal M, Wiltink J, Kirschner Y, Wild PS, Münzel T, et al. (2013) Differential associations of depressive symptom dimensions with cardio-vascular disease in the community: Results from the Gutenberg Health Study. PLoS ONE 8(8):e72014.
17. Marijnissen RM, Bus BA, Holewijn S, Franke B, Purandare N, et al. (2011) Depressive symptom clusters are differentially associated with general and visceral obesity. J Am Geriatr Soc 59:67–72.
18. Wiltink J, Michal M, Wild PS, Zwiener I, Blettner M, et al. (2013) Associations between subtypes of depression and different measures of obesity (BMI, WC, WHtR, WHR). BMC Psychiatry 13:223.
19. Stewart SM, Simmons A, White PC (2011) Somatic items in the assessment of depressive symptoms in pediatric patients with diabetes. J Behav Med 34:112–119.
20. Sultan S, Luminet O, Hartemann A (2010) Cognitive and anxiety symptoms in screening for clinical depression in diabetes: a systematic examination of diagnostic performances of the HADS and BDI-SF. J Affect Disord 123:332–336.
21. Wild PS, Zeller T, Beutel M, Blettner M, Dugi KA, et al. (2012) [The Gutenberg Health Study]. Bundesgesundheitsblatt Gesundheitsforschung Gesundheitsschutz 55:824–829.
22. Kroenke K, Spitzer RL, Williams JB (2001) The PHQ-9: validity of a brief depression severity measure. J Gen Intern Med 16:606–613.
23. Smolderen KG, Spertus JA, Reid KJ, Buchanan DM, Krumholz HM, et al. (2009) The association of cognitive and somatic depressive symptoms with depression recognition and outcomes after myocardial infarction. Circ Cardiovasc Qual Outcomes 2:328–337.
24. Hoen PW, Whooley MA, Martens EJ, Na B, van Melle JP, et al. (2010) Differential associations between specific depressive symptoms and cardiovascular prognosis in patients with stable coronary heart disease. J Am Coll Cardiol 56:838–844.
25. de Jonge P, Mangano D, Whooley MA (2007) Differential association of cognitive and somatic depressive symptoms with heart rate variability in patients with stable coronary heart disease: Findings from the heart and soul study. Psychosom Med 69:735–739.
26. Lampert T, Kroll LE (2009) Die Messung des sozioökonomischen Status in sozialepidemiologischen Studien. In *Gesundheitliche Ungleichheit*. ed. Richter M, Hurrelmann K: VS Verlag für Sozialwissenschaften, p. 309–334.
27. Spitzer RL, Kroenke K, Williams JB, Löwe B (2006) A brief measure for assessing generalized anxiety disorder: the GAD-7. Arch Intern Med 166:1092–1097.
28. Kroenke K, Spitzer RL, Williams JB, Monahan PO, Löwe B (2007) Anxiety disorders in primary care: prevalence, impairment, comorbidity, and detection. Ann Intern Med 146:317–325.
29. Löwe B, Gräfe K, Zipfel S, Spitzer RL, Herrmann-Lingen C, et al. (2003) Detecting panic disorder in medical and psychosomatic outpatients: comparative validation of the Hospital Anxiety and Depression Scale, the Patient Health Questionnaire, a screening question, and physicians' diagnosis. J Psychosom Res 55:515–519.
30. Connor KM, Kobak KA, Churchill LE, Katzelnick D, Davidson JR (2001) Mini-SPIN. A brief screening assessment for generalized social anxiety disorder. Depress Anxiety 14:137–140.
31. Seeley-Wait E, Abbott MJ, Rapee RM (2009) Psychometric properties of the mini-social phobia inventory. Prim Care Companion J Clin Psychiatry 11:231–236.
32. Hofmann M, Köhler B, Leichsenring F, Kruse J (2013) Depression as a risk factor for mortality in individuals with diabetes: a meta-analysis of prospective studies. PLoS One 8(11):e79809.
33. McGregor M, Lin EH, Katon WJ (2011) TEAMcare: an integrated multi-condition collaborative care program for chronic illnesses and depression. J Ambul Care Manage 34:152–162.
34. Katon WJ, Lin EH, Von Korff M, Ciechanowski P, Ludman EJ, et al. (2010) Collaborative care for patients with depression and chronic illnesses. N Engl J Med 363:2611–2620.

The Effects of Short-Term Synaptic Depression at Thalamocortical Synapses on Orientation Tuning in Cat V1

Aylin Cimenser[1,2]*, Kenneth D. Miller[3,4,5]

1 Harvard Medical School, Boston, Massachusetts, United States of America, 2 Department of Physics, Boston University, Boston, Massachusetts, United States of America, 3 Center for Theoretical Neuroscience, College of Physicians and Surgeons, Columbia University, New York, New York, United States of America, 4 Department of Neuroscience, College of Physicians and Surgeons, Columbia University, New York, New York, United States of America, 5 Swartz Program in Theoretical Neuroscience, College of Physicians and Surgeons, Columbia University, New York, New York, United States of America

Abstract

We examine the effects of short-term synaptic depression on the orientation tuning of the LGN input to simple cells in cat primary visual cortex (V1). The total LGN input has an untuned component as well as a tuned component, both of which grow with stimulus contrast. The untuned component is not visible in the firing rate responses of the simple cells. The suppression of the contribution of the untuned input component to firing rate responses is key to establishing orientation selectivity and its invariance with stimulus contrast. It has been argued that synaptic depression of LGN inputs could contribute to the selective suppression of the untuned component and thus contribute to the tuning observed in simple cells. We examine this using a model fit to the depression observed at thalamocortical synapses *in-vivo*, and compare this to an earlier model fit based on *in-vitro* observations. We examine the tuning of both the conductance and the firing rate induced in simple cells by the net LGN input. We find that depression causes minimal suppression of the untuned component. The primary effect of depression is to cause the contrast response curve to saturate at lower contrasts without differentially affecting the tuned vs. untuned components. This effect is slightly weaker for *in-vivo* vs. *in-vitro* parameters. Thus, synaptic depression of LGN inputs does not appreciably contribute to the orientation tuning of V1 simple cells.

Editor: Li I. Zhang, University of Southern California, United States of America

Funding: This study was supported by R01-EY11001 (http://report.nih.gov) to KM and by the Gatsby Charitable Foundation through the Gatsby Initiative in Brain Circuitry at Columbia University (http://www.gatsby.org.uk/en/Neuroscience.aspx). The funders had no role in study design, data collection and analysis, decision to publish, or preparation of the manuscript.

Competing Interests: The authors have declared that no competing interests exist.

* Email: aylin@nmr.mgh.harvard.edu

Introduction

Much of the stimulus selectivity of simple cells in layer 4 of cat primary visual cortex (V1), including their tuning for stimulus orientation, can be understood from the feedforward input they receive along with cellular and synaptic nonlinearities [1–27]. Factors that may play a role in determining orientation tuning include the pattern of inputs the cells receive from the lateral geniculate nucleus (LGN) of the thalamus [5]; feedforward inhibition driven by LGN inputs [20,24,26]; suppression of voltage variability with increasing stimulus contrast, which changes the cell's input/output function [17,19]; and synaptic depression [27,28]. Intracortical excitation affects the gain of simple-cell responses but does not seem to alter the orientation tuning induced by these other factors [6,7] (see also in rodents: [29,30]).

The arrangement of LGN inputs alone cannot account for orientation tuning. The net input driven by a simple cell's LGN cells can be decomposed into an orientation-untuned component and a tuned component, which for a drifting grating stimulus correspond respectively to the mean and the temporal modulation of the input [20,24]. Both components increase with contrast, so that the peak LGN input (mean plus modulation) in response to a high-contrast stimulus at the null orientation (orthogonal to the preferred) should be higher than that for a low-contrast preferred stimulus [20,26]. Yet most V1 cells respond little to a high-contrast null stimulus while responding robustly to a low-contrast preferred stimulus [17,31–33].

Two factors appear to suppress null relative to preferred responses. First, voltage responses to a null stimulus are weaker, relative to preferred, than predicted from the arrangement of LGN inputs. A null stimulus evokes depolarization that grows with contrast, but even at the highest contrast this depolarization is rarely if ever larger than the preferred-orientation voltage response at low (4%) contrast (Fig. 5A of [17]). Recurrent amplification of preferred responses may contribute to this. Considering LGN input alone, at any given contrast the mean LGN-induced input should be equal for the null and the preferred orientations [20]. Experimentally, the LGN-input-induced mean voltage response to the null is estimated to be only about 70% of that to the preferred (Fig. S3B of [19]). Second, the firing rate to a null stimulus is strongly suppressed relative to this voltage response, typically remaining slightly suppressed relative to spontaneous firing across all stimulus contrasts, so that the ratio of preferred to null firing rate strongly increases with stimulus contrast [17,31]. The suppression of null spiking response is largely explained by an observed reduction in voltage variability with increasing contrast, which causes the mean null voltage response to remain a constant number of standard deviations of the voltage noise below spike threshold, keeping spiking probability (the firing rate) constant across contrasts [17,19].

It has been argued that synaptic depression at geniculocortical synapses could suppress null voltage response and, along with the arrangement of LGN inputs, explain orientation tuning [28]. Here we reexamine this issue, using a model fit to the weaker synaptic depression seen *in-vivo* [34] as well as one fit to the stronger depression seen *in-vitro* [35].

Materials and Methods

We modeled the spatial arrangement of the relay cells in LGN that connect to a V1 simple cell as in previous studies [20]. We used measured LGN firing rates and included synaptic depression, either fit by us to *in-vivo* experimental studies [34] as described below, or using a previous fit [23] to an *in-vitro* experimental study [35]. We modeled the tuning of the total LGN input – the total LGN-evoked excitatory conductance – to a V1 simple cell under three conditions: 1. No depression at thalamocortical synapses, 2. Depression, using *in-vivo* fit parameters 3. Depression, using *in-vitro* fit parameters. We also modeled the tuning of simple-cell firing rates that would be elicited by these conductances. We focused only on tuning, ignoring response amplitude (that is, we present tuning curves normalized to the response at the preferred orientation and maximal contrast studied), because tuning but not amplitude seems to be determined simply by feedforward input and its processing at the synapse and the postsynaptic cell, independently of intracortical excitation [6,7,29,30] (excepting possible effects of intracortical excitation on voltage variability, which influences spike rate tuning, but this effect is incorporated in our spiking model as discussed further below).

Determining the LGN firing rate

To determine orientation tuning curves at varying contrasts, we used LGN firing rates from experimental data (Dataset S1) that is kindly provided to us by Chong Weng and Jose-Manuel Alonso (SUNY). These data consist of the responses of seven LGN X-cells to drifting sinusoidal gratings in anesthetized cat LGN. The temporal frequency of the gratings was 1.6 Hz and the spatial frequency of the grating was.28 cycles/degree. The sinusoidal gratings were presented at contrasts: 3%, 6%, 12%, 24%, 48%, 72% and 96%.

We took the firing rate for a given LGN cell in response to a grating of a given contrast to be given by the cell's cycle-averaged peri-stimulus time histogram (PSTH; the average firing rate as a function of time across one cycle of the drifting grating) for gratings of that contrast, averaged over 300 stimulus cycles. The phase of the PSTH for a grating of a given orientation was matched to the phase of the grating as it passed over the cell's receptive field center (locations of LGN receptive field centers are described below). We also compared the performance of a linear rectified model fit to the PSTH, constructed as follows. Rectified sinusoids of the form $|B+A\sin(2\pi ft)|_+$ were constructed, where B was the background firing rate, taken to be the mean firing rate at 3% contrast; f was the temporal frequency of the stimulus; A was the amplitude; and $|x|_+=x,\ x>0;\ |x|_+=0$ otherwise. The amplitude, A, was adjusted so that the rectified sinusoid and the cycle-averaged PSTH had the same Fourier amplitude at the stimulus frequency.

The LGN firing rates used in fitting the depression model are described below, in the Materials and Methods subsection "Fitting the synaptic depression model".

Constructing LGN spike trains

For a given time-dependent firing rate of an LGN cell, spike timings were constructed from an inhomogeneous Poisson process with an absolute refractory period of $t_{ref}=1$ msec (or a homogeneous Poisson process in the case of background firing, when firing rates are not changing in time). The problem of generating spike trains with a specified refractory period was first studied by [36] and further analysis was done by [37–41]. For an absolute refractory period, the correction is simple: if the firing rate at time t is $r(t)$, then the average fraction of trials that exhibit refractoriness at t is $\int_{t-t_{ref}}^{t} r(t')dt'$. Thus, if the firing rate when not refractory – the "free firing rate" – is $q(t)$, then the observed firing rate is equal to the free firing rate times the percentage of time not refractory:

$$r(t)=q(t)\ (1-\int_{t-t_{ref}}^{t} r(t')dt'). \tag{1}$$

We used a discretized version of this formula, given $r(t)$ from the data, to compute $q(t)$; computed the next spike time after the last refractory period from an inhomogeneous Poisson process with rate $q(t)$; and set spike probability to zero for $t_{ref}=1$ msec after each spike. Note that when the firing rate is a constant, the free firing rate can be written as:

$$\frac{1}{q}=\frac{1}{r}-t_{ref}. \tag{2}$$

For fitting the model to the data of Boudreau and Ferster [34], we used bins of 0.1 msec duration. For the remaining analysis, we estimated the firing rates using bins of 1 msec duration.

Spatial Organization of LGN

The LGN was constructed with four overlying sheets [42] as in [20]. Each sheet covered the same $6.8°\times6.8°$ area of the visual field. A sheet consisted of two lattices with 30×30 ON cells and 30×30 OFF cells. The two lattices were offset by one-half of the lattice spacing. A cell's receptive field center location corresponded to its lattice position.

Connections of relay cells in LGN to a simple cell in V1

A simple cell receptive field was modeled as a Gabor function [5,43]: a sinusoidal oscillation of 0.8 cycles/degree multiplied by Gaussian envelopes parallel to and perpendicular to the direction of oscillation. We used the "broadly tuned" receptive field parameters of [20]: letting x and y be the directions parallel and perpendicular to the oscillation, respectively, the Gaussians in the Gabor had standard deviations $\sigma_x=.24$ and $\sigma_y=.41$. This results in a receptive field with 1.85 subfields (defined as the ratio of the length of the Gaussian parallel to the oscillation to one half-cycle of the oscillation, where the length of a Gaussian is defined as the distance between the points where it takes 5% of its peak value). The orientation of the receptive field was aligned with the

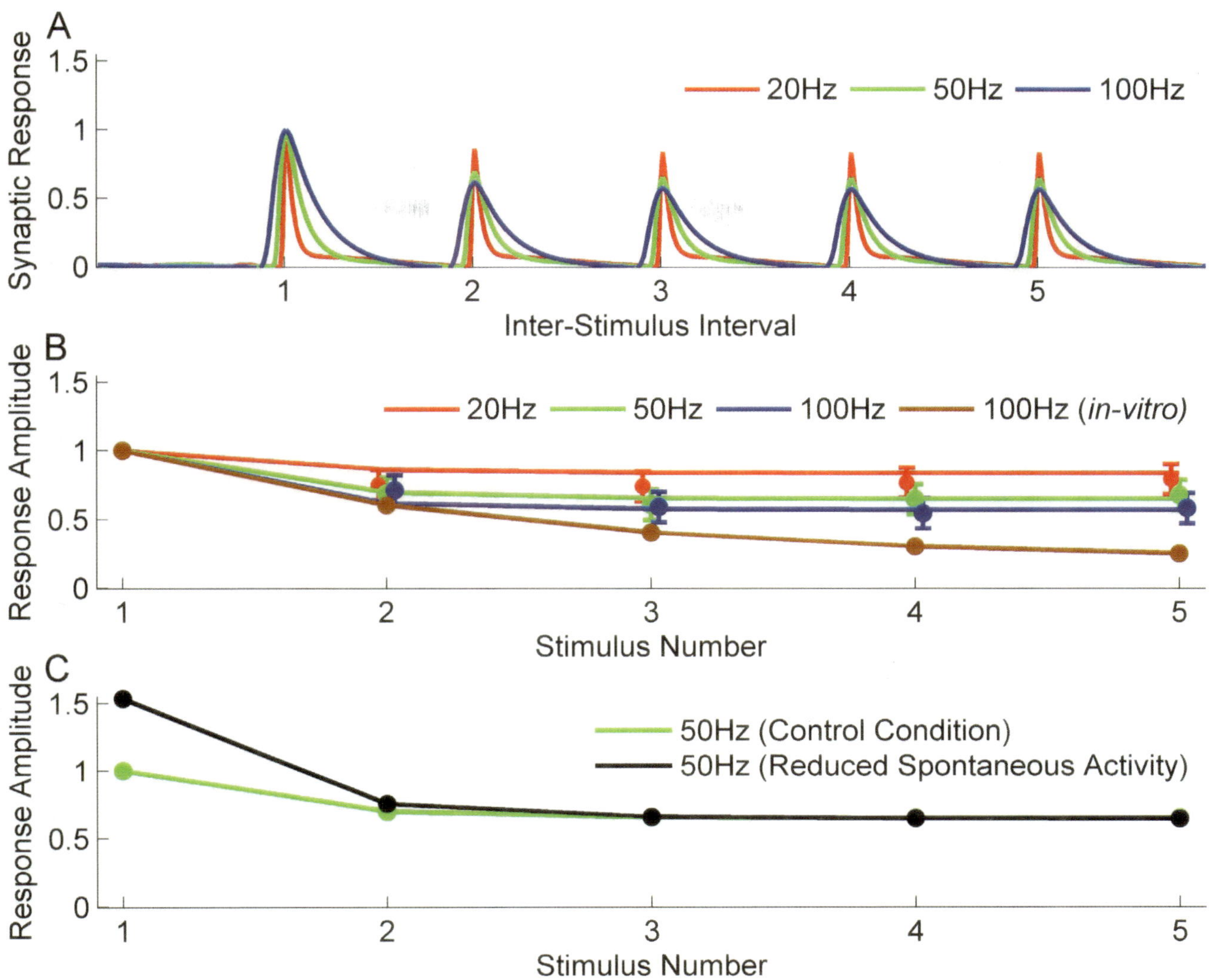

Figure 1. Results from our model of synaptic depression at visual thalamocortical synapses *in-vivo*, based on the model of Dittman and Regehr (1998). A) Model behavior: Dynamics of the normalized PSP's evoked in response to stimulation of a model synapse with different frequencies. Average responses are shown to delivery of 20 Hz, 50 Hz and 100 Hz trains of electrical stimuli to LGN following the background activity. The response is normalized to equal 1 at 90% of the peak value (see Materials and Methods). Note that peaks are aligned and the response to the first stimulus is identical to all three frequencies. The *x-axis* is scaled so that inter-stimulus interval is shown as equal at all frequencies. In units of time, inter-stimulus intervals are 50 msec, 20 msec and 10 msec for the red, green and blue curves. B) Comparison with experimental data: Smooth curves show model response amplitudes (90% of peak value from panel A) as a function of stimulus number at stimulation frequencies of 20 (red), 50 (green) and 100 (blue) Hz. Mean *in-vivo* response amplitudes measured by Boudreau and Ferster [34] are indicated by colored dots; error bars show the size of the data points in their figures, which they state are larger than the error bars and thus serve as an upper bound of the experimental error bars. For comparison, results obtained by using *in-vitro* depression parameters ($f-\tau$ model) are shown for the case of 100 Hz stimulation (brown circles and line). C) Effect of increased intraocular pressure. Green: control response to 50 Hz stimulation, identical to green line in (B). Black: responses when background LGN firing rates were reduced before stimulation from a mean value of 11.8 Hz for control condition to a mean value of 4.1 Hz, modeling effects of increase in intraocular pressure (see Materials and Methods). The response to the first stimulus when the LGN firing rates were low is 1.5 times the value when the LGN firing rates were high. The corresponding ratio from Boudreau and Ferster [34] is 1.45±0.11.

LGN grid. The Gabor function was chosen to be symmetric about the center of the receptive field.

We determined the thalamocortical connection strengths to the model simple cell from this Gabor function receptive field stochastically as in [20]. This gives a time-invariant strength g^j for the connection from the jth LGN neuron to the cortical cell. In addition, each strength is modulated by a time-varying factor $w^j(t)$ determined by synaptic depression, as explained below. The time dependence of the AMPA conductances for the jth synapse were modeled as differences of simple exponentials for each presynaptic spike, weighted by the value of the depression factor $w^j(t)$ at the time of the spike:

$$g^j_{AMPA}(t) = \sum_{\{t_i\}<t} w^j(t_i)\left(e^{-(t-t_i)\big/\tau^{fall}_{AMPA}} - e^{-(t-t_i)\big/\tau^{rise}_{AMPA}}\right) \quad (3)$$

with corresponding time constants $\tau^{rise}_{AMPA} = .25$ msec, $\tau^{fall}_{AMPA} = 1.75$ msec [20], where $\{t_i\} < t$ represents the presynaptic spike timings, $t_1, t_2, ..,$ up to time t. The time course of NMDA conductances was also modeled with exponentials, except that the decay of NMDA conductance was modeled as a double exponential with a fast and a slow time constant:

$$g^j_{NMDA}(t) = \sum_{\{t_i\}<t} w^j(t_i)\left(f_{fast} \cdot e^{-(t-t_i)/\tau^{fall}_{NMDA,fast}} + (1-f_{fast}) \cdot e^{-(t-t_i)/\tau^{fall}_{NMDA,slow}} - e^{-(t-t_i)/\tau^{rise}_{NMDA}}\right) \quad (4)$$

The values were chosen from [22] as $\tau^{rise}_{NMDA} = 5.5$ msec, $\tau^{fall}_{NMDA,fast} = 63$ msec, $\tau^{fall}_{NMDA,slow} = 200$ msec and $f_{fast} = 88\%$. Voltage dependence of the NMDA conductance was ignored. The total conductance evoked by the jth synapse was: $g^j_{TOTAL}(t) = g^j\left((1-\alpha)\frac{g^j_{AMPA}(t)}{\int \tilde{g}^j_{AMPA}(t)dt} + \alpha\frac{g^j_{NMDA}(t)}{\int \tilde{g}^j_{NMDA}(t)dt}\right)$ where $\tilde{g}^j_{AMPA}(t)$ is $g^j_{AMPA}(t)$ evaluated with a single presynaptic spike and $w^j = 1$, and similarly for $\tilde{g}^j_{NMDA}(t)$. $\alpha = 80\%$ is the ratio of NMDA to AMPA conductances.

Distribution of transmission delays from LGN to cortex

Boudreau and Ferster [34] classified cortical cells with response latencies less than 2.3 msec as monosynaptic cells, and provided a distribution of these response latencies. Reasoning that the difference in response latencies reflects differences in transmission delays between LGN and cortex, we randomly picked the transmission delay between a given LGN neuron and the model cortical neuron from the distribution mentioned above. This is accomplished by shifting the contribution to the PSP from an individual LGN neuron by the corresponding delay, and ensures that the response latency of the model cortical neuron is equal to the average latency of the monosynaptic cells studied in Boudreau and Ferster.

Modeling synaptic depression

Depression is modeled as a factor $w(t)$ for each synapse that varies between 0 and 1, reflecting the degree of depression.

In-vivo: Depression was modeled with a calcium-dependent recovery time as suggested in previous studies [44]. The idea behind this model is that as calcium accumulates, the time constant for recovery becomes smaller, thereby speeding up the process of recovery from depression. In mathematical terms, between two spikes, the change in Calcium concentration, $Ca(t)$, is given as:

$$\tau_{Ca}\frac{dCa(t)}{dt} = Ca_{rest} - Ca(t) \quad (5)$$

and the change in release ready sites, $N(t)$, is given as:

$$-\frac{dN(t)}{dt} = (N(t) - N_0)\frac{k_{\max}}{1 + K_N Ca_0/Ca(t)}. \quad (6)$$

During a spike, the change in Calcium concentration is:

$$Ca(t_+) = Ca(t_-) + Ca_0 \quad (7)$$

and the change in release ready sites is:

$$N(t_+) = (1 - p_o)N(t_-). \quad (8)$$

Here, t_- represents the time just before a spike and t_+ represents the time just after a spike. Ca_0 is the increase in calcium concentration after each spike. N_0 is the total number of ready sites. Initially, all the sites are release ready, $N(t_0-) = N_0$, and after each spike, a fraction p_0 of the release ready sites are used. The synaptic strength associated with a spike at time t is proportional to $p_0 N(t_-)$, so $w(t) = N(t_-)/N_0$.

Defining $\tilde{K}_N \equiv K_N Ca_0/Ca(t)$, experimental data suggests that small changes in Ca_0 lead to measurable changes in $\tilde{K}_N$ [44]. In order to allow the model to reproduce this behavior, K_N should be on the order of 1. We chose $K_N = 1$. Defining $k_0 \equiv \frac{k_{\max}}{1 + Ca_0/Ca_{rest}}$ and solving the above equations in between spikes, with t representing the time just after the last spike and $t' > t$ the time being solved for, the dynamics of the calcium concentration can be written as:

$$Ca(t') = Ca_{rest} + (Ca(t) - Ca_{rest})\exp(-(t'-t)/\tau_{Ca}) \quad (9)$$

while the available release ready sites can be written as:

$$N(t') = N_0 - (N_0 - N(t))\exp(-k_0(t'-t)) \left(\frac{Ca_0 + Ca(t)}{Ca_0 + Ca_{rest} + (Ca(t) - Ca_{rest})\exp(-(t'-t)/\tau_{Ca})}\right)^{-\tau_{Ca}(k_{\max} - k_0)} \quad (10)$$

In-vitro: We used the "$f-\tau$" model of synaptic depression [45,46]. Between spikes, w recovers toward 1 with time constant τ: $\tau\frac{dw}{dt} = 1 - w$. At each spike, a fraction $(1-f)$ of the synaptic resources are used: $w \rightarrow fw$. The depression parameter associated with a spike is equal to w just before the spike. In agreement with Boudreau and Ferster [34], we were not able to fit the *in-vivo* data with an $f-\tau$ model within the error bars given in Fig. 1A. As a comparison to the model described above fit to *in-vivo* data, we used the $f-\tau$ model with parameters that were fit in previous work [23] to *in-vitro* paired-pulse experiments in cat V1 slices [35]. These parameters are $f = .563$, $\tau = 99$ msec.

Quantifying the PSP amplitude

To fit the *in-vivo* depression model to the data of Boudreau and Ferster [34], we equate the relative amplitude of the conductance in our model with the relative PSP amplitude. This is based on the fact that, if the synaptic conductance is small relative to the background conductance, then a scaling of the synaptic conductance vs. time by a factor just scales the potential vs. time by the same factor. As in Ref. [34], depression is characterized by PSP amplitudes relative to the first amplitude in a train. To quantify the relative PSP amplitude in our model, we follow the procedures in the experiments of Boudreau and Ferster [34]. These authors observed that the incremental amplitude of the responses to individual stimuli in each train were superimposed on slow trends. To remove the slow trends, we first interpolate (by using spline interpolation; MATLAB; Mathworks, Natick, MA) the total LGN input (as conductance) measured at each stimulus onset and subtract the fit from the original total LGN input. Then, we define the amplitude of the cortical PSP to the first stimulus as the magnitude of the conductance at 90% of the peak relative to the baseline, where baseline is defined as the average response over $0.7 - 1.2$ msec after stimulus onset, as in Boudreau and Ferster [34]. Subsequent PSP amplitudes are measured at the same time relative to stimulus onset as the first PSP amplitude.

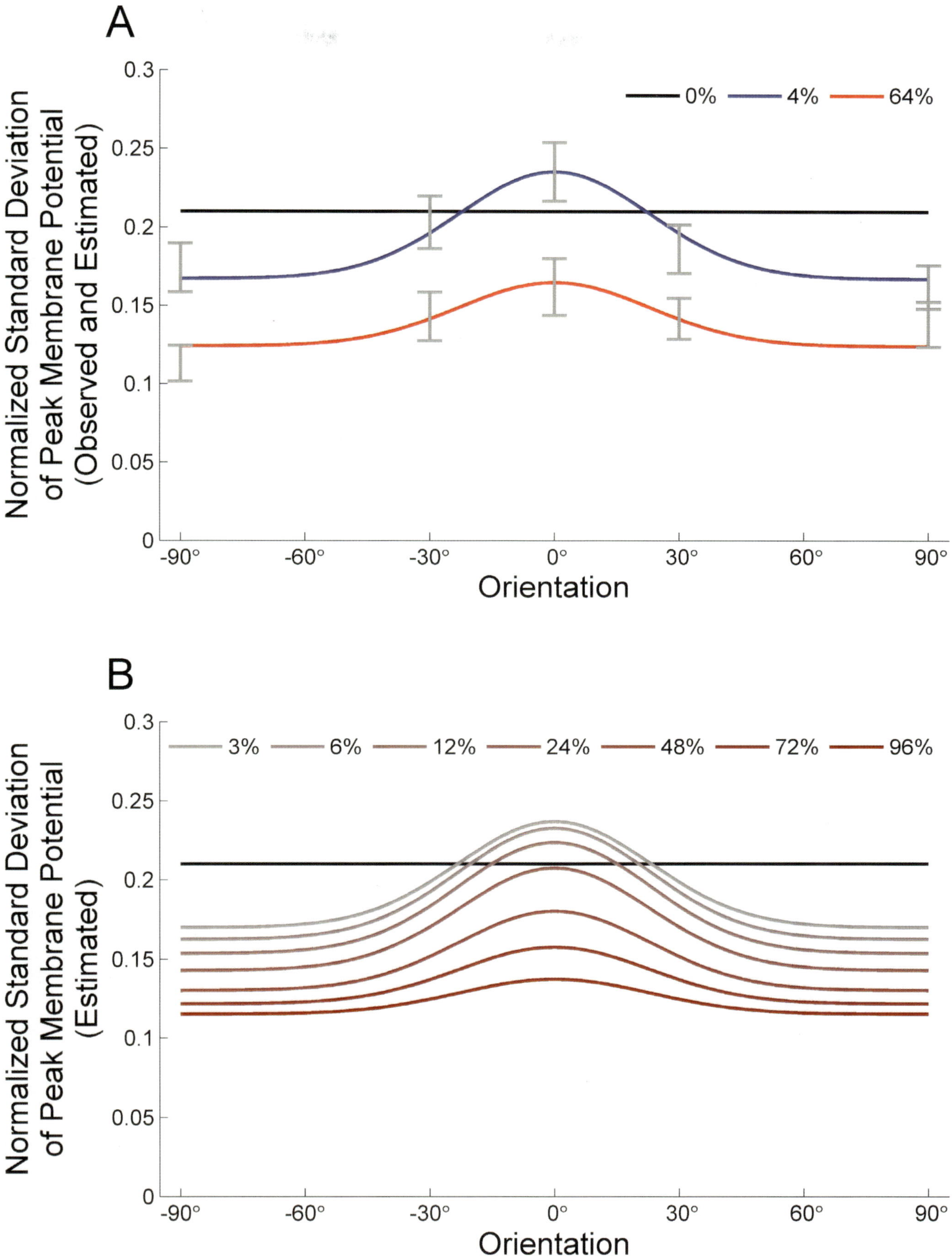
A
0.3
0.25
0.2
0.15
0.1
0.05
0
Normalized Standard Deviation of Peak Membrane Potential (Observed and Estimated)
0%
4%
64%
-90°
-60°
-30°
0°
30°
60°
90°
Orientation
B
0.3
0.25
0.2
0.15
0.1
0.05
0
Normalized Standard Deviation of Peak Membrane Potential (Estimated)
3%
6%
12%
24%
48%
72%
96%
-90°
-60°
-30°
0°
30°
60°
90°
Orientation

Figure 2. Tuning of the standard deviation of the peak membrane potential normalized to the mean peak membrane potential at 64% contrast preferred orientation. A) Data from Finn et al. [17] (data points and error bars) and our fits to them (smooth curves). Observed normalized standard deviation for the background (0% contrast) is 0.21. For 4% and 64% contrasts observed values are shown as error bars at orientations −90°,−30°,0°,30° and 90°. Estimated normalized standard deviation values are shown as smooth curves that are fit to the data by considering a single function, $f(contrast,orientation)$, (Eq. 12), which is constrained to give observed experimental values (see Materials and Methods). $f(contrast,orientation)$ is shown here for 0% contrast (black curve), 4% contrast (blue curve) and 64% contrast (red curve). B) The estimated normalized standard deviation values, *f(contrast, orientation)*, that we use in our simulations for contrasts 0%, 3%, 6%, 12%, 24%, 48%, 72% and 96%.

Fitting the synaptic depression model

Boudreau and Ferster [34] allowed the system to recover for periods of 1.75 sec between successive trains of stimuli. However, even with recovery between successive trains of stimuli, spontaneous activity can cause synaptic depression and affect the response of the cortical neurons to stimulation. In order to study this effect, Boudreau and Ferster used increased intraocular pressure as a means to reduce spontaneous LGN activity and studied its effect on response properties of cortical neurons. They reported that LGN spontaneous rates were 11.8±2.9 spikes/sec in the control condition and 4.1±1.4 spikes/sec in the condition of increased intraocular pressure.

We replicated these experiments in our simulations as follows: For each set of depression parameters, all of the LGN neurons in the model were made to fire spontaneously for a period of 1.75 sec. Following this, stimulus trains at 20, 50 or 100 Hz were presented (all of the LGN neurons fire synchronously, but note they have varying transmission delays as described above), and the resulting PSP's in the cortical neuron were monitored. Each simulation leads to estimates of the train of cortical PSP amplitudes (quantified as discussed previously) at the corresponding stimulus frequency. For the control condition, we took the spontaneous firing rates of the LGN cells to be 11.8 spikes/sec. To model the effect of reduced spontaneous activity, we again allowed the LGN neurons to fire with a background rate of 11.8 spikes/sec for a period of 1.75 sec and then with a background rate of 4.1 spikes/sec for 5 sec, as in the experiments. At the end of this period, a stimulus train was presented at 50 Hz, and the resulting PSP's in the cortical neuron were monitored. We compared the cortical PSP amplitudes from the control conditions (20, 50 and 100 Hz) and the first PSP amplitude from the reduced spontaneous activity case with the experimental data. For the reduced spontaneous activity case, Boudreau and Ferster [34] reported that the first PSP amplitude increased by 44.9±0.11% (mean±stan-standard error) relative to control, and that subsequent PSP amplitudes were not significantly different from control. Their standard error corresponds to an error bar of ±0.11 in the relative units of our Fig. 1. For the control condition, Boudreau and Ferster referred to error bars that were smaller than their displayed data points (their Fig. 4D); their data points had a radius of 0.11 in the same relative units. We use this value of 0.11 in relative units for all error bars in our Fig. 1B and for the error bar (not shown in our Fig. 1C) for the first PSP for the reduced spontaneous activity. We searched the parameter space for p_o within $0<p_o<1$, $k_{\max}$ within $0<k_{\max}<100$, $k_0/k_{\max}$ within $0<k_0/k_{\max}<1$, and τ_{Ca} within $0\text{msec}<\tau_{Ca}<20\text{msec}$, and determined parameters that agreed with the experimental data (produced values within error bars for all data points). We chose from among those the values $p_o=0.85$, $k_{\max}=84\,\text{sec}^{-1}$, $k_0/k_{\max}=0.03$ and $\tau_{Ca}=3msec$, which were the parameters giving the minimum value for the maximum absolute error over the 5 stimulus trains for the spontaneous case (at 20, 50 and 100 Hz) and the first stimulus for the control case.

Estimating the firing rate of a simple cell

To determine whether spike threshold might alter or amplify tuning effects of synaptic depression, we estimated the tuning of firing rate that would be induced by the LGN inputs. To do so, we make the simplifying assumption that voltage is linear in the excitatory conductance. For large voltage excursions, voltage response can be sublinear in the excitatory conductance [47], but the assumption of linearity can be justified for two reasons (i) From resting potential to spike threshold, i.e ~20 mV, the relationship can be reasonably approximated as linear [47]. (ii) To the degree that voltage response is sublinear in the excitatory conductance, the problem with tuning will get worse, i.e. the difference between null and preferred responses will be weaker, so linearity is a conservative assumption for purposes of our study, which focuses on whether synaptic depression can enhance the difference between null and preferred responses.

Given the assumption that voltage response is linear in the conductance, we estimate the normalized firing rate of simple cells from the LGN input using the results of Finn et al [17]. These authors found that the firing rate of simple cells is related to mean membrane potential and its standard deviation across trials through the following power law relationship.

$$R(v_m,v_s)=constant\ x\ |v_m+k*v_s|_+^{\,p} \tag{11}$$

Here, $|x|_+=x,x>0;\ =0$, otherwise. v is the membrane potential relative to the resting potential, $v_m=mean(v)$, $v_s=std(v)$, $k=0.68$ and p was found by fitting Fig. 7B of [17] to Eq. 11, giving the exponent $p=3.62$.

Supplementary Fig. 1C of [17] (replotted in our Fig. 2A, data points with error bars) shows the tuning of the normalized standard deviation of the peak voltages for three contrasts (0%, 4% and 64%) and five orientations (−90°, −30°, 0°, 30°, 90°), averaged over 52 simple cells in cat V1. For each cell, the preferred orientation was set to 0°, and the tuning curve was normalized by the cell's peak voltage at 64% contrast at the preferred orientation. To estimate the standard deviation values for other values of contrast, c, and orientation, o, we first fit the data (Supplementary Fig. 1C of [17]) to a smooth function that we found could well fit the data, given by.

$$f(c,o)=f_{background}+(a_1c^{1/4}-a_2c^{1/2})\exp\left(-(o/o_s)^2/2\right)-a_3c^{1/4} \tag{12}$$

Here, $f_{background}\equiv f(c=0,o)$ corresponds to the value at zero contrast, $f_{background}=0.21$ [17]. We fit the remaining constants: $a_1=0.26$, $a_2=0.24$, $a_3=0.096$ and $o_s=23°$. This function is shown as the smooth curves in Fig. 2A which are fits to the data of Supplementary Fig. 1C of [17]. The curves fall within the experimentally reported range. Next, we estimated the standard deviations at contrasts (3%, 6%, 12%, 24%, 48%, 72% and 96%; curves for these contrasts shown in Fig. 2B) and orientations (−90° to 90° with 10° intervals) to use in our simulations as follows: For each contrast c and orientation o, we generated many trials of simple cell responses and determined the mean, c_m, and standard deviation, c_s, of the conductance response at each time across the

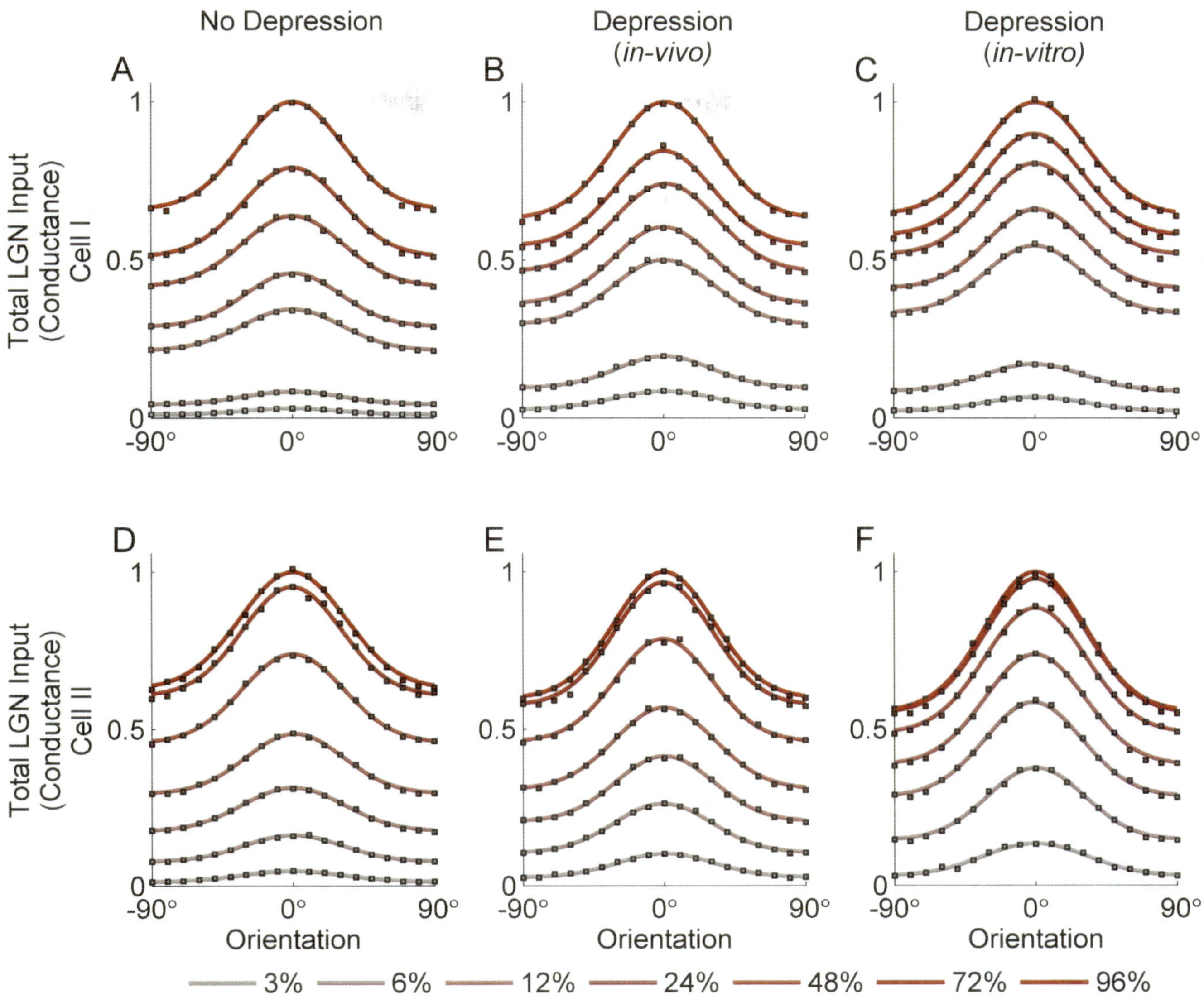

Figure 3. Orientation tuning of the peak LGN input to the simple cell (in terms of conductance) over a cycle in response to drifting grating stimuli of varying contrasts. Results are shown for two different models of LGN response time course, each based on the response time course of a measured LGN cell: Cell I (A–C) and Cell II (D–F). In each figure, the colored circles show peak input for 6 different contrast levels (3%, 6%, 12%, 24%, 48%, 72% and 96%) and 19 orientation angles (from −90° to 90° with steps of 10°). The colored smooth curves show fits of a Gaussian plus baseline to these tuning curves at the different contrasts. Each fit is normalized to the value of the fit at the preferred orientation at highest contrast (96%), which is set to 1. Orientation tuning curves are calculated for the cases: No Depression (A, D), Depression using *in-vivo* (B, E) fit parameters, Depression using *in-vitro* (C, F) fit parameters.

cycle. We then took v_m at each time equal to the corresponding value of c_m. We took the values of v_s across the cycle to be the corresponding values of c_s scaled so that, at the peak of the cycle, the value of v_s, relative to the peak v_m at 64% contrast and preferred orientation, was given by $f(c,o)$ (Eq. 12). That is, we used Eq. 12 to determine v_s at the peak of the cycle, relative to the peak v_m at 64% contrast and preferred orientation as determined by our simulations; and used our simulations to determine the relative values of v_s at other points in the cycle (relative to the v_s at the peak of the cycle). Then, using the v_m and v_s values at each point in the cycle, we used Eq. 11 to determine the normalized firing rates at each time across the cycle (normalized to the peak response across orientations and contrasts).

It is important to note that we are interested only in tuning properties and so we model normalized firing rates, ignoring absolute response levels. Given that (1) intracortical excitation does not alter mean voltage orientation tuning [6,7,29,30] and (2) our model of the voltage standard deviation implicitly includes the effects of intracortical excitation (because the voltage standard deviation at the cycle peak, relative to the peak mean voltage at 64% contrast, preferred orientation, is fit to empirical measurements of voltage noise in simple cells *in-vivo*), explicitly incorporating intracortical excitation into our model would not alter spiking orientation tuning. Hence, we neglect modeling intracortical excitation in determining the spike-rate tuning that would be induced by the LGN input. Note also that, if all conductances were multiplied by a factor k, then using the above procedure all spike rates would be multiplied by the factor k^p. Thus, only the relative conductances across contrasts and orientations, and not the absolute conductance amplitudes, influence the normalized spiking tuning that we present here.

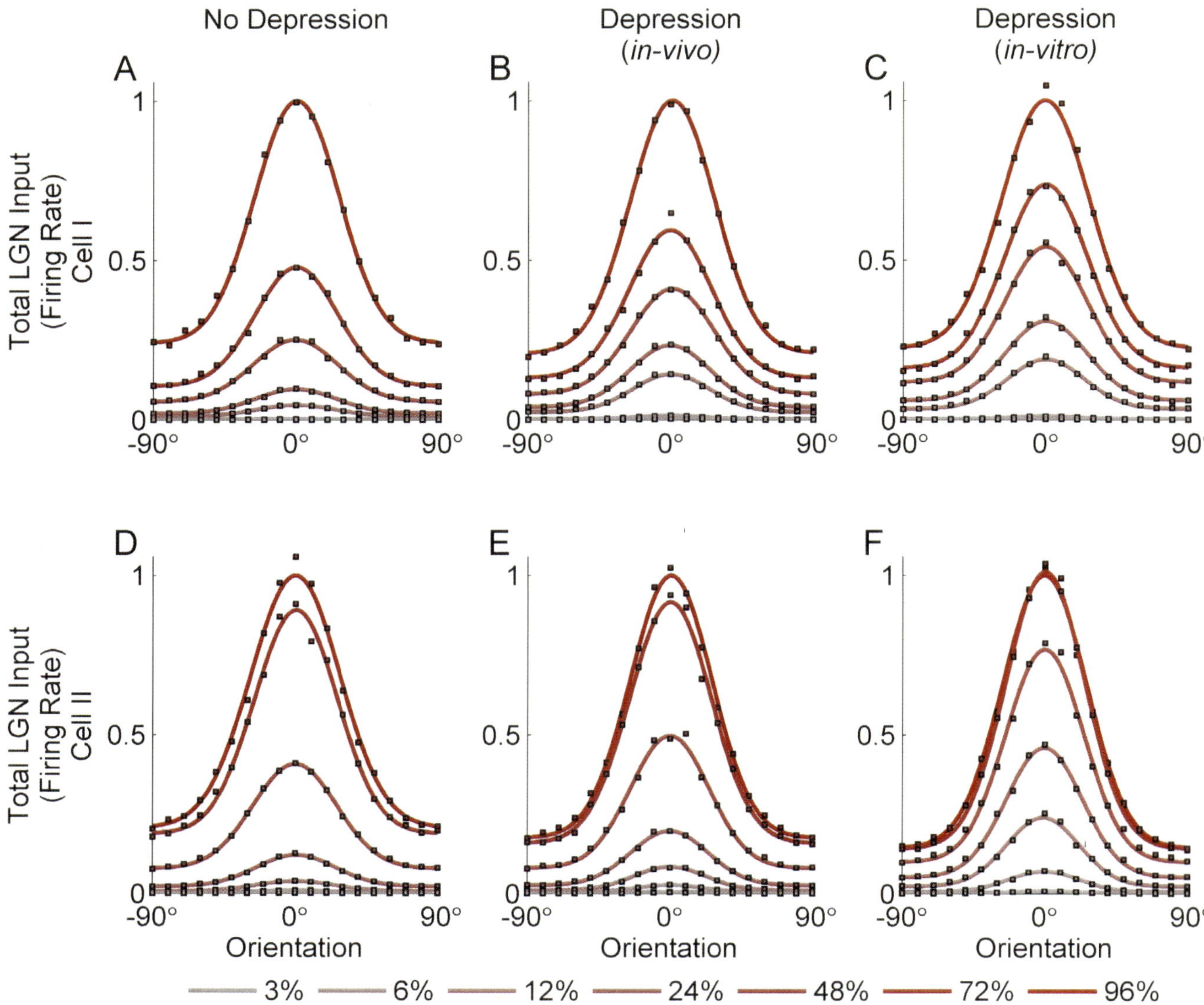

Figure 4. Orientation tuning of the peak LGN input to the simple cell (in terms of firing rate) over a cycle in response to drifting grating stimuli of varying contrasts. Results are shown for two different models of LGN response timecourse, each based on the response timecourse of a measured LGN cell: Cell I (A–C) and Cell II (D–F). In each figure, the colored circles show peak input for 6 different contrast levels (3%, 6%, 12%, 24%, 48%, 72% and 96%) and 19 orientation angles (from -90° to 90° with steps of 10°). The colored smooth curves show Gaussian fits to these tuning curves at the different contrasts. Each fit is normalized to the value of the fit at the preferred orientation at highest contrast (96%), which is set to 1. Orientation tuning curves are calculated for the cases: No Depression (A, D), Depression using *in-vivo* (B, E) fit parameters, Depression using *in-vitro* (C, F) fit parameters.

Quantifying orientation tuning width

We quantify orientation tuning as the half-width at half-height [17], where half-height is defined as half the distance between the maximum response and baseline (as shown in Supplementary Fig. 2 of [17]). Baseline is meant to indicate firing rate in the absence of a stimulus. We defined the baseline as the cortical-cell response when LGN-cell firing rates were set to their mean firing rates at 3% contrast, i.e. the weakest stimulus for which we had data. The rationale for this choice is that such weak stimuli typically modulate the firing rate of LGN cells linearly, without rectification. Consequently, the firing rate of LGN cells in the absence of a stimulus is approximately identical to their mean firing rate in response to a drifting grating with a 3% contrast. If the cortical cell's response to a stimulus orthogonal to the preferred was greater than the half-height, we set the half-width at half-height to be 90°.

Results

In order to assess depression of thalamocortical synapses *in-vivo*, Boudreau and Ferster [34] recorded intracellularly from V1 simple cells receiving direct input from the LGN, as judged by the short latency and low timing jitter of LGN-evoked PSP's. They delivered trains of electrical stimuli to the LGN, and examined the change over time in the resulting PSP amplitudes recorded in the simple cell. They observed that the second PSP amplitude (*i.e.*, in response to the second stimulus in the train) was strongly reduced relative to the first PSP amplitude, with relatively little further reduction for subsequent PSP's (see Fig. 1B). They tried to fit their data with a simple $''f-\tau''$ model, in which a synapse's strength is

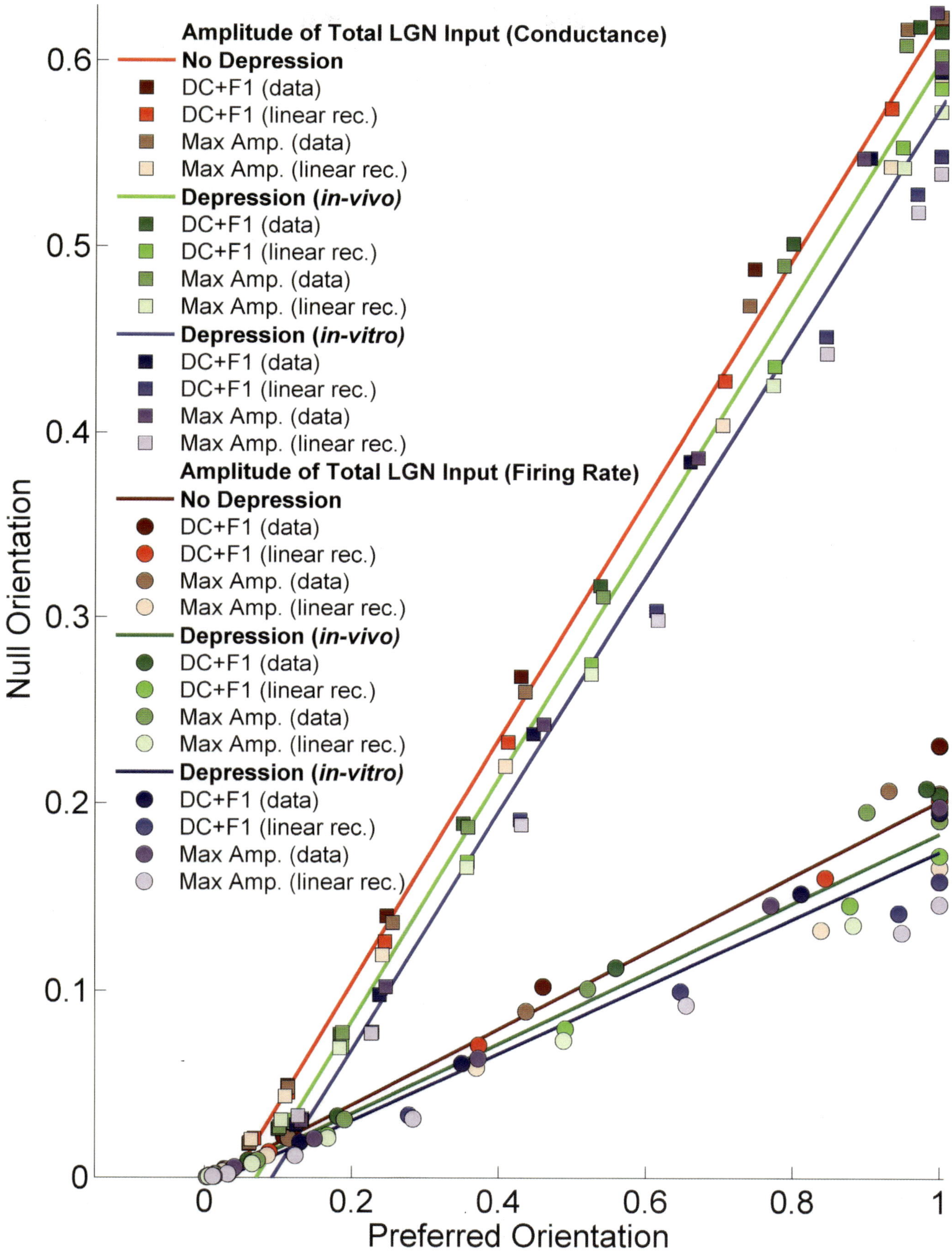
Amplitude of Total LGN Input (Conductance)
No Depression
DC+F1 (data)
DC+F1 (linear rec.)
Max Amp. (data)
Max Amp. (linear rec.)
Depression (in-vivo)
DC+F1 (data)
DC+F1 (linear rec.)
Max Amp. (data)
Max Amp. (linear rec.)
Depression (in-vitro)
DC+F1 (data)
DC+F1 (linear rec.)
Max Amp. (data)
Max Amp. (linear rec.)
Amplitude of Total LGN Input (Firing Rate)
No Depression
DC+F1 (data)
DC+F1 (linear rec.)
Max Amp. (data)
Max Amp. (linear rec.)
Depression (in-vivo)
DC+F1 (data)
DC+F1 (linear rec.)
Max Amp. (data)
Max Amp. (linear rec.)
Depression (in-vitro)
DC+F1 (data)
DC+F1 (linear rec.)
Max Amp. (data)
Max Amp. (linear rec.)
Null Orientation
Preferred Orientation
0
0.1
0.2
0.3
0.4
0.5
0.6
0
0.2
0.4
0.6
0.8
1

Figure 5. Amplitude of the conductance and the firing rate at the null orientation as a function of amplitude at the preferred orientation. The cases shown are: No Depression (red), Depression using *in-vivo* (green) or *in-vitro* (blue) fit parameters. Amplitudes are means across the 7 models of LGN timecourse, where for each model of LGN timecourse and depression the amplitude is scaled so that input to the preferred orientation at highest contrast is 1. Four different response measures are shown: either the actual experimental PSTH is used ("data") or a linear rectified approximation to it (see Materials and Methods); and there are two different measures of the size of this response (maximum amplitude over a cycle or DC+F1, where DC is mean over a cycle and F1 is Fourier amplitude of the first harmonic). Results from all contrast levels are pooled together and displayed for each of model of depression and response measure. Linear fits (minimizing sum-squared error) to each model are also shown (See color insets).

multiplied by $f<1$ after each spike and, between spikes, relaxes toward that synapse's maximal strength with time constant τ. Such models have been successfully used to model cortical synaptic depression as observed in many *in-vitro* experiments [23,45,46]. Boudreau and Ferster [34] observed that, because of the transient character of the synaptic depression observed *in-vivo*, this model underestimated the initial depression and overestimated the depression that occurred later in the train and so gave very poor fits.

In a different set of experiments, studying the climbing fiber synapse in cerebellum, Dittman and Regehr [44] showed that recovery from depression was accelerated by accumulation of presynaptic residual calcium. They suggested a modification to the "$f-\tau$" model in which the recovery time, τ, is not constant but instead is calcium dependent. This dependence leads to maintenance of synaptic efficacy under conditions that would otherwise deplete the available transmitter pool.

We find that the [44] depression model allows good fits to the *in-vivo* experimental data on monosynaptic cells obtained by Boudreau and Ferster [34] (Fig. 1). From the time course of model response to presynaptic trains of stimuli at 20 Hz, 50 Hz and 100 Hz (Fig. 1A), we can extract the amplitude of response to each stimulus. The model amplitudes (Fig. 1B, 20 Hz (red), 50 Hz (green) and 100 Hz (blue)) show reasonable matches to the experimental observations and fall within an upper bound estimate of the experimental error (Fig. 1B, error bars) for all stimulus frequencies. The model successfully captures the large initial reduction in amplitude, evident on the 2nd stimulus of the train, and the small changes in amplitude over subsequent stimuli. For comparison, using parameters obtained from the "$f-\tau$" model fit from *in-vitro* experiments, we observe a much more gradual decrease in amplitude with stimulus number (Fig. 1B, 100 Hz (brown)), as noted by [34], and we found that this was true of this model for any parameters that produced significant depression.

Hereafter, we will refer to the [44] model, which uses the depression parameters from the fit to the *in-vivo* geniculocortical data of [34], as the "*in-vivo*" model, and to the "$f-\tau$" model, which uses the depression parameters from the fit of [23] to *in-vitro* geniculocortical data [35], as the "*in-vitro*" model.

The stimulus-induced depression observed by [34] was weak relative to that typically observed *in-vitro*. They speculated that this may be due to synapses already being partially depressed due to spontaneous activity, as had been suggested in the somatosensory thalamocortical system [48,49]. To test this, they reduced LGN spontaneous firing rates by about 65% by applying intraocular pressure. Consistent with pre-existing depression, they found that this increased the amplitude of response to the first stimulus in a 50 Hz train by 45±11% on average, but had little effect on responses to subsequent stimuli in the train. We replicated this experiment by lowering the LGN firing rates by the same amounts as in the experiments, as discussed in the Materials and Methods section. The results for the *in-vivo* model closely parallel the experimental observations (Fig. 1C). Reduced spontaneous activity (Fig. 1C, 50 Hz (black)) results in increased amplitude of response to the first stimulus and has little effect on the remaining stimuli compared to spontaneous activity obtained from the control condition (Fig. 1C, 50 Hz (green)). In Fig. 1 we assume that the simple cell receives LGN inputs with weights stochastically sampled from a Gabor function (see Materials and Methods), [20], but the fit does not depend on this choice: we obtain similar results if constant weights are assigned to all LGN ON and OFF-center inputs (not shown).

Having a successful model of the depression observed *in-vivo* in cat V1, we now use this to model the effects of depression on the total LGN input received by a layer 4 simple cell at various orientations and contrasts. We assume that the simple cell receives LGN inputs with weights stochastically sampled from a Gabor function [20]. We assume that all LGN inputs have the same periodic timecourse of response to a drifting sinusoidal luminance grating of a given contrast, except that the LGN inputs vary in the phase of their response according to their positions relative to the grating and the orientation of the grating. As a model of the timecourse of LGN response, we use the responses of a single measured LGN cell to gratings of various orientations and contrasts. We study the model for eight different choices of measured LGN cell and thus eight different models of the timecourse of LGN response. Alternatively, we could have let each LGN input be modeled by a different LGN cell, but this would have tended to average out the variations; we choose the more extreme alternative in order to see the largest range of possible variations in LGN input. To study the effect of depression at thalamocortical synapses, we simply model the net LGN input to a simple cell, and do not model any cortical mechanisms, such as inhibition, that might combine with this input to produce cortical responses. To characterize the tuning of the net LGN input, we use two measures, as described in Materials and Methods. First, we characterize the tuning of the total LGN-induced conductance as a direct measure of the net input. Second, to determine whether spike threshold effects might reveal stronger effects of synaptic depression on tuning, we estimate the tuning of the simple-cell firing rate responses that would be induced by this LGN input. Note that we are only interested in tuning, which is independent of intracortical excitation [6,7,29,30], and not the response amplitude, which depends on intracortical excitation [6,7,29,30], so we ignore amplitude and report only normalized responses (normalized to the response at optimal orientation and largest contrast studied).

Figs. 3 and 4 show the tuning of the peak LGN input conductance to a simple cell (Fig. 3) and of the firing rate this conductance would evoke in the simple cell (Fig. 4), for two models of LGN timecourse, each based on the response of a different measured LGN cell (cell 1: Fig. 3A-C and Fig. 4A–C; cell 2: Fig. 3D-F and Fig. 4D–F). For the conductance (Fig. 3), the input in response to the null orientation (defined as the orientation orthogonal to the preferred) grows strongly with contrast, so that the null input at high contrast is much larger than the input to the preferred orientation at low contrasts. This is true whether the synapses are modeled without depression (Fig. 3A,D) or with depression modeled as in the *in-vivo* model (Fig. 3 B,E) or the *in-vitro* model (Fig. 3 C,F). With depression, low-contrast input is

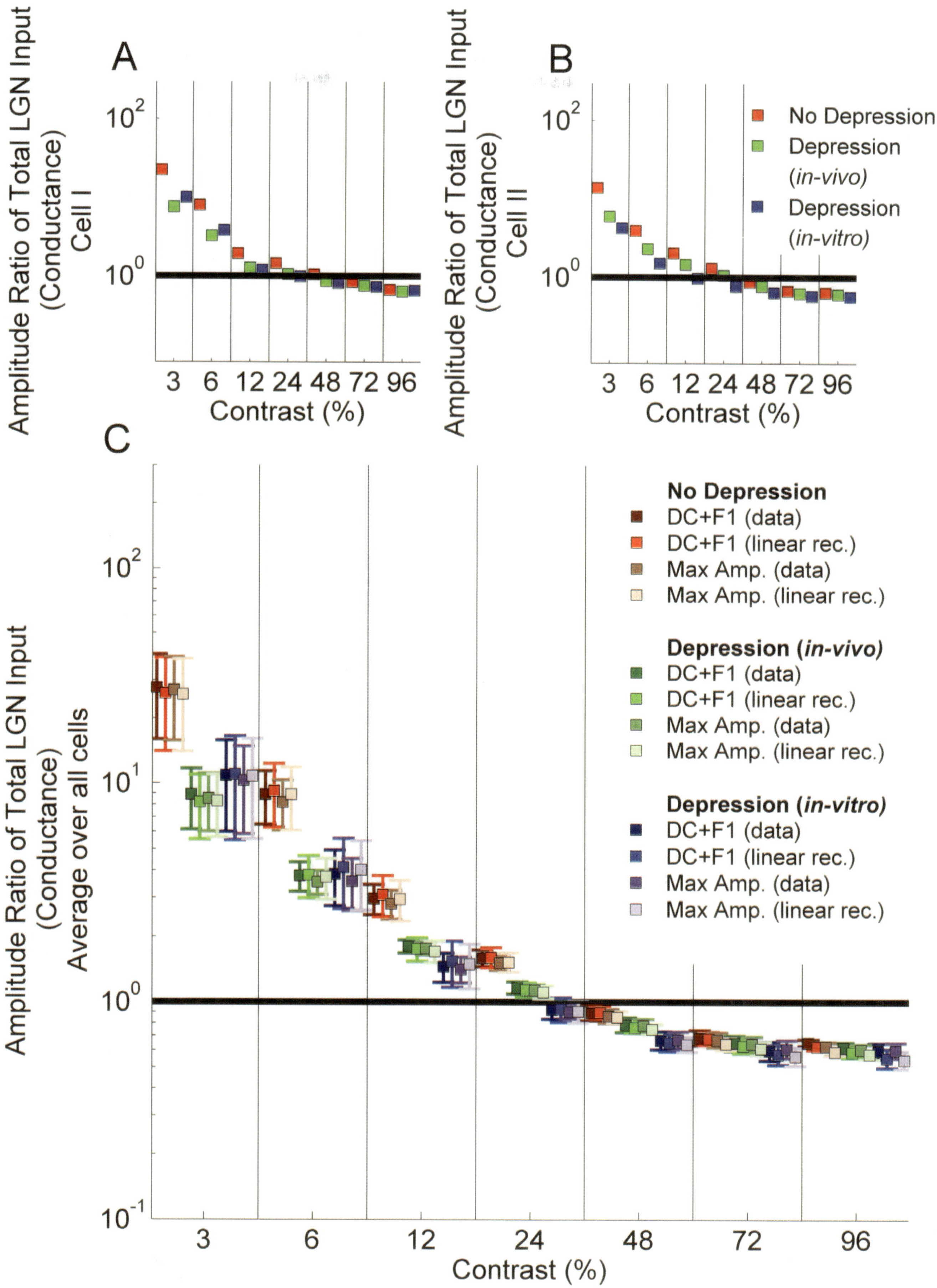
A
Amplitude Ratio of Total LGN Input (Conductance) Cell I
10^2
10^0
3 6 12 24 48 72 96
Contrast (%)
B
Amplitude Ratio of Total LGN Input (Conductance) Cell II
10^2
10^0
3 6 12 24 48 72 96
Contrast (%)
No Depression
Depression (in-vivo)
Depression (in-vitro)
C
Amplitude Ratio of Total LGN Input (Conductance) Average over all cells
10^2
10^1
10^0
10^{-1}
3 6 12 24 48 72 96
Contrast (%)
No Depression
DC+F1 (data)
DC+F1 (linear rec.)
Max Amp. (data)
Max Amp. (linear rec.)
Depression (in-vivo)
DC+F1 (data)
DC+F1 (linear rec.)
Max Amp. (data)
Max Amp. (linear rec.)
Depression (in-vitro)
DC+F1 (data)
DC+F1 (linear rec.)
Max Amp. (data)
Max Amp. (linear rec.)

Figure 6. Ratio of the amplitude of the tuning curve in Fig. 3 (normalized conductance) at the null orientation (the orientation orthogonal to the preferred) at 96% contrast to that at the preferred orientation (*x-axis*; 3%, 6%, 12%, 24%, 48%, 72% and 96%). Black horizontal line indicates amplitude ratio 1. The cases shown are: No Depression (red), Depression using *in-vivo* (green) fit parameters, Depression using *in-vitro* (blue) fit parameters. A) Amplitude ratios for Cell I of Fig. 2; B) Amplitude ratios for Cell II of Fig. 2; C) Amplitude ratios averaged over all 7 experimentally measured LGN cells (mean ± std error). In C, four different response measures are shown: either the actual experimental PSTH is used ("data") or a linear rectified approximation to it (see Materials and Methods); and there are two different measures of the size of this response (maximum amplitude over a cycle or DC+F1, where DC is mean over a cycle and F1 is Fourier amplitude of the first harmonic); see inset for colors corresponding to these 4 measures. All points between each pair of vertical bars represent the same contrast: for different response measures, results for each contrast are offset relative to each other for ease of visualization.

larger relative to high-contrast input than without depression. This corresponds to the fact that synaptic depression induces saturation of input at lower contrasts. That is, with depression, a given low contrast is a larger percentage of the saturating contrast and hence behaves, relative to the largest contrast, as does a higher contrast without depression (note that each panel in Fig. 3 is normalized so that 1 represents the preferred input to high contrast). However, for a curve with a given size of preferred input, the size of the null input is about the same with or without depression, though slightly reduced by depression. Results for firing rate tuning curves (Fig. 4) are similar in these respects, although the tuning curves for the firing rate are narrower and the null firing rate much lower relative to preferred firing rate than was the case for membrane potential (Fig. 3). Overall, as shown in Fig. 5, the ratio of null input to preferred input changes little across contrasts, both in terms of membrane potential and firing rate, and synaptic depression of either form causes only a very slight reduction in this ratio. Depression fit to the *in-vitro* data causes about twice the reduction in this ratio as does depression fit to the *in-vivo* model, but both reductions are slight.

To better assay the effect of the null-orientation response on orientation tuning, we examine the ratio of the response to the null orientation at the highest contrast to that at the preferred orientation at a given contrast (Fig. 6, membrane potential; Fig. 7, firing rate; contrast of preferred-orientation stimulus is given on the *x-axis*; different measures of response in figures discussed further below). As noted in the Introduction, in real neurons this ratio generally stays below 1 even for the lowest-contrast preferred-orientation stimulus. It must stay below 1 to explain the observation that cells show spike responses to the preferred orientation at the lowest responsive contrast but not to the null orientation even at the highest contrast. For the two LGN cells examined in Figs. 3,4 (Figs. 6A,B and Figs. 7A,B) and more generally on average across the eight LGN cells used as models of LGN time course (Figs. 6C, 7C), the results using *in-vivo* vs. *in-vitro* depression models are very close (see error bars in Figs. 6C, 7C). Depression improves the results (reduces the ratio) at any given preferred-orientation contrast, but ratios remain greater than 1 for low preferred-orientation contrasts under all depression models (for contrasts of 12% or less for the *in-vitro* depression model, and contrasts of 24% or less for the *in-vivo* depression model or for no depression). Although the contrast levels at which the ratio is less than 1 for firing rate responses (Fig. 7) are similar to those for conductance responses (Fig. 6), the range of the ratio for different contrasts is much broader for firing rate responses.

As discussed in the Introduction, the relative suppression of response to null-orientation stimuli, which is critical to observed orientation tuning, also manifests as a value significantly less than 1 for the ratio of the mean LGN-induced conductance to a null-orientation stimulus to that for a preferred-orientation stimulus, at least at high contrast. We examined this for our various models. We found that the ratio remains very close to 1 across all contrasts and regardless of the absence or, if present, the form of geniculocortical depression (Fig. 8). In this figure, at each contrast we averaged only over LGN cells for which the DC component of the null-orientation response and the DC component of the preferred-orientation response were both >0.05, in units in which the peak conductance to the highest-contrast preferred orientation is 1 (as in Fig. 3). When these mean responses were smaller, the ratios of the two responses could be poorly behaved, but the absolute difference between the two mean responses was never greater than 0.02 across the excluded cases.

Finally, we examined the dependence on contrast of the half-width at half-height (Materials and Methods) of the tuning curve (Fig. 9). Experimentally, half-width is invariant to stimulus contrast for firing rate responses [17,32,33,50], while for voltage responses it broadens moderately with contrast (this broadening, along with the changing input/output relationship due to decreasing voltage variance, produces the contrast-invariant spiking response) [17,19,50]. For conductance responses, the half-width increases dramatically with contrast, reaching a plateau near 90° for contrasts of 24% and above, reflecting the lack of suppression of the untuned component of the LGN input (Fig. 9A). This increase is slightly less with synaptic depression, with a greater reduction for *in-vitro* than for *in-vivo* depression, but the reductions due to depression are slight. As a result, firing-rate tuning widths increase significantly with contrast (Fig. 9B). The tuning widths are slightly lower with synaptic depression, but the increase in width with contrast is similar with or without depression.

Previous modeling efforts have used a linear rectified model of LGN input and have used the DC+F1 as a surrogate for the peak input [24]. To determine whether these approximations affect any of our results, in Figs. 5–9, we computed results both with and without these approximations. To model the response of an LGN cell, we considered the cycle-averaged PSTH (referred to as "data" in Fig. 6C, 7C), or a linear-rectified fit to this PSTH consisting of a sinusoidal modulation plus a constant, with negative values set to zero (see Materials and Methods). For each of these two models, we considered two measures of the total input to the simple cell: the peak input over a cycle, or the sum of the mean (DC) and first harmonic (F1) over a cycle, which would be equal to the peak if there were no higher harmonics. As can be seen in the figures, these alternative choices for measures of LGN response or of the summed LGN input make very little difference to the results.

Discussion

We find that synaptic depression as measured *in-vivo* in thalamocortical synapses [34] can be well fit by a model of depression that incorporates a calcium-dependent change in the time constant of recovery from depression [44]. Using this "*in-vivo*" model as well as an earlier, simpler model [45,46] fit to *in-vitro* data [35], we find that thalamocortical depression in either form has little impact on the orientation tuning of the LGN input to V1 simple cells or its contrast dependence, other than to induce response saturation at lower contrasts. Thus, the contrast-

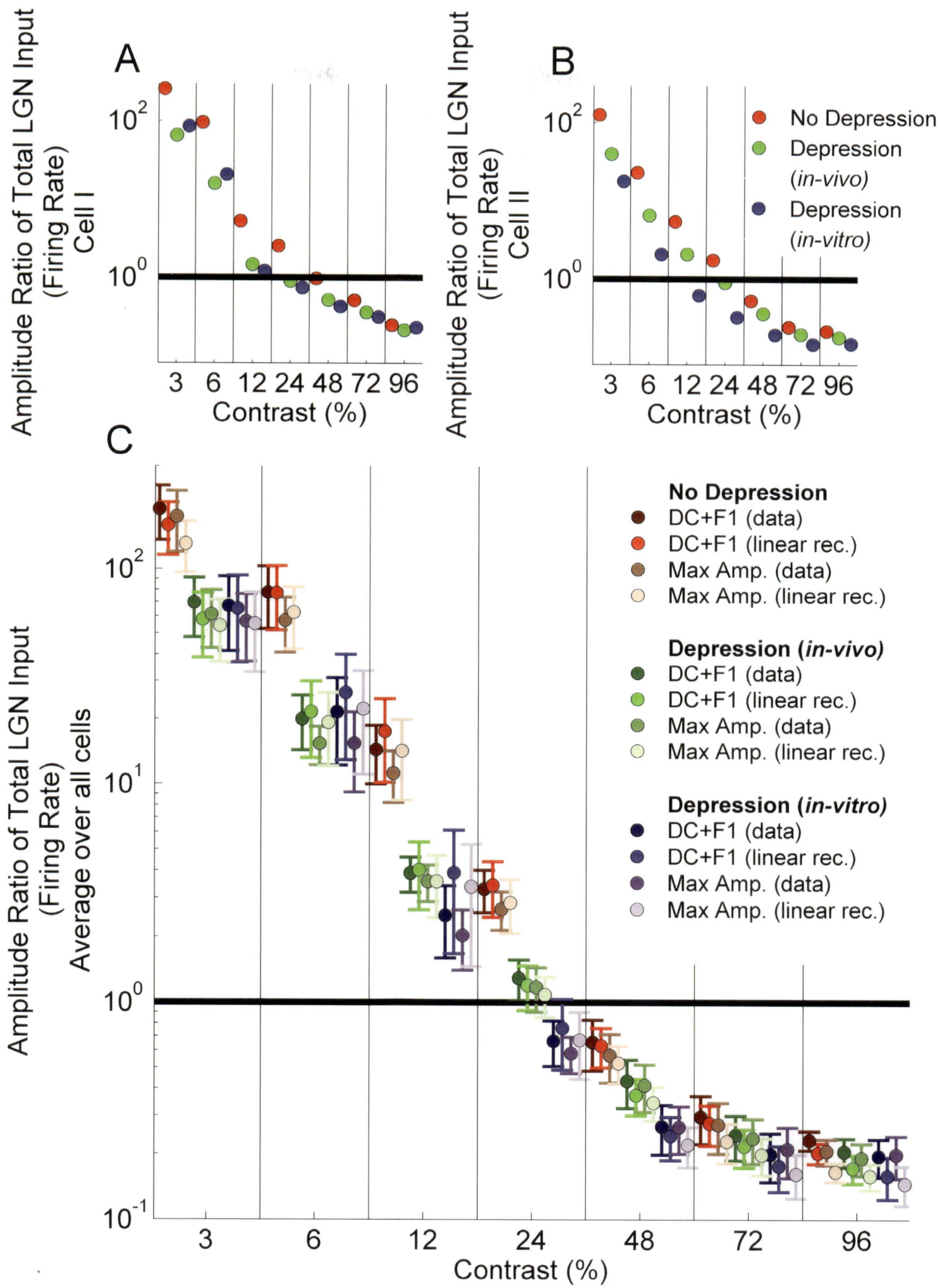
A
Amplitude Ratio of Total LGN Input
(Firing Rate)
Cell I
10^2
10^0
3 6 12 24 48 72 96
Contrast (%)
B
Amplitude Ratio of Total LGN Input
(Firing Rate)
Cell II
10^2
10^0
3 6 12 24 48 72 96
Contrast (%)
No Depression
Depression (in-vivo)
Depression (in-vitro)
C
Amplitude Ratio of Total LGN Input
(Firing Rate)
Average over all cells
10^2
10^1
10^0
10^{-1}
3 6 12 24 48 72 96
Contrast (%)
No Depression
DC+F1 (data)
DC+F1 (linear rec.)
Max Amp. (data)
Max Amp. (linear rec.)
Depression (in-vivo)
DC+F1 (data)
DC+F1 (linear rec.)
Max Amp. (data)
Max Amp. (linear rec.)
Depression (in-vitro)
DC+F1 (data)
DC+F1 (linear rec.)
Max Amp. (data)
Max Amp. (linear rec.)

Figure 7. Ratio of the amplitude of the orientation tuning curve in Fig. 4 (normalized firing rate) at the null orientation (the orientation orthogonal to the preferred) at 96% contrast to that at the preferred orientation at varying contrasts (*x-axis*; 3%, 6%, 12%, 24%, 48%, 72% and 96%). Black horizontal line indicates amplitude ratio 1. The cases shown are: No Depression (red), Depression using *in-vivo* (green) fit parameters, Depression using *in-vitro* (blue) fit parameters. A) Amplitude ratios for Cell I of Fig. 2; B) Amplitude ratios for Cell II of Fig. 2; C) Amplitude ratios averaged over all 7 experimentally measured LGN cells (mean ± std error). In C, four different response measures are shown: either the actual experimental PSTH is used ("data") or a linear rectified approximation to it (see Materials and Methods); and there are two different measures of the size of this response (maximum amplitude over a cycle or DC+F1, where DC is mean over a cycle and F1 is Fourier amplitude of the first harmonic); see inset for colors corresponding to these 4 measures. All points between each pair of vertical bars represent the same contrast: for different response measures, results for each contrast are offset relative to each other for ease of visualization.

invariance of the orientation tuning of simple cell responses [17,32,33,50] must depend on cortical mechanisms beyond the LGN synapse, e.g. feedforward inhibition driven by LGN excitation of cortical inhibitory cells [20,25,26,51] and/or effects of spike threshold and its interaction with voltage fluctuations [17,26,50].

Modeling synaptic depression

In our fit to the *in-vivo* data with the calcium-dependent recovery model, we found the exponential decay time constant for calcium to be $\tau_{Ca} = 3msec$, which is very low in comparison with/ found by Dittman and Regehr [44], at the climbing fiber to purkinje cell synapse (or $\tau_{Ca} = 20msec$ when EGTA-AM was added to the presynaptic terminals). In addition to the difference in the synapses being studied, one possible contributor to the difference is temperature: Dittman and Regehr's experiments were conducted at 24 C, whereas Boudreau and Ferster's were at 38.3 C. A more accurate model of synaptic depression may also include the dependence of temperature as observed experimentally [52]. It also may be that the model, including the time constant necessary to fit the thalamocortical data, does not accurately represent the underlying biophysical mechanisms at the thalamocortical synapse, but is simply a phenomenological model that is able to fit the data.

The Role of Synaptic Depression in V1 Responses

We have found that synaptic depression causes little change in the ratio of null-orientation to preferred-orientation LGN input to a simple cell (Fig. 5) and thus has little effect on orientation tuning, other than to cause saturation to occur at lower contrasts as reported previously [23,27].

It is not surprising that synaptic depression causes similar suppression of response to all orientations at a given contrast, and thus has little effect on orientation tuning. Individual LGN cells are not tuned for the orientation of a drifting grating, and thus depression has the same effect on an individual LGN cell's output for any stimulus orientation. The LGN response is confined to and peaks within a particular portion of the stimulus cycle. Synaptic depression changes the temporal waveform over a cycle of the input from an LGN cell, relative to its firing rate, by suppressing later portions of the response relative to earlier portions (e.g., [23] (Fig. 5)). Orientation tuning arises from the fact that a preferred-orientation stimulus tends to drive all of a simple cell's LGN inputs to peak near the same phase of the stimulus cycle, whereas in response to a null grating LGN responses are dispersed across the stimulus cycle [20]. The total LGN input to a simple cell over time is predicted to be well approximated, as we have verified here, by the rectified sum of a mean (the zeroeth harmonic) and a sinusoid (the first harmonic or F1; the temporal modulation of the input at the same temporal frequency as the stimulus), in essence because the Gabor-function receptive field filters out higher harmonics in the time course of individual LGN cells [24]. The mean is untuned for orientation, and represents the sum of the means of the individual LGN inputs. The F1 is the orientation-tuned component, and represents the tendency of the LGN cells to all modulate their firing rates at roughly the same phase for preferred but not for null stimuli. For synaptic depression to differentially affect response to different orientations, the change in the LGN input waveform that it induces must either change the size of the DC relative to the F1 (*e.g.*, a thinner pulse of input has a smaller individual DC/F1 ratio) and/or change the tuning of the F1 (*i.e.*, lead to greater decrease in the net F1 for a given degree of phase desynchronization). Both effects are apparently small, even for strong depression.

Previous papers have studied the effects of synaptic depression on orientation selectivity. Carandini et al. [27] assumed perfect push-pull inhibition, i.e. that for each LGN cell driving excitatory input to a simple cell, an identical LGN cell except of opposite center type drives equal-strength inhibitory input. This eliminates the untuned component of the LGN input, leaving only the tuned component, so that in particular the input to a null-orientation stimulus is zero. Given a nearly-zero spike threshold, this solves the problem of achieving contrast-invariant orientation tuning [20], leaving synaptic depression simply to solve the problem of causing earlier contrast saturation in cortex than in LGN without altering orientation tuning.

Our results and conclusions significantly differ from Banitt et al. [28], who also studied the effect of synaptic depression on orientation tuning. First, we focused on the effects of thalamocortical synaptic depression as measured *in-vivo* by Boudreau and Ferster [34]. We fit our model to the full set of *in-vivo* data (including 20, 50, and 100 Hz pulse train data taking into account prior spontaneous activity, as well as the case of reduced spontaneous activity). The "moderate depression" model of Banitt et al. [28] was said to be fit to this *in-vivo* data, and in agreement with our findings it failed to suppress non-preferred responses. However their moderate depression model, while reasonably fitting the *in-vivo* data for 50 Hz pulse trains, failed to fit the data for 20 Hz pulse trains (their Fig. 6; conversely, their "strong depression" model in that figure reasonably fit the first two ISI's for 20 Hz *in-vivo* data, but failed to fit the 50 Hz *in-vivo* data); they did not illustrate model fits to 100 Hz *in-vivo* data. It also appears that their fitting to the *in-vivo* data was done assuming an undepressed state as the initial condition, rather than a partially depressed state due to prior spontaneous activity as in the data, as no mention of spontaneous activity was made for this protocol.

Second, Banitt et al. [28] primarily focused on a "strong depression" model that was said to be based on a fit to the *in-vitro* depression data of Stratford et al [35] (Fig. 1g). They reported that this strong depression could largely suppress depolarization at orientations far from the preferred and achieve contrast-invariant spiking tuning, unlike our findings using a depression model fit to the same *in-vitro* data. However, they appear to have used a different strong depression model to study orientation tuning than was used to fit the *in-vitro* data, and both appear to differ from the strong depression model as defined parametrically, even though all are identified as the same strong depression model. After a

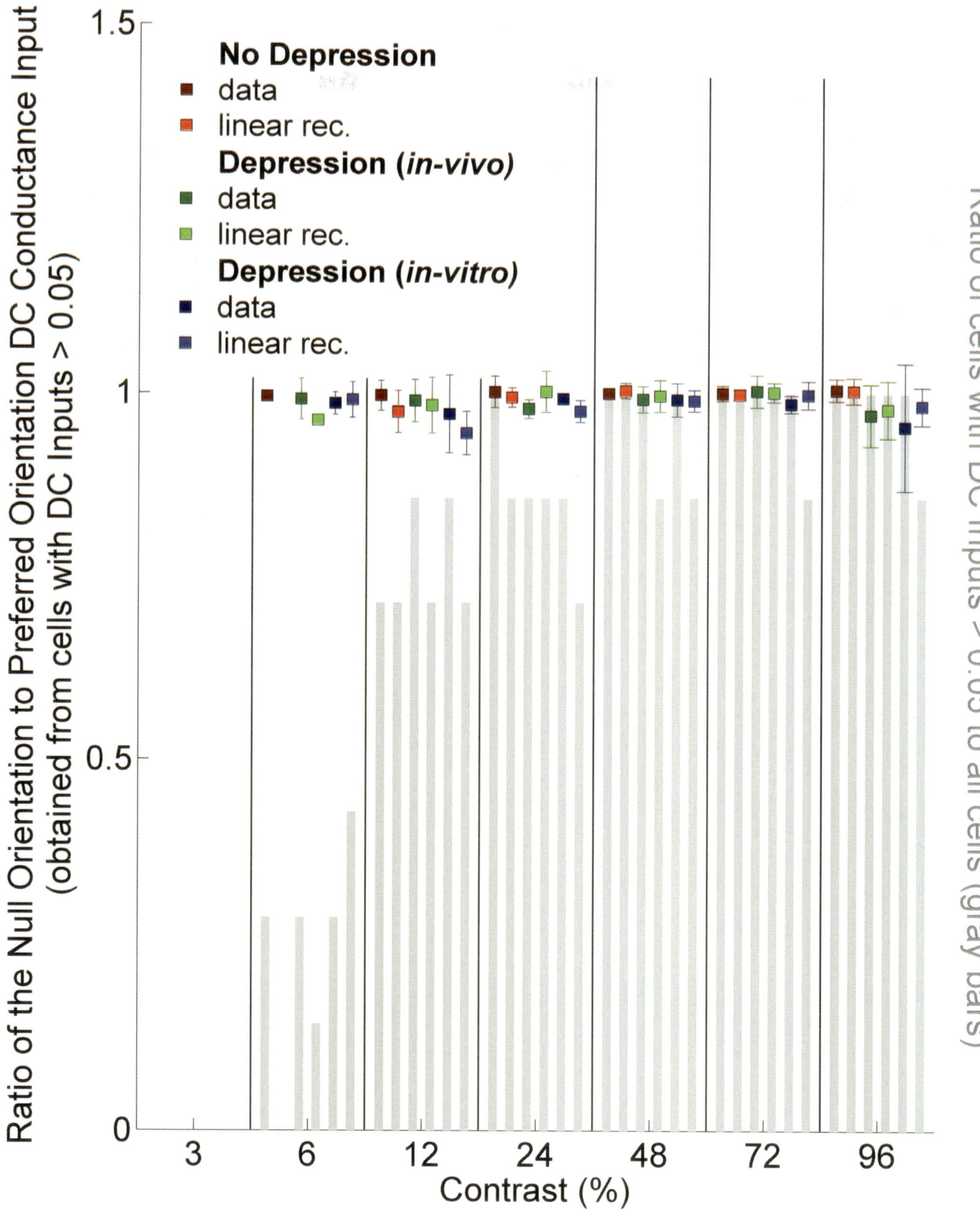

Figure 8. Ratio of the null orientation DC input to preferred orientation DC input averaged over LGN cells, across contrasts. Only cells for which both DC's were greater than 0.05 are included in the calculation; mean ratios (squares) and the standard deviations (error bars) are shown. The cases shown are: No Depression (red), Depression using *in-vivo* (green) or *in-vitro* (blue) fit parameters. For each case, two different response measures are shown: either the actual experimental PSTH is used ("data") or a linear rectified approximation to it (see Fig. 7 legend and Materials and Methods). For a given response measure and contrast (3%, 6%, 12%, 24%, 48%, 72% or 96%), ratio of number of cells that have both DC inputs >0.05 to total number of cells is shown as gray bars.

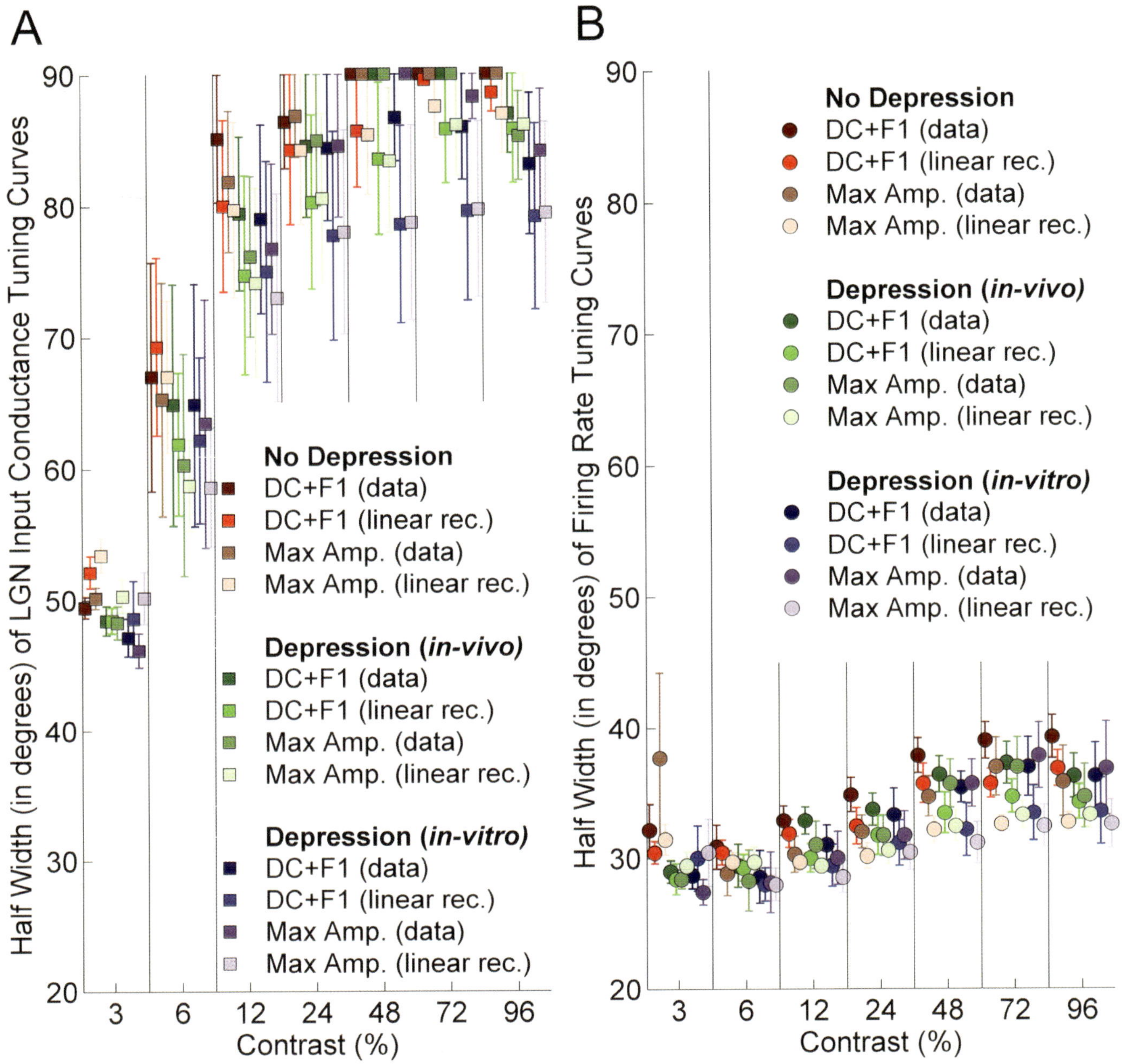

Figure 9. Half-width of tuning curves at half-height (i.e., difference between orientation giving peak response and orientation giving 50% of peak response) obtained from the tuning curves of total LGN input: A) Conductance B) Firing Rate. Each half-width is calculated at a specific contrast (*x-axis*; 3%, 6%, 12%, 24%, 48%, 72% and 96%). Half-widths are averaged over the experimentally measured LGN cells, mean ± std error (*y-axis*). If null-orientation response was greater than 50% of the peak response, the half-width is undetermined (half-width >90°, See Supplementary Fig. 2 of [17]; in such cases we set the half-width to 90°. Four different response measures are shown, as described in legend of Fig. 7. Conventions as in Fig. 7.

20 msec ISI beginning from an undepressed state, their model fit to the *in-vitro* data matched the observed depression to 62% of initial strength (their Fig. 3C); their model used in studying orientation tuning depressed to 44% of initial strength (their Fig. 6B); and it is easy to calculate that the parameters they gave for the strong depression model would produce synaptic depression to about 30% of initial strength, which should manifest as a similar level of EPSP depression (because their model was linear except for somatic voltage-dependent conductances and reversal potential effects, none of which should have led to significant deviations from linearity for the small depolarizations of an EPSP). These discrepancies were not noted or explained. It is also puzzling that their moderate depression model (their Fig. 9A) produced more hyperpolarized voltages than their strong depression model (their Fig. 8C) for non-preferred orientations at low contrasts (3% and 10%), even though their moderate depression model appeared to always produce less synaptic depression at the thalamocortical synapses than their strong depression model (*e.g.*, their Fig. 6). Without knowing the models they actually used to study orientation tuning, we find it difficult to compare their

findings to ours. In sum, we conclude that depression models matched to either *in-vivo* or *in-vitro* physiological data, which we have constructed, do not significantly impact orientation tuning.

Thalamocortical synaptic depression has also been postulated to contribute to other V1 response properties, including band-pass rather than low-pass responses to sinusoidal stimuli, nonlinear differences in the responses to broadband or transient stimuli vs. the responses to sinusoidal stimuli, contrast adaptation, and direction selectivity [53]; contrast-dependent changes in temporal frequency tuning [23] and in the temporal phase of response to drifting grating stimuli [23,53]; and the suppression of responses to preferred stimuli by superimposed mask stimuli [27]. It will be of interest to revisit these issues with a model matched to the thalamocortical depression observed *in-vivo*.

Applicability to Rodents

We have based our model on a large number of studies in cat V1 (see references in Introduction) that have established the classic "Hubel-Wiesel" model of the arrangement of LGN inputs to layer 4 simple cells, the dependence of spiking tuning for orientation and contrast on the tunings of the voltage mean and voltage standard deviation and on feedforward vs. intracortical input, and the properties of synaptic depression *in-vivo* and *in-vitro*. While we expect our basic finding, that synaptic depression does not significantly impact orientation tuning or its contrast dependence, will carry over to rodents, many of these details may differ in rodent V1. In particular, it is already known that ON-center and OFF-center excitatory inputs appear to be more strongly overlapping in rodent [54] vs. cat [10,14,55] simple cells, with spatially "intervening inhibition" playing an important role in segregating ON from OFF subregions in rodents [54]; cats have a "push-pull" arrangement between excitatory and inhibitory input, whereas in rodents the arrangement appears to be "push-push" [47,56]; and the difference between orientation tuning in LGN and V1 is much less marked in rodents than in cats [57]. Further investigation is needed to determine the degree to which the mechanisms of orientation selectivity and its contrast invariance differ between carnivores and rodents.

Origins of Contrast Invariance of Orientation Selectivity

As summarized in the Introduction, the origin of contrast-invariant orientation tuning in thalamic-recipient simple cells in middle layers of anesthetized cat V1, in response to drifting gratings, can be attributed to: (1) the Gabor-function arrangement of LGN inputs to a simple cell [5], which causes the net LGN input to be composed of an orientation-untuned DC and an orientation-tuned F1 [20,24]; (2) some degree of suppression of the voltage response to a null-orientation stimulus relative to that to a preferred-orientation stimulus, relative to the levels expected from LGN input alone [17,19]; and (3) contrast-dependent suppression of voltage noise, causing the mean voltage in response to a null stimulus to stay the same number of standard deviations from threshold across contrasts and thus preventing spiking response to the null orientation [17,19]. Sadogapan and Ferster [19] presented evidence that (3) is substantially due to a corresponding decrease in the variability of the LGN input to simple cells with increasing stimulus contrast. Several network mechanisms that could cause such variability of suppression have also been proposed [58–60]. The mechanism responsible for (2) is not known. One postulated mechanism for (2) is an untuned component of feedforward inhibition that grows with contrast [20,24,26,27], which might also contribute to (3) by decreasing input resistance. The present work demonstrates that thalamocortical synaptic depression matched to physiological measurements does not substantially contribute to (2) or more generally to contrast-invariant orientation tuning.

Supporting Information

Dataset S1 LGN Firing Rates (Hz). Each.csv file is from a single LGN cell. Each file contains a matrix. Rows: Time (Duration: 625 msec (1 cycle)). Columns: Contrast (Total 7:96%, 72%, 48%, 24%, 12%, 6%, 3%).

Author Contributions

Analyzed the data: AC KM. Contributed reagents/materials/analysis tools: AC KM. Contributed to the writing of the manuscript: AC KM.

References

1. Hubel DH, Wiesel TN (1962) Receptive fields, binocular interaction and functional architecture in the cat's visual cortex. J Physiol 160: 106–154.
2. Bullier J, Mustari MJ, Henry GH (1982) Receptive-field transformations between LGN neurons and S-cells of cat-striate cortex. J Neurophysiol 47: 417–438.
3. Tanaka K (1983) Cross-correlation analysis of geniculostriate neuronal relationships in cats. J Neurophysiol 49: 1303–1318.
4. Saul AB, Humphrey AL (1992) Evidence of input from lagged cells in the lateral geniculate nucleus to simple cells in cortical area 17 of the cat. J Neurophysiol 68: 1190–1208.
5. Reid RC, Alonso JM (1995) Specificity of monosynaptic connections from thalamus to visual cortex. Nature 378: 281–284.
6. Ferster D, Chung S, Wheat H (1996) Orientation selectivity of thalamic input to simple cells of cat visual cortex. Nature 380: 249–252.
7. Chung S, Ferster D (1998) Strength and orientation tuning of the thalamic input to simple cells revealed by electrically evoked cortical suppression. Neuron 20: 1177–1189.
8. Ferster D, Miller KD (2000) Neural mechanisms of orientation selectivity in the visual cortex. Annu Rev Neurosci 23: 441–471.
9. Alonso JM, Usrey WM, Reid RC (2001) Rules of connectivity between geniculate cells and simple cells in cat primary visual cortex. J Neurosci 21: 4002–4015.
10. Lampl I, Anderson JS, Gillespie DC, Ferster D (2001) Prediction of orientation selectivity from receptive field architecture in simple cells of cat visual cortex. Neuron 30: 263–274.
11. Hirsch JA, Martinez LM, Alonso JM, Desai K, Pillai C, et al. (2002) Synaptic physiology of the flow of information in the cat's visual cortex in vivo. J Physiol 540: 335–350.
12. Kara P, Pezaris JS, Yurgenson S, Reid RC (2002) The spatial receptive field of thalamic inputs to single cortical simple cells revealed by the interaction of visual and electrical stimulation. Proc Natl Acad Sci U S A 99: 16261–16266.
13. Martinez LM, Alonso JM, Reid RC, Hirsch JA (2002) Laminar processing of stimulus orientation in cat visual cortex. J Physiol 540: 321–333.
14. Martinez LM, Wang Q, Reid RC, Pillai C, Alonso JM, et al. (2005) Receptive field structure varies with layer in the primary visual cortex. Nat Neurosci 8: 372–379.
15. Priebe NJ, Ferster D (2005) Direction selectivity of excitation and inhibition in simple cells of the cat primary visual cortex. Neuron 45: 133–145.
16. Priebe NJ, Ferster D (2006) Mechanisms underlying cross-orientation suppression in cat visual cortex. Nat Neurosci 9: 552–561.
17. Finn IM, Priebe NJ, Ferster D (2007) The emergence of contrast-invariant orientation tuning in simple cells of cat visual cortex. Neuron 54: 137–152.
18. Priebe NJ, Ferster D (2012) Mechanisms of neuronal computation in Mammalian visual cortex. Neuron 75: 194–208.
19. Sadagopan S, Ferster D (2012) Feedforward origins of response variability underlying contrast invariant orientation tuning in cat visual cortex. Neuron 74: 911–923.
20. Troyer TW, Krukowski AE, Priebe NJ, Miller KD (1998) Contrast-invariant orientation tuning in cat visual cortex: thalamocortical input tuning and correlation-based intracortical connectivity. J Neurosci 18: 5908–5927.
21. Lauritzen TZ, Krukowski AE, Miller KD (2001) Local correlation-based circuitry can account for responses to multi-grating stimuli in a model of cat V1. J Neurophysiol 86: 1803–1815.
22. Krukowski AE, Miller KD (2001) Thalamocortical NMDA conductances and intracortical inhibition can explain cortical temporal tuning. Nat Neurosci 4: 424–430.

23. Kayser A, Priebe NJ, Miller KD (2001) Contrast-dependent nonlinearities arise locally in a model of contrast-invariant orientation tuning. J Neurophysiol 85: 2130–2149.
24. Troyer TW, Krukowski AE, Miller KD (2002) LGN input to simple cells and contrast-invariant orientation tuning: an analysis. J Neurophysiol 87: 2741–2752.
25. Lauritzen TZ, Miller KD (2003) Different roles for simple-cell and complex-cell inhibition in V1. J Neurosci 23: 10201–10213.
26. Palmer SE, Miller KD (2007) Effects of inhibitory gain and conductance fluctuations in a simple model for contrast-invariant orientation tuning in cat V1. J Neurophysiol 98: 63–78.
27. Carandini M, Heeger DJ, Senn W (2002) A synaptic explanation of suppression in visual cortex. J Neurosci 22: 10053–10065.
28. Banitt Y, Martin KA, Segev I (2007) A biologically realistic model of contrast invariant orientation tuning by thalamocortical synaptic depression. J Neurosci 27: 10230–10239.
29. Li YT, Ibrahim LA, Liu BH, Zhang LI, Tao HW (2013) Linear transformation of thalamocortical input by intracortical excitation. Nat Neurosci 16: 1324–1330.
30. Lien AD, Scanziani M (2013) Tuned thalamic excitation is amplified by visual cortical circuits. Nat Neurosci 16: 1315–1323.
31. Alitto HJ, Usrey WM (2004) Influence of contrast on orientation and temporal frequency tuning in ferret primary visual cortex. J Neurophysiol 91: 2797–2808.
32. Sclar G, Freeman RD (1982) Orientation selectivity in the cat's striate cortex is invariant with stimulus contrast. Exp Brain Res 46: 457–461.
33. Skottun BC, Bradley A, Sclar G, Ohzawa I, Freeman RD (1987) The effects of contrast on visual orientation and spatial frequency discrimination: a comparison of single cells and behavior. J Neurophysiol 57: 773–786.
34. Boudreau CE, Ferster D (2005) Short-term depression in thalamocortical synapses of cat primary visual cortex. J Neurosci 25: 7179–7190.
35. Stratford KJ, Tarczy-Hornoch K, Martin KA, Bannister NJ, Jack JJ (1996) Excitatory synaptic inputs to spiny stellate cells in cat visual cortex. Nature 382: 258–261.
36. Johnson DH, Swami A (1983) The transmission of signals by auditory-nerve fiber discharge patterns. J Acoust Soc Am 74: 493–501.
37. Jones K, Tubis A, Burns EM (1985) On the extraction of the signal-excitation function from a non-Poisson cochlear neural spike train. J Acoust Soc Am 78: 90–94.
38. Miller MI (1985) Algorithms for removing recovery-related distortion from auditory-nerve discharge patterns. J Acoust Soc Am 77: 1452–1464.
39. Bi Q (1989) A closed-form solution for removing the dead time effects from the poststimulus time histograms. J Acoust Soc Am 85: 2504–2513.
40. Berry MJ, 2nd, Meister M (1998) Refractoriness and neural precision. J Neurosci 18: 2200–2211.
41. Paninski L (2004) Maximum likelihood estimation of cascade point-process neural encoding models. Network 15: 243–262.
42. Worgotter F, Koch C (1991) A detailed model of the primary visual pathway in the cat: comparison of afferent excitatory and intracortical inhibitory connection schemes for orientation selectivity. J Neurosci 11: 1959–1979.
43. Jones JP, Palmer LA (1987) The two-dimensional spatial structure of simple receptive fields in cat striate cortex. J Neurophysiol 58: 1187–1211.
44. Dittman JS, Regehr WG (1998) Calcium dependence and recovery kinetics of presynaptic depression at the climbing fiber to Purkinje cell synapse. J Neurosci 18: 6147–6162.
45. Abbott LF, Varela JA, Sen K, Nelson SB (1997) Synaptic depression and cortical gain control. Science 275: 220–224.
46. Tsodyks MV, Markram H (1997) The neural code between neocortical pyramidal neurons depends on neurotransmitter release probability. Proc Natl Acad Sci U S A 94: 719–723.
47. Liu BH, Li YT, Ma WP, Pan CJ, Zhang LI, et al. (2011) Broad inhibition sharpens orientation selectivity by expanding input dynamic range in mouse simple cells. Neuron 71: 542–554.
48. Castro-Alamancos MA (2004) Absence of rapid sensory adaptation in neocortex during information processing states. Neuron 41: 455–464.
49. Castro-Alamancos MA, Oldford E (2002) Cortical sensory suppression during arousal is due to the activity-dependent depression of thalamocortical synapses. J Physiol 541: 319–331.
50. Anderson JS, Carandini M, Ferster D (2000) Orientation tuning of input conductance, excitation, and inhibition in cat primary visual cortex. J Neurophysiol 84: 909–926.
51. Hirsch JA, Martinez LM, Pillai C, Alonso JM, Wang Q, et al. (2003) Functionally distinct inhibitory neurons at the first stage of visual cortical processing. Nat Neurosci 6: 1300–1308.
52. Fuhrmann G, Cowan A, Segev I, Tsodyks M, Stricker C (2004) Multiple mechanisms govern the dynamics of depression at neocortical synapses of young rats. J Physiol 557: 415–438.
53. Chance FS, Nelson SB, Abbott LF (1998) Synaptic depression and the temporal response characteristics of V1 cells. J Neurosci 18: 4785–4799.
54. Liu BH, Li P, Sun YJ, Li YT, Zhang LI, et al. (2010) Intervening inhibition underlies simple-cell receptive field structure in visual cortex. Nat Neurosci 13: 89–96.
55. Ferster D (1988) Spatially opponent excitation and inhibition in simple cells of the cat visual cortex. J Neurosci 8: 1172–1180.
56. Tan AY, Brown BD, Scholl B, Mohanty D, Priebe NJ (2011) Orientation selectivity of synaptic input to neurons in mouse and cat primary visual cortex. J Neurosci 31: 12339–12350.
57. Scholl B, Tan AY, Corey J, Priebe NJ (2013) Emergence of orientation selectivity in the Mammalian visual pathway. J Neurosci 33: 10616–10624.
58. Rajan K, Abbott LF, Sompolinsky H (2010) Stimulus-dependent suppression of chaos in recurrent neural networks. Phys Rev E Stat Nonlin Soft Matter Phys 82: 011903.
59. Rubin DB, Miller KD (2011) Normalization in a simple circuit model of visual cortex explains stimulus-induced reduction in shared variability. Program No. 428.10. 2011 Neuroscience Meeting Planner. Washington, DC: Society for Neuroscience, 2011. Online.
60. Litwin-Kumar A, Doiron B (2012) Slow dynamics and high variability in balanced cortical networks with clustered connections. Nat Neurosci 15: 1498–1505.

6

Altered Functional Connectivity between Emotional and Cognitive Resting State Networks in Euthymic Bipolar I Disorder Patients

Giannis Lois, Julia Linke, Michèle Wessa*

Department of Clinical Psychology and Neuropsychology, Institute of Psychology, Johannes Gutenberg-University Mainz, Mainz, Germany

Abstract

Bipolar disorder is characterized by a functional imbalance between hyperactive ventral/limbic areas and hypoactive dorsal/cognitive brain regions potentially contributing to affective and cognitive symptoms. Resting-state studies in bipolar disorder have identified abnormal functional connectivity between these brain regions. However, most of these studies used a seed-based approach, thus restricting the number of regions that were analyzed. Using data-driven approaches, researchers identified resting state networks whose spatial maps overlap with frontolimbic areas such as the default mode network, the frontoparietal networks, the salient network, and the meso/paralimbic network. These networks are specifically engaged during affective and cognitive tasks and preliminary evidence suggests that functional connectivity within and between some of these networks is impaired in bipolar disorder. The present study used independent component analysis and functional network connectivity approaches to investigate functional connectivity within and between these resting state networks in bipolar disorder. We compared 30 euthymic bipolar I disorder patients and 35 age- and gender-matched healthy controls. Inter-network connectivity analysis revealed increased functional connectivity between the meso/paralimbic and the right frontoparietal network in bipolar disorder. This abnormal connectivity pattern did not correlate with variables related to the clinical course of the disease. The present finding may reflect abnormal integration of affective and cognitive information in ventral-emotional and dorsal-cognitive networks in euthymic bipolar patients. Furthermore, the results provide novel insights into the role of the meso/paralimbic network in bipolar disorder.

Editor: Andreas Reif, University of Wuerzburg, Germany

Funding: The study was funded by the Deutsche Forschungsgemeinschaft (SFB 636/C6). The funders had no role in study design, data collection and analysis, decision to publish, or preparation of the manuscript.

Competing Interests: The authors have declared that no competing interests exist.

* Email: wessa@uni-mainz.de

Introduction

Bipolar disorder (BD) is a heterogeneous disease characterized by acute dysfunctional mood states, alternating between mania (BD-I) or hypomania (BD-II) and depression, and related to dysfunctional emotion generation and regulation [1]. Further, BD patients suffer from cognitive impairments such as impaired verbal memory, deficits in executive functions and attentional deficits which are also present during remission [2,3].

It has been proposed that the neural mechanisms underlying dysfunctional emotion regulation as well as cognitive impairments in BD are related to hypoactive ventral prefrontal areas that exert diminished top-down control on limbic brain structures resulting in hyperactivity of these structures [1,4–7]. This disturbed frontolimbic functional connectivity (FC) has been shown during cognitive tasks [8], emotional tasks [9–11], and during resting state [12–16] in both symptomatic and euthymic BD patients.

Two main approaches to investigate functional brain connectivity are the seed-based analysis (SBA) and independent component analysis (ICA). SBA is a hypothesis-driven approach that correlates the time-series of the blood-oxygen-level-dependent (BOLD) signal of one brain region "seed" with the time-series of all other brain regions, resulting in a map that defines the functional connections of the predefined brain region. In contrast, ICA is a data-driven approach that identifies temporally coherent patterns of BOLD signal that are maximally independent from each other. ICA takes into account the BOLD signal from the whole brain to generate functional maps of different brain networks [17].

Studies that employed ICA to investigate functional connectivity during resting state were able to delineate a dozen of resting state networks (RSNs) that are consistent across subjects and sessions [18,19] and show high concordance with measures of structural connectivity [20]. Additionally, the recently developed functional network connectivity (FNC) technique provides the possibility to quantify functional interactions between RSNs.

Interestingly, some of the identified RSNs are engaged during tasks that target affective and cognitive processes [17,21]. For instance, the meso/paralimbic network (MPN) [22,23] or else described as the medial temporal lobe network [24], composed of amygdala, hippocampus, parahippocampal gyrus, and temporal poles, is implicated in processing of emotional information and interoceptive awarenenss [21,24], whereas the left and right frontoparietal networks (FPNs) are implicated in cognitive control and attention (right FPN) or language processes and working memory (left FPN) [17,21] and are comprised of lateral prefrontal regions and inferior parietal cortex [25,26]. Moreover, the salient network (SN) involved in the detection of salient stimuli [27] is mainly composed of the anterior insula and the anterior cingulate cortex [28]. The SN and the FPNs are broadly engaged during a wide range of cognitively demanding tasks [28]. In contrast to these networks, the default mode network (DMN), which is comprised of posterior cingulate cortex/precuneus, ventro-medial prefrontal cortex (vmPFC) and bilateral angular gyri, is strongly associated with self-referential activities and is deactivated during tasks that are directed towards external stimuli [29,30]. Despite the differences between these RSNs, recent findings showed that the SN, the DMN and the FPNs functionally interact with each other [28,31] and that deficits in engagement and disengagement of these 3 networks may be relevant to cognitive and affective dysfunctions [27,32]. Taking into account the association of these RSNs with affective and cognitive functions known to be impaired in BD and given the overlap between the spatial maps of these RSNs and frontolimbic areas that are affected in BD, it can be argued that patterns of functional connectivity within or between these networks may be impaired in BD.

The majority of RS-fMRI studies in BD demonstrated abnormal ventral PFC connectivity with amygdala [14,33] or other subcortical areas (i.e. thalamus, striatum) [12] using SBA. To date, only 4 RS-fMRI studies have employed ICA and investigated within or between-networks connectivity in adult BD-I patients. One study focused on the DMN and reported reduced engagement of the medial PFC within the DMN in manic BD patients [34]. Another RS-fMRI study compared within-network functional connectivity between psychotic BD patients, schizophrenia patients, their respective first degree relatives and healthy subjects using the ICA as a tool to explore potential psychosis endophenotypes [22]. They identified networks that may be implicated in BD (e.g. DMN, MPN, SN and FPNs) and they reported aberrant connectivity in psychotic BD patients within the posterior DMN and the MPN. These abnormalities were shared with schizophrenia patients but not BD relatives suggesting that these findings may be related to the common psychotic symptoms between the two clinical groups. Using a largely overlapping sample, the same research group investigated inter-networks connectivity in BD [23]. They found increased connectivity between the MPN and the SN in psychotic BD patients. This increased connectivity uniquely distinguished this group from healthy BD relatives and schizophrenia patients and correlated positively with the negative mood symptoms of BD patients [23]. Finally, a recent RS-fMRI study investigating both within- and between-network connectivity in BD and borderline personality disorder patients revealed aberrant connectivity patterns in BD between networks implicated in self-referential processing [35]. However, this study did not examine subcortical networks (i.e. MPN).

Given the sparse empirical evidence of RS-fMRI studies that employed a data-driven approach in BD, the present study sought to investigate functional connectivity within and between RSNs in BD using ICA. Our study extends prior work that used similar methodology by examining euthymic BD patients with minimum residual mood symptoms and no current psychotic symptoms. We focused on the DMN, the FPNs (i.e. right and left), the SN, and the MPN as these networks or brain regions within these networks have been previously implicated in BD [5,22,23,34,36,37]. Based on the neurobiological model of BD and previous findings from RS-fMRI studies in BD, we expected to find altered functional connectivity within and between these RSNs that may reflect the underlying pathophysiology of the disorder. To further investigate whether abnormal functional connectivity patterns are affected by the clinical course of the disease, we examined the relationship between functional connectivity measures and some aspects of the history of the disease (i.e. onset of illness, time in remission, number of manic and depressive episodes, and history of psychotic symptoms) and medication. We focused on these variables as they describe sufficiently the clinical course of BD and some of them seem to correlate with behavioral variables [38,39] and with brain activation and connectivity patterns [5,13] within euthymic BD patients.

Materials and Methods

Ethical statement

The ethics committee of the Medical Faculty Mannheim of the University Heidelberg approved the study and all participants gave written informed consent before study participation. Participants/patients having legal guardians or caretakers were excluded from study participation. Only participants/patients, whose capacity to consent was not compromised were investigated in the present study. The capacity to consent was evaluated by senior clinicians as part of the diagnostic interview as well as by cognitive testing (forward and backward digit-span task, Culture Fair Intelligence Test (CFT-20)), which was in the normal range for all participants. All potential participants who declined to participate or otherwise did not participate were not disadvantaged in any other way by not participating in the study. The study has been conducted according to the principles expressed in the Declaration of Helsinki.

Participants

We assessed 30 patients with bipolar I disorder (BD) who were recruited through epidemiological studies at the Central Institute of Mental Health in Mannheim, Germany, or local support groups. Thirty five healthy controls (HC) were recruited from the registry office of the city of Mannheim. Demographic differences between groups were not statistically significant (Table 1). Exclusion criteria for all participants were age under 18, neurological disorder or head trauma with unconsciousness, and common MRI exclusion criteria. Patients were also excluded if they fulfilled criteria of another Axis-I mental disorder as defined by the DSM-IV within the last 6 months and if they had lifetime diagnosis of rapid cycling, schizoaffective disorder or schizophrenia. To increase ecological validity of the patient sample, patients with lifetime (not current) Axis-I disorders were not excluded. More specifically, 7 patients met the criteria for lifetime history of substance abuse or dependence, and 3 patients met the criteria for lifetime anxiety and eating disorders (i.e. agoraphobia, social anxiety disorder, and bulimia). HCs were excluded if they fulfilled the criteria for any lifetime or current DSM-IV axis I mental disorder or took any psychotropic medication. The ethics committee of the Medical Faculty of Mannheim of the University Heidelberg approved the study and all participants gave written informed consent before study participation.

Diagnostic assessment

Main and comorbid diagnoses (for patients) and exclusion criteria (for HCs) were evaluated based on the Structured Clinical Interview for DSM-IV Axis I Disorders. The Young Mania Rating Scale, the Hamilton Rating Scale for Depression (HAM-D), and the Beck Depression Inventory (BDI) were administered to assess residual mood symptoms. Based on the clinical interview, patients were euthymic for at least two months before testing and had minimum residual symptoms (Table 1).

Variables describing the clinical course of the disease such as the number of past depressive and manic episodes, the age at illness

Table 1. Demographic and Clinical Characteristics of Participants.

Characteristics	BD (N = 30)	HC (N = 35)	Statistics	p-value
Gender (Female/Male)	17/13	20/15	$\chi^2 = 0.34$	0.853
Age, years, mean (SD)	40.83 (9.43)	41.94 (8.36)	T(65) = 0.5	0.62
Years of education, mean (SD)	14.97 (2.58)	14.89 (2.31)	T(65) = 0.6	0.54
Current Symptoms, [range], mean (SD)				
YMRS[a] Score	[0–5] 1.3 (1.6)	[0–2] 0.11 (0.40)	T(65) = 3.9	0.00
BDI[b] Score	[0–20] 6.7 (5.94)	[0–12] 1.26 (2.44)	T(65) = 5.5	0.00
HAM-D[c] Score	[0–5] 0.83 (1.17)	[0–2] 0.14 (0.43)	T(65) = 3.2	0.02
History of illness				
No. of past depressive episodes, mean (SD)	3.63 (3.12)			
No. of past manic episodes, mean (SD)	2.66 (2.48)			
Age at illness onset, years, mean (SD)	23.73 (9.51)			
Time in remission, years, mean (SD)	3.08 (3.44)			
Medication load, mean (SD)	3.10 (2.35)			
History of psychotic symptoms (Yes/No)	13/17			

[a]YMRS = Young Mania Rating Scale,
[b]BDI = Beck Depression Inventory,
[c]HAM-D = Hamilton Depression Rating Scale.

onset, the time in remission, and the presence of psychotic symptoms were acquired for every patient. We also verified that the medication status of all patients had been stable during the past 6 months. Among the patients 4 did not take any medication, 25 patients took mood stabilizers (lithium: n = 6, valproate: n = 11, lamotrigin: n = 6, carbamazepin: n = 2), 11 patients took antidepressants (venlaflaxin: n = 3, citalopram: n = 2, sertralin: n = 2, duloxetin: n = 1, clomipramin: n = 1, mirtazapin: n = 1, opipramol: n = 1) and 11 patients took antipsychotic medication (quetiapin: n = 7, perazin: n = 1, risperidon: n = 1, olanzapin: n = 1, aripiprazol: n = 1) at the time of scanning. In accordance to previous studies [11], we coded the number and dosage of each medication and calculated a composite measure of total medication load. For antidepressants and mood stabilizers, we categorized each medication into low-dose (1 or 2 levels) or high-dose (3 or 4 levels) groupings as previously performed [40]. We added a no-dose subtype for those not taking these medications. Using a similar procedure, we estimated the clinical equivalency of the antipsychotic medication to Chlorpromazine dose equivalent, coding them as 0 (no medication), 1 (equal to or below the chlorpromazine dose equivalent), or 2 (above the chlorpromazine dose equivalent) [41]. A composite measure of medication load was generated by summing all individual medication codes for the two categories for each individual participant. The demographic and clinical characteristics of the two groups of participants are shown in Table 1.

Data Acquisition

Data were acquired on a 3-T whole body scanner (Magnetom Trio, Siemens Medical Solutions, Erlangen, Germany). We conducted one high-resolution T1-weighted 3 dimensional MRI sequence (slice thickness = 1.1 mm, field of view = 256×240×176 mm^3, TR = 2.3 s, TE = 2.98 ms). We acquired 40 gradient-echo T2*-weighted slices (slice thickness = 2.3 mm) per volume with the following parameters: TR = 2.7 s, flip angle = 90°, TE = 27 ms, field of view = 220 mm^2, matrix = 96×96, voxel size = 2.3 mm×2.3 mm×2.3 mm. During acquisition of resting-state, participants were instructed to lie still with their eyes closed and not to fall asleep for 5 minutes. 120 whole-brain volumes were acquired with the initial 4 images being discarded to allow for T2 stabilization effects.

Data Analysis

Pre-Processing. Imaging data were preprocessed according to standard procedures using SPM8 (http://www.fil.ion.ucl.ac.uk/spm). Preprocessing involved realignment to the mean image of each run, slice-timing, and normalization into Montreal Neurological Institute standardized space (http://www.mni.mcgill.ca). During normalization, the images were resampled every 3 mm using sinc interpolation and smoothed with a 9×9×9 mm Gaussian kernel to decrease spatial noise. One BD patient and one HC were excluded from the initial sample (i.e. 31 BD patients and 36 HC) due to excessive movement during the fMRI scans (i.e. more than 3 mm translation or 3 degrees rotation and 2 mm or degrees in the first derivatives of motion parameters). In order to exclude the possible confound of different motion artefacts in the compared groups, we additionally estimated the maximum absolute displacement of each brain volume as compared to the previous volume from the translation parameters in the x (left/right), y (anterior/posterior), and z (superior/inferior) directions [42]. No group differences were present in the maximum motion (t = 1,32, df = 65, p = 0.19). This variable was used as nuisance regressor in the group comparisons.

Group-ICA. The Group ICA of fMRI toolbox (GIFT; version 1.3i; http://icatb.sourceforge.net) [43] was used to carry out a group ICA in the preprocessed and normalized data. Using the minimum description length criteria to determine the number of independent components (ICs), we were not able to identify all the RSNs of interest. It has been shown that increasing the number of ICs yields refined components that correspond to known anatomical and functional segmentations [17,44,45]. Following previous procedures [44,45], we gradually increased the number of ICs to 40 until all networks of interest were identified. An initial data reduction step used principal component analysis on the subject-specific data and was followed by an IC estimation that produced 40 time courses and spatial maps with the Infomax algorithm [46]. This algorithm was repeated 20 times in Icasso, each time with different initial conditions. Resulting components of different runs were clustered to estimate the reliability of the decomposition [47]. The index *Iq*, which ranges from 0 to 1, reflects the difference between intra-cluster and extra-cluster similarity [47]. Each of the 40 components had a cluster quality index greater than 0.8. Group-level spatial maps were estimated as the centrotypes of component clusters to reduce sensitivity to initial algorithm parameters. These components were identified in the group of 65 subjects without differentiating between HCs and BD patients to ensure that the same components are identified in each group. Group-level ICs (both spatial maps and time courses) were then back-reconstructed for each subject using the GIGA method [43,48]. Therefore, the subject-specific time course of each component represented a pattern of synchronized brain activity, whose coherency pattern across voxels was represented in the associated spatial map. Component intensity values were then z-scaled to provide normalized scores across subjects.

Based on previous ICA studies and to validate our results, we repeated the Group ICA analysis with 75 ICs components; this high model order yield refined components that correspond to known anatomical and functional segmentation (see Analysis S1).

Identifying Valid RSNs. To identify valid RSNs, we first estimated the voxel-wise spatial overlap of the ICs with SPM's standard tissue-type probability maps for gray matter, white matter and cerebrospinal fluid (http://imaging.mrc-cbu.cam.ac.uk/imaging/Templates) using Pearson's correlation (Table S1). Subsequently, group-level ICs were spatially sorted in GIFT toolbox using templates of the RSNs of interest (i.e. DMN, right and left FPN, SN, MPN; Table S1). These templates were based on whole-brain task-based co-activation networks, which were derived from ICA analyses on peak activation coordinates archived in a large neuroimaging database (i.e. BrainMap Database) [21]. On the basis of their spatial overlap with the templates, 6 ICs were identified as RSNs of interest. The DMN was divided into an anterior (aDMN) and a posterior component (pDMN) (Figure 1A and B) and the FPNs comprised of two lateralized components (i.e. right and left) (Figure 1C and D). The MPN and SN were each identified as a single component (Figure 1E and F). The highest voxel-wise spatial overlap between the 6 ICs and the corresponding templates were similar to previously reported values (r = 0.31–0.55; [49,50]). The last step in the selection procedure was to examine the spectral characteristics of the 6 selected ICs using the same procedure as in Allen and colleagues [18]. For each group-level IC, we estimated the difference between the peak spectral power and minimum spectral power at frequencies to the right of the peak (i.e. dynamic range), and the ratio of the integral of power below 0.10 Hz to the integral of power between 0.15 and 0.25 Hz (i.e. low frequency to high frequency power ratio). Visual inspection of the scatter plot of low frequency to high frequency power ratio versus dynamic range confirmed that all 6 ICs are dominated by frequency fluctuations inside the 0.01–0.1 Hz window (Figure S1).

Within-network connectivity analysis. Statistical inference was carried out on the subject-specific *z*-maps of the 6 RSNs of interest using SPM8. For each group, we computed one-sample *t*-test to create statistical maps of the 6 components of interest (Figure 1). Threshold for the one-sample t-test was set at $p<0.05$ (Family-wise error, FWE correction) to select only the core nodes of each RSN. Subsequently, we created a binary representation of the conjunction of the statistical maps of the two groups, obtained from the one-sample *t* test results, which was further masked to exclude the non-gray matter voxels (Table S2). Group comparisons were restricted to voxels within these binary masks. Two-sample *t*-tests were performed to compare the 6 RSNs between the two groups ($p<0.05$ FWE correction). In addition, to account for type I error inflation for testing 6 RSNs, voxels were only considered significant if they survived a subsequent Bonferroni

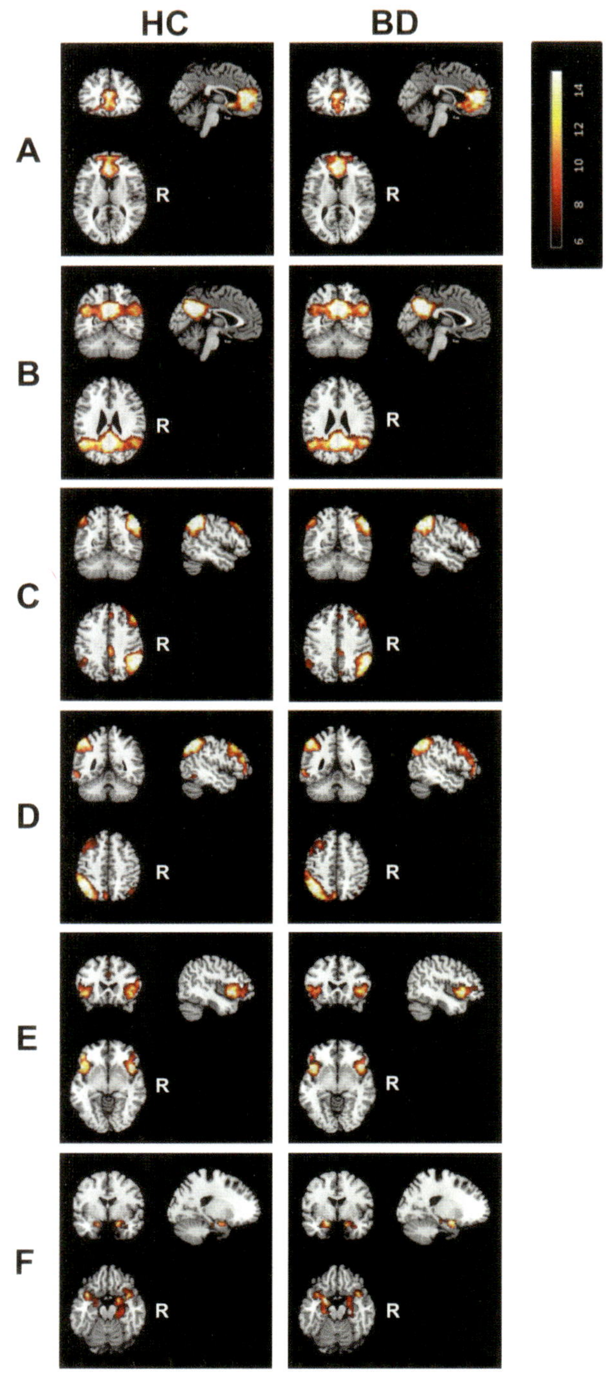

Figure 1. Resting state networks of interest. Illustration of one-sample-t-test maps of the anterior and posterior default mode network, right and left frontoparietal network, the salience network, and the meso/paralimbic network identified in the control (left column) and patient (right column) group. Maps are thresholded at P<0.05 (whole-brain FWE corrected). R, Right.

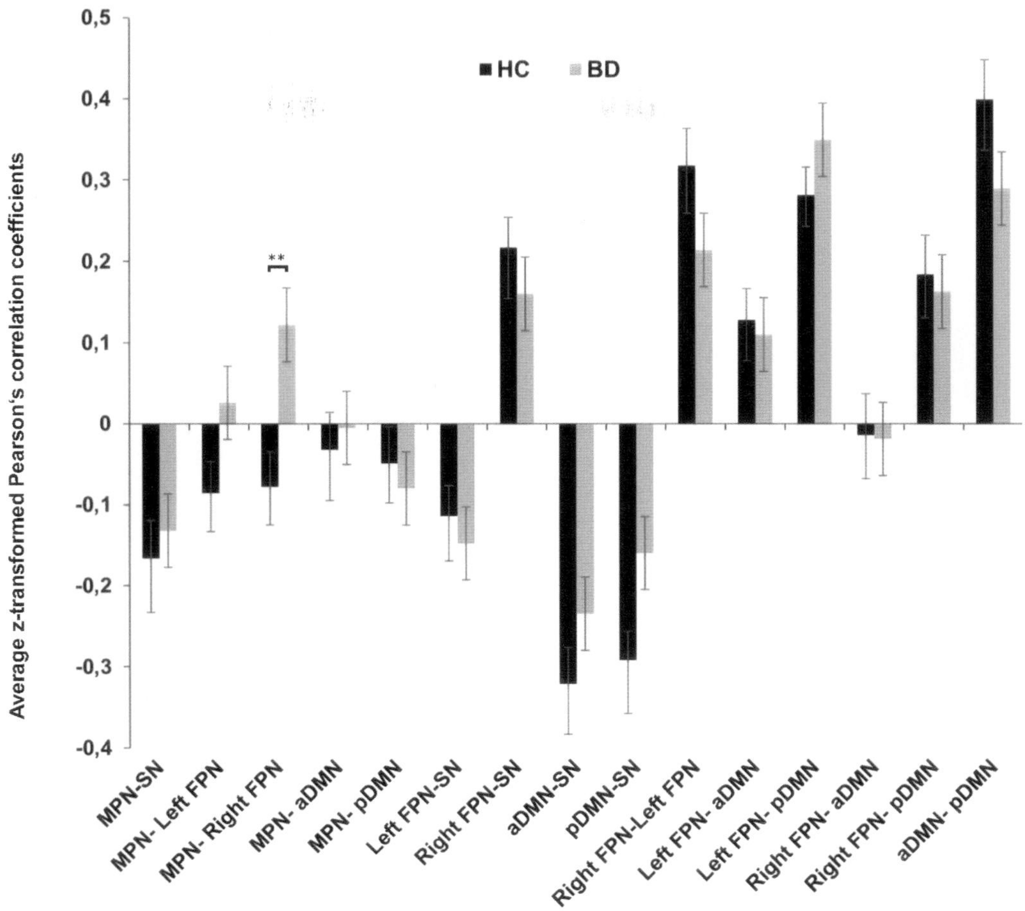

Figure 2. Functional network connectivity (FNC) between components. Average Fisher's z-transformed Pearson's correlation coefficients from FNC analysis reflecting connectivity between the 6 components of interest (15 possible pairs of components) for the healthy control (HC) and patient group (BD). Error bars represent the standard error of the mean (SEM). Asterisks (**) depict FDR significant finding.

correction for multiple testing at $p<0.008$ (0.05/6). Age, gender and maximum motion were used as nuisance variables in the analysis.

Between-networks connectivity analysis. The subject-specific time courses of each RSN were entered in the FNC analysis (http://mialab.mrn.org/software). The FNC estimates the Pearson's correlation coefficient between pairs of time courses with a maximal lagged correlation approach (i.e. −3 to +3 s lag) [32]. Time course data were first band-pass filtered with a Butterworth filter with cutoff frequencies of.01–.1 Hz [51] and then pairwise correlations were computed between the time courses of the 6 RSNs of interest, resulting in 15 total pairwise correlations for each subject. Resulting Pearson's correlation coefficients were transformed to Fisher's z values and within-group correlations between networks as well as between-group differences in correlation coefficients were estimated. To control for multiple comparisons, p-values were thresholded according to a false discovery rate (FDR) of 0.05. Age gender and maximum motion were used as nuisance variables in the analysis.

Correlations with variables related to the clinical course of the disease. Additionally, we tested the effect of variables related to the clinical course of the disease on abnormal within- and between-networks functional connectivity. Using the MarsBaR toolbox (http://marsbar.sourceforge.net) we extracted the mean subject-specific *z*-values of the clusters showing significant between-group differences ($p<.05$, FDR correction) in the within-network connectivity and subsequently we conducted bivariate Pearson's correlations between the extracted values and the illness-related variables within the patient group. Similarly, bivariate Pearson's correlations were conducted between correlation coefficients estimating FNC between the MPN and right FPN (aberrant pair of networks) and variables related to the clinical course of the disease within the BD group.

To address the question whether the history of psychotic symptoms influences abnormal connectivity patterns, we divided the patient group into patients with ($n = 13$) and without ($n = 17$) history of psychotic symptoms and we performed a two-sample T-test to examine between-group differences in functional connectivity within- and between-networks (limited to aberrant connectivity).

Results

Components of interest and statistical comparison of RSNs

The 6 RSNs of interest were identified separately for the HC and BD group by performing one-sample-t-tests on the subject specific *z*-maps ($p<0.05$, FWE-corrected, Figure 1). Consistent with previous studies that used a high order model, the DMN was divided into an anterior part (aDMN) that covers the medial PFC/ACC (BA 10/32/24) and a posterior part (pDMN) that covers the precuneus/posterior cingulate cortex and angular gyri (BA 23/39)

Table 2. Pearson's correlation coefficients and p values from FNC analysis.

Component combination	HC	BD	Between groups *p* (FDR corrected)
MPN-SN	−0.166*	−0.132*	0.835
MPN- Left FPN	−0.086	0.026	0.069
MPN- Right FPN	−0.078	0.122*	0.001§
MPN- aDMN	−0.032	−0.005	0.890
MPN- pDMN	−0.049	−0.080	0.794
Left FPN-SN	−0.114*	−0.148*	0.579
Right FPN-SN	0.217*	0.160*	0.335
aDMN-SN	−0.322*	−0.235*	0.219
pDMN-SN	−0.292*	−0.160	0.122
Right FPN-Left FPN	0.318*	0.214*	0.098
Left FPN- aDMN	0.128*	0.110*	0.829
Left FPN- pDMN	0.282*	0.350*	0.216
Right FPN- aDMN	−0.014	−0.019	0.838
Right FPN- pDMN	0.184*	0.163*	0.566
aDMN- pDMN	0.400*	0.290*	0.205

* Denotes significant ($p<0.05$ FDR corrected) Pearson's coefficient correlations between components within each group.
§Denotes significant ($p<0.05$ FDR corrected) group differences in the magnitude of the correlation between components.

(Figure 1A and 1B). The right and left fronto-parietal networks mainly covered the inferior parietal cortex (BA 39/40) dorsolateral PFC (BA 45/9) and ventrolateral PFC (BA 46/47) (Figure 1C and 1D). The SN encompassed the anterior insula/lateral orbitofrontal cortex (BA 38/45/47) and the supramarginal gyrus (BA 40) (Figure 1E). The MPN included the amygdala, hippocampus, parahippocampal gyrus, temporal poles, and a part of insular cortex (BA 28/30/34/38) (Figure 1F). The location of the FC peaks and corresponding z-scores of every network are presented in Table S3.

There were no significant between-group differences within the 6 RSN of interest. An exploratory analysis without Bonferroni correction for testing multiple components also yielded no significant between-group differences.

Between network connectivity

The 15 possible pairwise network combinations were tested for significant maximal-lagged correlations in each group (Figure 2 and Table 2). As expected, both groups showed strong positive connectivity between the right and left FPN and between the pDMN and aDMN. The SN showed positive FNC with the right FPN and negative FNC with the left FPN and the two DMNs. Both groups showed positive connectivity between the pDMN and the two lateralized fronto-parietal networks as well as between the aDMN and the left fronto-parietal network. We observed significant group differences in FNC between the MPN and the right FPN (p = .001, FDR-corrected; Figure 2 and 3). Whereas this combination of networks showed a tendency towards negative FNC in the HC group (r = −0.078), there was significant positive FNC between the two networks in the BD group (r = 0.122). Mean lag times did not differ between groups for any of the 15 combinations.

Relationship with variables related to the clinical course of the disease

We conducted bivariate Pearson's correlations to investigate the relationship between abnormal functional connectivity and variables related to the clinical course of the disease or medication load within the BD group. There was no correlation between illness-related variables or medication load and abnormal between-networks connectivity patterns even when no correction for multiple testing was applied. Furthermore, the two-sample T-test revealed no differences in functional connectivity between patients with and without history of psychotic symptoms.

Discussion

The present study extends previous knowledge by investigating functional connectivity within and between RSNs that have not been examined in detail despite their potential relevance for both affective and cognitive dysfunctions in BD. Compared to previous RS-fMRI studies in BD that employed an exploratory multivariate method, the present study comprised a larger sample of euthymic BD-I patients without current psychotic symptoms. Analysis of between-network connectivity revealed that in contrast to HC subjects where activity of the executive network does not correlate with activity of the MPN, BD patients display an increased interaction between the MPN and the right FPN.

To better interpret this finding, we drew upon evidence from meta-analytic studies that compared activation maps of different behavioral paradigms with ICA-derived spatial maps of RSNs [17,21]. In this context, the positive FNC between the MPN and the right FPN in the BD group may reflect abnormal communication between a limbic-paralimbic network implicated in emotional processing and a right-lateralized dorsal network involved in executive functions and cognitive control [21]. In line with this assumption, neurobiological models of BD proposed that impaired emotion regulation in BD may result from a functional imbalance between a dorsal-cognitive network (i.e. dorsal ACC, dorsal PFC, inferior parietal cortex), and a ventral-emotional network (i.e. amygdala, parahippocampal gyrus, striatum, subgenual cingulate cortex, orbitofrontal cortex) [1,4,52]. In this respect, it is noteworthy that a trend-level group-related effect was also observed for the MPN-left FPN pair (p = .069) in the same

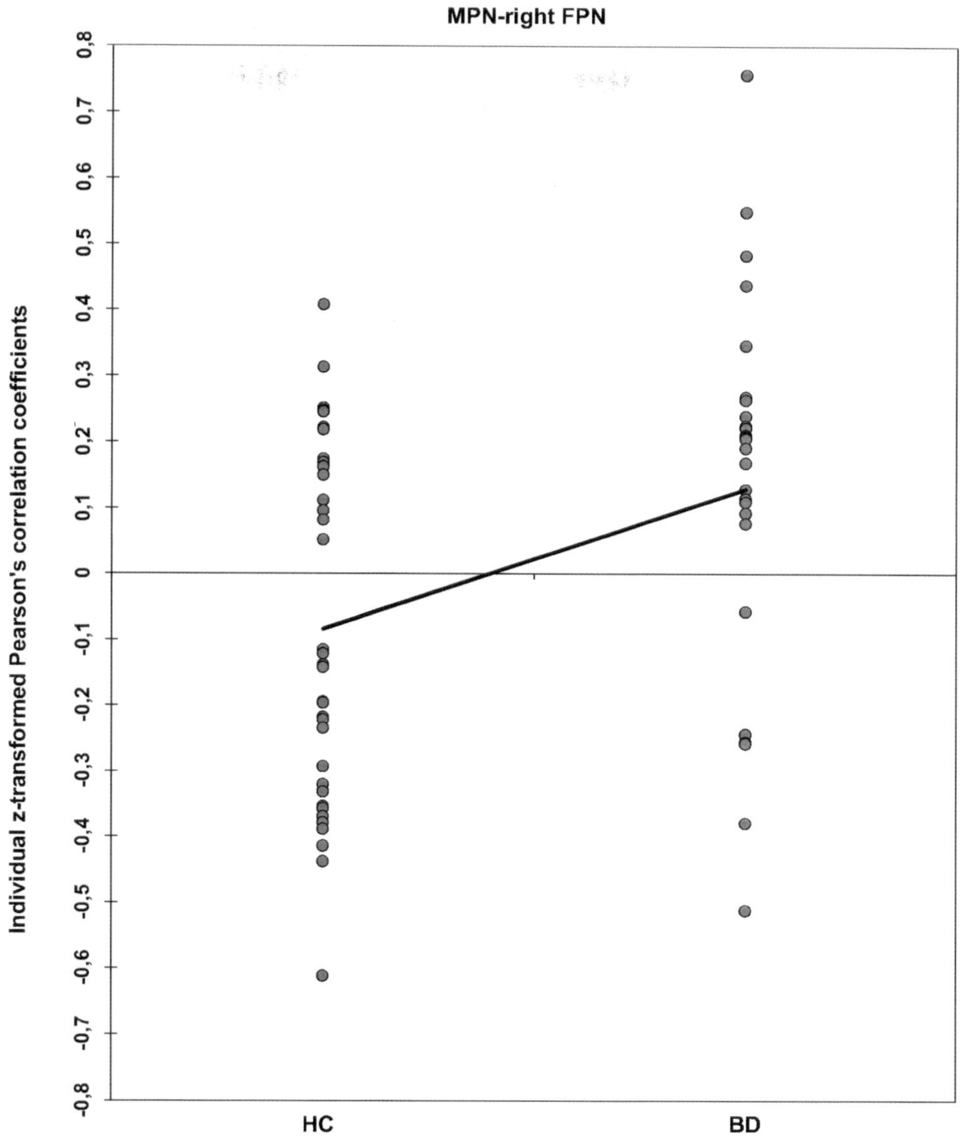

Figure 3. Functional network connectivity (FNC) between MPN-right FPN in the individual level. Fisher's z-transformed Pearson's correlation coefficients depicting individual FNC values for the MPN-right FPN pair. Both samples are normally distributed and have equal variance. The line connects the average FNC values of the two groups.

direction as the main MPN-right FPN finding. Both findings suggest a general functional imbalance of the limbic network with fronto-parietal/cognitive networks in BD.

The present finding may be interpreted as impaired top-down control or abnormally increased bottom-up interference between these networks through the reciprocal connections between limbic-paralimbic structures and lateral PFC regions [53]. Independent of the direction of the interaction (i.e. top-down or bottom-up), this result supports previous evidence from seed-based studies showing abnormal FC between limbic structures, such as amygdala, and right PFC at rest [13,16] or during emotional tasks [9,54,55]. Our results are also in line with a recent meta-analysis showing increased ventral-limbic activation and decreased right-lateralized PFC activation during emotional processing in BD patients [37].

Aberrant FNC between the MPN and the right FPN in the BD group did not correlate with medication load or variables characterizing the clinical course of the disease, namely, the number of manic and depressive episodes, the age of illness onset, the time in remission, and the history of psychotic symptoms. Previous research has shown that some of these clinical characteristics of BD patients correlate with behavioral variables [38,39] and with brain activation and connectivity patterns [5,13]. The absence of significant correlations in the present sample of euthymic BD patients with minimum residual mood symptoms and no current psychotic symptoms indicates that aberrant FNC between the MPN and the right FPN may constitute a trait marker of BD. Emerging questions, for future studies to address, focus on whether this FC abnormality reflects a developmental failure to establish healthy prefrontal–limbic modulation early in life which may later result in the onset of the disease [5] and may be present in healthy populations at high risk for developing BD or represents common state- and mood-independent effects of previous BD episodes.

Contrary to our hypothesis, we did not observe abnormal within-network FC in any of the 6 RSNs of interest also when no correction for multiple comparisons was applied. In line with the lack of significant within-network FC findings in the present study, a recent RS-fMRI study showed significant BD-related impairments in between- but not in within-network FC [35]. This evidence leads to the assumption that BD like schizophrenia may be mainly characterized by dysconnectivity in large-scale networks [56,57].

Based on our hypotheses, abnormal FC within and between the RSNs of interest may underlie affective and cognitive symptoms of the disorder. Therefore, these abnormalities would more likely characterize symptomatic rather than euthymic patients. In line with this idea, previous ICA studies that investigated functional connectivity patterns in BD at rest reported altered connectivity within the DMN in manic [34] or psychotic [22,23] BD patients. The assumption that these alterations are state-dependent is further supported by evidence that these abnormal FC patterns are either shared by schizophrenic patients [22] or correlate with negative mood symptoms [23].

Another plausible explanation for the lack of BD-related abnormal FC in the present study may be the context-dependent nature of these abnormalities, which may only be present or more pronounced during cognitive and emotional tasks that engage these networks and not at rest. Future ICA studies comparing rest and task conditions should investigate this possibility.

The present findings have to be interpreted in the light of some limitations. First, inherent to the nature of the ICA, there is no optimal way to estimate the number of ICs (problem of dimensionality). Yet, the number of ICs has a significant impact on the spatial characteristics of the RSNs [58]. Most studies use the Minimum Description Length criteria as standard criteria to determine the number of ICs. However, using these criteria, we were not able to identify all common RSNs that were of interest for the present study. As previous studies showed that detection of some RSNs requires higher dimensionality models [44], we decided to gradually increase the dimensionality until the point that all the networks of interest were identified [44]. The aim was to find the minimum number of components in which our hypotheses could be tested. Additionally, we performed the same analysis with a standard high model order ICA (i.e. 75 ICs), as previous studies have demonstrated that this model order yield refined components that correspond to known anatomical and functional segmentations [17,44,45]. Importantly, we found similar results concerning the MPN with both 40 and 75 ICs (see Analysis S1).

A second limitation is related to the correlation analysis between abnormal FC patterns and clinical characteristics. The absence of correlations may also be related to the lack of power as the sample was relatively small for this type of analysis and patients investigated here were relatively healthy leading to little variance with regard to symptomatic variables.

Furthermore, medication load was assessed as a composite measure assuming synergistic rather than antagonistic effects of the different types of medication namely antidepressants, mood stabilizers, and antipsychotics. It is rather unlikely that the effects of different classes of medication on brain connectivity are synergistic and independent from each other. Therefore, category-specific medication effects may still confound the present findings. However, due to possible pharmacological interactions between different types of medication the independent impact of every class of medication on connectivity cannot be directly assessed in the present sample. Future studies using medication-based selection criteria for the patient group and a drug-free baseline are more suitable to address questions about potential pharmacological effects on brain connectivity.

Finally, the interpretation of resting state data in light of previous task-related neuroimaging studies has to be made with caution. It still remains an open question to what extent task-based differences in specific brain regions in BD are reflected in different connectivity patterns of their respective brain networks at rest. Furthermore, to date, there is very sparse evidence linking RSNs with behavior and cognitive or emotional processes which could provide functional interpretations of widely observed RSNs.

In conclusion, the present study substantially extends prior work in BD by employing a data-driven multivariate approach to examine euthymic BD-I patients without current psychotic symptoms. We showed abnormal interactions between the MPN and the right FPN in BD at rest. This abnormality may underlie impaired integration of affective and cognitive processes leading to dysfunctional emotion regulation. Furthermore, the present results highlight the importance of the MPN in this disorder.

Supporting Information

Figure S1 Scatter plot of low frequency (LF) to high frequency (HF) power ratio versus dynamic range for all components. Red squares represent the 6 components of interest selected in the present study.

Table S1 Voxel-wise spatial overlap (Pearson's r) of RSNs of interest with gray matter, white matter, cerebrospinal fluid masks and templates of RSNs.

Table S2 Number of voxels before and after excluding non-gray matter voxels.

Table S3 Peak within-network functional connectivity for both groups.

Analysis S1 Group Independent component analysis with 75 ICs.

Acknowledgments

The authors thank Johanna Forneck, Janine Heissler, Manuela Glasbrenner, Katja Nitsche, Kristina Schaffer, Claudia Stief, and Birgül Sarun for their assistance in data acquisition.

Author Contributions

Conceived and designed the experiments: JL MW. Performed the experiments: JL. Analyzed the data: GL. Contributed reagents/materials/analysis tools: GL JL MW. Wrote the paper: GL JL MW.

References

1. Phillips ML, Ladouceur CD, Drevets WC (2008) A neural model of voluntary and automatic emotion regulation: implications for understanding the pathophysiology and neurodevelopment of bipolar disorder. Mol Psychiatry 13: 829, 833–857.

2. Mann-Wrobel MC, Carreno JT, Dickinson D (2011) Meta-analysis of neuropsychological functioning in euthymic bipolar disorder: an update and investigation of moderator variables. Bipolar Disord 13: 334–342.
3. Sole B, Bonnin CM, Torrent C, Martinez-Aran A, Popovic D, et al. (2012) Neurocognitive impairment across the bipolar spectrum. CNS Neurosci Ther 18: 194–200.
4. Phillips ML, Drevets WC, Rauch SL, Lane R (2003) Neurobiology of emotion perception II: Implications for major psychiatric disorders. Biol Psychiatry 54: 515–528.
5. Strakowski SM, Adler CM, Almeida J, Altshuler LL, Blumberg HP, et al. (2012) The functional neuroanatomy of bipolar disorder: a consensus model. Bipolar Disord 14: 313–325.
6. Wessa M, Kanske P, Linke J (2013) Bipolar disorder: A neural network perspective on a disorder of emotion and motivation. Restor Neurol Neurosci.
7. Wessa M, Linke J (2009) Emotional processing in bipolar disorder: behavioural and neuroimaging findings. Int Rev Psychiatry 21: 357–367.
8. Pompei F, Dima D, Rubia K, Kumari V, Frangou S (2011) Dissociable functional connectivity changes during the Stroop task relating to risk, resilience and disease expression in bipolar disorder. Neuroimage 57: 576–582.
9. Foland LC, Altshuler LL, Bookheimer SY, Eisenberger N, Townsend J, et al. (2008) Evidence for deficient modulation of amygdala response by prefrontal cortex in bipolar mania. Psychiatry Res 162: 27–37.
10. Townsend JD, Torrisi SJ, Lieberman MD, Sugar CA, Bookheimer SY, et al. (2013) Frontal-amygdala connectivity alterations during emotion downregulation in bipolar I disorder. Biol Psychiatry 73: 127–135.
11. Versace A, Thompson WK, Zhou D, Almeida JR, Hassel S, et al. (2010) Abnormal left and right amygdala-orbitofrontal cortical functional connectivity to emotional faces: state versus trait vulnerability markers of depression in bipolar disorder. Biol Psychiatry 67: 422–431.
12. Anand A, Li Y, Wang Y, Lowe MJ, Dzemidzic M (2009) Resting state corticolimbic connectivity abnormalities in unmedicated bipolar disorder and unipolar depression. Psychiatry Res 171: 189–198.
13. Anticevic A, Brumbaugh MS, Winkler AM, Lombardo LE, Barrett J, et al. (2013) Global prefrontal and fronto-amygdala dysconnectivity in bipolar I disorder with psychosis history. Biol Psychiatry 73: 565–573.
14. Chai XJ, Whitfield-Gabrieli S, Shinn AK, Gabrieli JD, Nieto Castanon A, et al. (2011) Abnormal medial prefrontal cortex resting-state connectivity in bipolar disorder and schizophrenia. Neuropsychopharmacology 36: 2009–2017.
15. Mamah D, Barch DM, Repovs G (2013) Resting state functional connectivity of five neural networks in bipolar disorder and schizophrenia. J Affect Disord.
16. Torrisi S, Moody TD, Vizueta N, Thomason ME, Monti MM, et al. (2013) Differences in resting corticolimbic functional connectivity in bipolar I euthymia. Bipolar Disord 15: 156–166.
17. Smith SM, Fox PT, Miller KL, Glahn DC, Fox PM, et al. (2009) Correspondence of the brain's functional architecture during activation and rest. Proc Natl Acad Sci U S A 106: 13040–13045.
18. Allen EA, Erhardt EB, Damaraju E, Gruner W, Segall JM, et al. (2011) A baseline for the multivariate comparison of resting-state networks. Front Syst Neurosci 5: 2.
19. Damoiseaux JS, Rombouts SA, Barkhof F, Scheltens P, Stam CJ, et al. (2006) Consistent resting-state networks across healthy subjects. Proc Natl Acad Sci U S A 103: 13848–13853.
20. Greicius MD, Supekar K, Menon V, Dougherty RF (2009) Resting-state functional connectivity reflects structural connectivity in the default mode network. Cereb Cortex 19: 72–78.
21. Laird AR, Fox PM, Eickhoff SB, Turner JA, Ray KL, et al. (2011) Behavioral interpretations of intrinsic connectivity networks. J Cogn Neurosci 23: 4022–4037.
22. Khadka S, Meda SA, Stevens MC, Glahn DC, Calhoun VD, et al. (2013) Is Aberrant Functional Connectivity A Psychosis Endophenotype? A Resting State Functional Magnetic Resonance Imaging Study. Biol Psychiatry.
23. Meda SA, Gill A, Stevens MC, Lorenzoni RP, Glahn DC, et al. (2012) Differences in resting-state functional magnetic resonance imaging functional network connectivity between schizophrenia and psychotic bipolar probands and their unaffected first-degree relatives. Biol Psychiatry 71: 881–889.
24. Damoiseaux JS, Beckmann CF, Arigita EJ, Barkhof F, Scheltens P, et al. (2008) Reduced resting-state brain activity in the "default network" in normal aging. Cereb Cortex 18: 1856–1864.
25. Corbetta M, Shulman GL (2002) Control of goal-directed and stimulus-driven attention in the brain. Nat Rev Neurosci 3: 201–215.
26. Vincent JL, Kahn I, Snyder AZ, Raichle ME, Buckner RL (2008) Evidence for a frontoparietal control system revealed by intrinsic functional connectivity. J Neurophysiol 100: 3328–3342.
27. Menon V (2011) Large-scale brain networks and psychopathology: a unifying triple network model. Trends Cogn Sci 15: 483–506.
28. Seeley WW, Menon V, Schatzberg AF, Keller J, Glover GH, et al. (2007) Dissociable intrinsic connectivity networks for salience processing and executive control. J Neurosci 27: 2349–2356.
29. Greicius MD (2003) Neuroimaging in developmental disorders. Curr Opin Neurol 16: 143–146.
30. Raichle ME, MacLeod AM, Snyder AZ, Powers WJ, Gusnard DA, et al. (2001) A default mode of brain function. Proc Natl Acad Sci U S A 98: 676–682.
31. Sridharan D, Levitin DJ, Menon V (2008) A critical role for the right fronto-insular cortex in switching between central-executive and default-mode networks. Proc Natl Acad Sci U S A 105: 12569–12574.
32. Jafri MJ, Pearlson GD, Stevens M, Calhoun VD (2008) A method for functional network connectivity among spatially independent resting-state components in schizophrenia. Neuroimage 39: 1666–1681.
33. Chepenik LG, Raffo M, Hampson M, Lacadie C, Wang F, et al. (2010) Functional connectivity between ventral prefrontal cortex and amygdala at low frequency in the resting state in bipolar disorder. Psychiatry Res 182: 207–210.
34. Ongur D, Lundy M, Greenhouse I, Shinn AK, Menon V, et al. (2010) Default mode network abnormalities in bipolar disorder and schizophrenia. Psychiatry Res 183: 59–68.
35. Das P, Calhoun V, Malhi GS (2014) Bipolar and borderline patients display differential patterns of functional connectivity among resting state networks. Neuroimage.
36. Chen CH, Suckling J, Lennox BR, Ooi C, Bullmore ET (2011) A quantitative meta-analysis of fMRI studies in bipolar disorder. Bipolar Disord 13: 1–15.
37. Houenou J, Frommberger J, Carde S, Glasbrenner M, Diener C, et al. (2011) Neuroimaging-based markers of bipolar disorder: evidence from two meta-analyses. J Affect Disord 132: 344–355.
38. Linke J, Sonnekes C, Wessa M (2011) Sensitivity to positive and negative feedback in euthymic patients with bipolar I disorder: the last episode makes the difference. Bipolar Disord 13: 638–650.
39. Wright KA, Lam D, Brown RG (2008) Dysregulation of the behavioral activation system in remitted bipolar I disorder. J Abnorm Psychol 117: 838–848.
40. Sackeim HA (2001) The definition and meaning of treatment-resistant depression. J Clin Psychiatry 62 Suppl 16: 10–17.
41. Gardner DM, Murphy AL, O'Donnell H, Centorrino F, Baldessarini RJ (2010) International consensus study of antipsychotic dosing. Am J Psychiatry 167: 686–693.
42. Van Dijk KR, Sabuncu MR, Buckner RL (2012) The influence of head motion on intrinsic functional connectivity MRI. Neuroimage 59: 431–438.
43. Calhoun VD, Adali T, Pearlson GD, Pekar JJ (2001) A method for making group inferences from functional MRI data using independent component analysis. Hum Brain Mapp 14: 140–151.
44. Abou-Elseoud A, Starck T, Remes J, Nikkinen J, Tervonen O, et al. (2010) The effect of model order selection in group PICA. Hum Brain Mapp 31: 1207–1216.
45. Kiviniemi V, Starck T, Remes J, Long X, Nikkinen J, et al. (2009) Functional segmentation of the brain cortex using high model order group PICA. Hum Brain Mapp 30: 3865–3886.
46. Bell AJ, Sejnowski TJ (1995) An information-maximization approach to blind separation and blind deconvolution. Neural Comput 7: 1129–1159.
47. Himberg J, Hyvarinen A, Esposito F (2004) Validating the independent components of neuroimaging time series via clustering and visualization. Neuroimage 22: 1214–1222.
48. Erhardt EB, Rachakonda S, Bedrick EJ, Allen EA, Adali T, et al. (2011) Comparison of multi-subject ICA methods for analysis of fMRI data. Hum Brain Mapp 32: 2075–2095.
49. Assaf M, Jagannathan K, Calhoun VD, Miller L, Stevens MC, et al. (2010) Abnormal functional connectivity of default mode sub-networks in autism spectrum disorder patients. Neuroimage 53: 247–256.
50. von dem Hagen EA, Stoyanova RS, Baron-Cohen S, Calder AJ (2013) Reduced functional connectivity within and between 'social' resting state networks in autism spectrum conditions. Soc Cogn Affect Neurosci 8: 694–701.
51. Cordes D, Haughton VM, Arfanakis K, Carew JD, Turski PA, et al. (2001) Frequencies contributing to functional connectivity in the cerebral cortex in "resting-state" data. AJNR Am J Neuroradiol 22: 1326–1333.
52. Strakowski SM, Adler CM, Holland SK, Mills NP, DelBello MP, et al. (2005) Abnormal FMRI brain activation in euthymic bipolar disorder patients during a counting Stroop interference task. Am J Psychiatry 162: 1697–1705.
53. Mayberg HS, Liotti M, Brannan SK, McGinnis S, Mahurin RK, et al. (1999) Reciprocal limbic-cortical function and negative mood: converging PET findings in depression and normal sadness. Am J Psychiatry 156: 675–682.
54. Perlman SB, Almeida JR, Kronhaus DM, Versace A, Labarbara EJ, et al. (2012) Amygdala activity and prefrontal cortex-amygdala effective connectivity to emerging emotional faces distinguish remitted and depressed mood states in bipolar disorder. Bipolar Disord 14: 162–174.
55. Vizueta N, Rudie JD, Townsend JD, Torrisi S, Moody TD, et al. (2012) Regional fMRI hypoactivation and altered functional connectivity during emotion processing in nonmedicated depressed patients with bipolar II disorder. Am J Psychiatry 169: 831–840.
56. Uhlhaas PJ, Singer W (2012) Neuronal dynamics and neuropsychiatric disorders: toward a translational paradigm for dysfunctional large-scale networks. Neuron 75: 963–980.
57. Uhlhaas PJ (2013) Dysconnectivity, large-scale networks and neuronal dynamics in schizophrenia. Curr Opin Neurobiol 23: 283–290.
58. Cole DM, Smith SM, Beckmann CF (2010) Advances and pitfalls in the analysis and interpretation of resting-state FMRI data. Front Syst Neurosci 4: 8.

7

Transcutaneous Auricular Vagus Nerve Stimulation Triggers Melatonin Secretion and Is Antidepressive in Zucker Diabetic Fatty Rats

Shaoyuan Li[1,2]¶, Xu Zhai[1]¶, Peijing Rong[1]*, Michael F. McCabe[3], Jingjun Zhao[1], Hui Ben[1], Xing Wang[2], Shuxing Wang[1,2,3]*

1 Department of Physiology, Institute of Acupuncture and Moxibustion, China Academy of Chinese Medical Sciences, Beijing, China, **2** Department of Anatomy, Xinxiang Medical University, Xinxiang, Henan Province, China, **3** Department of Anesthesia, Critical Care, and Pain Medicine, Massachusetts General Hospital, Harvard Medical School, Boston, Massachusetts, United States of America

Abstract

Decreased circulating melatonin is implicated in depression. We recently found that Zucker diabetic fatty rats (ZDF, fa/fa) develop depression-like behaviors and that transcutaneous auricular vagus nerve stimulation (taVNS) is antidepressive in ZDF rats. Here we studied whether the ZDF rats could be used as a depression rodent model and whether the antidepressive effect of taVNS is mediated through modulation of melatonin secretion. Adult male ZDF and Zucker lean (ZL, fa/+) littermates were used. 30 min-taVNS procedures (2/15 Hz, 2 mA) were administered once daily under anesthesia for 34 consecutive days in pineal intact ZDF (n = 8) and ZL (n = 6) rats, as well as in pinealectomized ZDF rats (n = 8). Forced swimming test (FST) was used to determine depression-like behavior and ELISA to detect plasma melatonin concentration on day 35. We found that naïve ZDF rats had a longer immobility time in FST and that long-term (34 days) taVNS treatment ameliorated the depression-like behavior. In both pineal intact and pinealectomized ZDF rats, taVNS induced acute melatonin secretion, both during and after the taVNS session. A low melatonin level is related to the poor FST performance in ZDF rats ($R = -0.544$) in contrast to ZL rats ($R = 0.247$). In conclusion, our results show that ZDF rats are ideal candidates of innate depression and that taVNS is antidepressive through triggering melatonin secretion and increasing its production.

Editor: David A. Slattery, University of Regensburg, Germany

Funding: This work was supported by National Natural Science Foundation of China-81271243, 81473780; Natural Science Foundation of Beijing, 7111007; National Basic Research Program of China (973 Program)-2012CB518503; and Project Supported National Science and Technology Ministry-2012BAF14B10. The funders had no role in study design, data collection and analysis, decision to publish, or preparation of the manuscript.

Competing Interests: The authors have declared that no competing interests exist.

* Email: rongpj@hotmail.com (PR); wshuxing@mgh.harvard.edu (SW)

¶ These authors contributed equally to this work.

Introduction

A craving for the understanding of major depressive disorder makes the search for additional animal models highly necessary. Proper animal models would accelerate the understanding of the etiology of depression and development of therapeutic approaches. Our recent studies found that Zucker diabetic fatty rats (ZDF, fa/fa) innately develop depression-like behaviors and that transcutaneous auricular vagus nerve stimulation (taVNS) is antidepressive in ZDF rats [1,2].

Melatonin (N-acetyl-5-methoxytryptamine) is the hormone that functions as the mediator of photoperiodic information to the central nervous system in vertebrates and allows a central circadian regulation of numerous physiological homeostasis including circadian rhythms, sleep, and mood [3]. Importantly, decreased level of circulating melatonin [4,5] and dysfunction of melatonin receptor type 1 [3] is contributable to depression. On the contrary, complementary with melatonin is associated with reduced depression in rats [4,5] and patients [6,7]. However, the melatonin effect was shorter lasting [8], finding approaches that can maintain melatonin secretion will be helpful to clinical patients.

As a kind of complementary and alternative medicine, acupuncture is a generally beneficial, well-tolerated, and safe monotherapy for depression in animal models, clinical patients, and eldercare facility residents [2,9]. The mechanism for the antidepressive effect of acupuncture may be its stimulation to the vagus nerve [1,10–14]. The taVNS stimulates the afferent auricular branches of vagus nerve that project to solitary nucleus [2]. Neurons in solitary nucleus further project, mono- or multi-synaptically, to the limbic and the autonomic nervous system structures, including the pineal gland, ventral tegmental area, the hypothalamus, amygdala, anterior cingulate cortex, nucleus accumbens, and the lateral prefrontal cortex [2]. Fibers from the solitary nucleus also project to the locus ceruleus and dorsal raphe nucleus, respectively major nuclei related to noradrenergic and serotonergic innervations of the entire brain cortex. The serotonergic, dopaminergic, and noradrenergic systems may be involved in the pathophysiology of depression and in the neuromechanisms of action of antidepressants [2]. However, it is

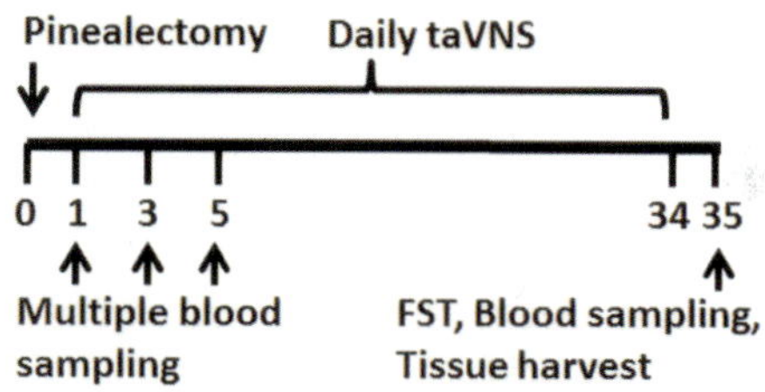

Figure 1. Illustration of experimental time in days. Showing time points for pinealectomy operation, taVNS, blood sampling, FST, and tissue harvest. Pinealectomy operation was done on day 0 (before taVNS sessions). Once daily taVNS administration began on day 1 and continued to day 34. Multiple blood sampling happened on day 1, 3, and 5 of taVNS sessions. On day 35, FST, blood and tissue sampling were done.

not clear whether the antidepressive mechanism of taVNS is mediated through the modulation of melatonin secretion. Based on the existence of overt depression in Zucker diabetic fatty (ZDF) rats [2] as well as the increasingly prevalent comorbidity of obesity and depression [15], in this study we show that ZDF rats are ideal depression animal model and that the mechanism of the antidepressive effect of taVNS is due to an enhanced tidal release of pineal and extrapineal melatonin.

Materials and Methods

Animal model

Male ZDF (n = 29) and ZL littermates (n = 18) were purchased from Vital River Laboratories International Inc. (Beijing, China). The animal room was maintained at 22±1°C artificially lighted from 7:00a.m. to 7:00p.m with light intensity similar to daylight. Littermates from the same or foster mother were housed in one large cage with water and normal food pellets available ad libitum except during taVNS session. The rats entered the experimental procedure at 8 weeks of age and separated into ZDF and ZL groups. At the start of the study the initial body weight was 300±30 grams for ZDF and 200±20 for ZL rats. The rats were raised in groups of three to four. The cages and beddings were changed every other day. The person in charge of the animal's welfare was also the same person who carried out the experiments. We used only male ZDF rats for the study to avoid a possible confounding effect from gender differences on the endogenous melatonin level and other possible hormone variation. The experimental protocol was approved by Institutional Animal Care and Use Committee in China Academy of Chinese Medical Sciences.

Administration of taVNS

All the time points recorded in this study are in accordance with the taVNS occurrences, i.e. the beginning of taVNS is day 1. Under 2% isoflurane inhalation anesthesia, two opposite magnetic electrodes (+/−) were placed over the right side auricular concha region, two opposite magnetic electrodes (+/−) were placed over the right side auricular concha region, inside and outside respectively so that electronic current can conduct through the tissue, including the vagus nerve fibers. Saline was applied between an electrode and the skin to improve electronic conduction. A 30 min taVNS procedure at a frequency of 2/15 Hz (2 and 15 Hz, switched every second) and an intensity of 2 mA was administered once daily via an electrical stimulator (HANS-100, Nanjing, China). The parameters had been proven effective previously [16]. The procedures were given in the afternoon between 2–5pm for 34 consecutive days. On day 1, 3, and 5, the taVNS was given after last blood sample collection. Auricular margin were used as sham acupoint (ZDF-Sham, n = 4).

Pinealectomy

To find out the role of pineal gland in depressive behavior and to explore whether there is another melatonin source, the effect of taVNS were also examined in pinealectomized (Px) rats. Pineal gland was removed from rats by referring to a reported method [17]. Briefly, 10 male ZDF rats were weighted and anesthetized intraperitoneally with 50 mg/kg sodium pentobarbital. The animal was fastened to a stereotaxic apparatus; an incision along the skull middle line was made to expose the lambda. The skull at the lambda was opened with a dental drill with a circle bit (0.5 cm Outside Diameter) so that the superior sagittal sinus was directly under view. The superior sagittal sinus was ligated with 5-0 silk suture at the rostral side for two ligations, cut between, and carefully pulled back. The pineal gland, located under the venous sinus, was removed in a single piece using tweezers and the bone fragment was returned to its place, the surgical layers were

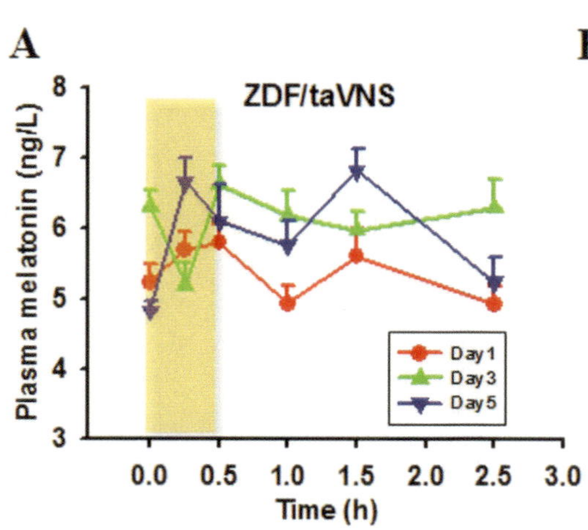

Figure 2. Acute plasma melatonin concentration change upon taVNS. Showing that each taVNS administration (shielded area) would trigger acute and tidal melatonin secretion in pineal intact (A) and pinealectomized ZDF rats (B). Note that the melatonin secretion tides existing both during and after tsVNS session and that the after-taVNS tides tended to be higher (A and B) or more frequent (B) with the increase of treatment days.

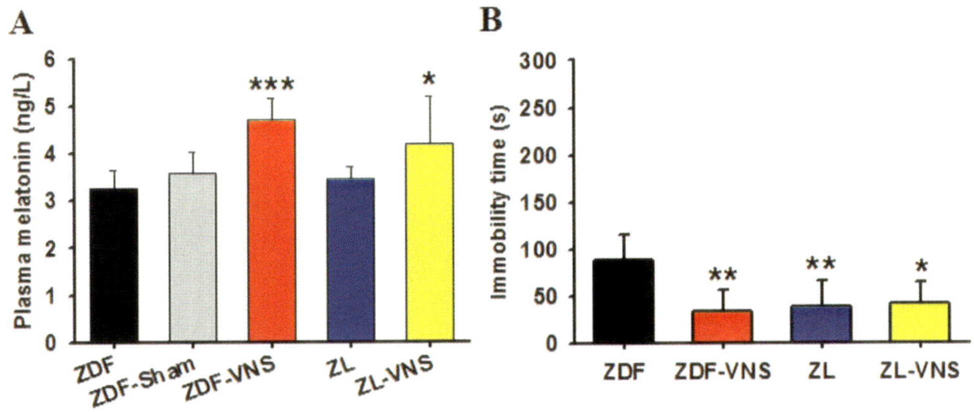

Figure 3. Plasma melatonin concentration and the immobility time in FST on day 35. The total production of melatonin in taVNS treated rats may be higher since the melatonin concentrations were still higher upon sacrifice on day 35, about 22 hours after the last taVNS session on day 34. This may represent the long term effect of taVNS on melatonin secretion (A). In the forced swimming session, a longer immobility time exists in naïve ZDF rats, in contrast to that in taVNS treated ZDF rats or naïve ZL rats (B). *, **, *** *P*<0.05, 0.01, 0.001 *vs.* ZDF, respectively.

sutured. Three of the eleven rats exhibiting postoperative poor grooming were euthanazied by intraperitoneal injection of sodium pentobarbital (200 mg/kg) and excluded from further experiments.

Forced swimming test

FST was performed only once on day 35 between 1 PM and 5 PM. The FST procedure was modified from a previously described method but omitted the pretest session [4,5], which we found to be a confounding factor to the final results such that the pre-tested rats tended to stay still in formal test and the immobility time was extremely prolonged and obscuring the difference between animal groups. Briefly, a rat was placed in a clear plastic tank (45×35×60 cm) containing 30 cm of water (24±0.5°C) for 5 min. The total duration of non-swimming within the 5-min session was recorded with a stopwatch as immobility scores (in seconds). A rat was judged to be non-swimming when no attempt was made to escape from the tank and the rat was hunched forward (a floating position). Following FST session, a rat was removed from the water tank, dried with paper towel and returned to the home cage. All sessions were observed by the same experimenter blinded to the group assignment to minimize between-experimenter and between-session variations.

Collection of plasma and ELISA

To determine the acute effect of taVNS on melatonin secretion, plasma samples were collected on days 1, 3, and 5, and at 6 points each day, including immediately before, 15 min during, 0, 30, 60 and 120 min after a taVNS procedure. In order to analyze the chronic trend of melatonin concentration, plasma was collected on day 35, around 22 hours after the last taVNS session.

Under 2% isoflurane anesthesia, 100 μl of blood was collected from tail vein of each rat, each time. The blood sample was centrifuged for 10 min at 110 g, and 60 μl plasma was collected. All plasma samples were stored in −80°C until use. The concentration of melatonin in plasma was analyzed by using enzyme linked immunosorbent assay (ELISA) kit (R&D system Inc. Beijing, China). The plasma melatonin concentration was calculated based on the standard curve and presented in nanograms per liter (ng/L).

Time points for all the above experiments were collectively shown in Figure 1.

Statistical analysis

By running GraphPad InStat version 3 for Windows, raw data from FST and ELISA were compared using One-way ANOVA to detect differences among treatment groups, followed

Table 1. Plasma melatonin concentration in rats on day 35.

Rat groups	Naïve ZDF	ZDF-taVNS	Naïve ZL	ZL-taVNS
Mean	3.273	4.712	3.458	4.2
Standard deviation (SD)	0.385	0.459	0.271	0.999
Sample size (N)	6	8	8	6
Std. error of mean(SEM)	0.157	0.162	0.096	0.408
Lower 95% conf. limit	2.869	4.328	3.231	3.151
Upper 95% conf. limit	3.678	5.095	3.685	5.249
P value vs. Naïve ZDF (Tukey-Kramer)		<0.001	=0.930	=0.043
DF	3			
Residual	24			
F	10.050			

Table 2. Immobility time in rats on day 35.

Rat group	Naïve ZDF	ZDF-taVNS	Naïve ZL	ZL-taVNS
Mean	87.833	33.625	39.25	41.333
Standard deviation (SD)	28.032	22.753	27.639	22.651
Sample size (N)	6	8	8	6
Std. error of mean(SEM)	11.444	8.044	9.772	9.247
Lower 95% conf. limit	58.411	14.600	16.139	17.559
Upper 95% conf. limit	117.26	52.650	62.361	65.108
P value vs. Naïve ZDF, (Tukey-Kramer)		=0.003	=0.008	=0.020
DF	3			
Residual	24			
F	6.231			

by Tukey-Kramer Multiple Comparisons Test to determine sources of differences. Data were presented as means ±standard deviation. Differences were considered to be statistically significant at the level of $\alpha = 0.05$. The correlation between melatonin concentration and immobility time was acquired by linear regression.

Results

Tidal melatonin secretion upon taVNS treatment

The acute effect of taVNS on melatonin level is shown in figure 2. As detected by ELISA on day 1,3, and 5 and from the 6 time points around taVNS procedure, the melatonin concentration changes in a parabolic manner during the taVNS session in ZDF rats. Even after the ending of the taVNS procedure, more parabolic melatonin tides occurs (Fig. 2). As compared between the during- and after-taVNS tides, taVNS session may trigger an acute melatonin increase. The taVNS triggered acute and tidal melatonin secretion exists in pineal intact (Fig. 2A) and pinealectomized ZDF rats (Fig. 2B), indicating that taVNS triggers melatonin secretion from extrapineal sources.

As compared between days, the melatonin tides on day 1 return to pre-stimulation level quickly. The tides tend to be higher or more frequent as each experimental day is completed (Fig. 2A,B).

Effects of long term taVNS on melatonin secretion and depression-like behavior in ZDF rats

As judged upon sacrifice on day 35, about 22 hours after the last taVNS administration, the melatonin concentration in taVNS treated rats is significantly higher (Fig. 3A, Table 1, One-way ANOVA $P = 0.0002$). Considering the short half-life of melatonin [8], these concentrations represent the long-term effect of taVNS on melatonin level.

As determined by the FST on day 35, the naïve ZDF rats performed poorly in the tank with an immobility time of 87.83 ± 28.03 (mean ± SD, $n = 6$). This immobility time is much longer than that of ZL rats and of taVNS treated ZDF rats (Fig. 3B, Table 2, One-way ANOVA $P = 0.0028$).

The antidepressive effect of taVNS was evaluated in both ZDF and ZL rats. While it is antidepressive in ZDF rats, the taVNS shows no antidepressive effect in ZL rats, possibly due to a relatively shorter immobility time in these rats (Fig. 3, Table 2, $P > 0.05$).

The correlation between the immobility time and melatonin level on day 35 is shown in Figure 4. The Fig. 4 clearly shows that lower melatonin level is related to the poor FST performance in ZDF rats. As analyzed in linear regression, a strong negative correlation is reached in ZDF ($R = -0.544$), in contrast to ZL rats ($R = 0.247$) in which no overt correlation was shown (Fig. 4, Table 3).

Discussion

ZDF (*fa/fa*) rats are widely used for diabetes and obesity research. Here we recommend ZDF rats as good candidates for depression studies based on our results that the ZDF rats have innate depression behavior as detected by FST.

ZDF rats develop type 2 diabetes, in which hyperinsulinemia is usually involved. There are studies suggesting that insulin increases sympathetic nerve activity in obese and diabetic rats by increasing glutamatergic drive to rostral ventrolateral medulla [18,19]. Moreover, the glutamatergic system has been implicated in the pathophysiology of depression and in the action mechanism of antidepressants [20]. Furthermore, melatonin and dextromethorphan, an N-methyl-D-aspartic acid (NMDA) receptor antagonist, have synergism in another depression rodent model, the Wistar-Kyoto rats [21]. Taken together, these results suggest that a

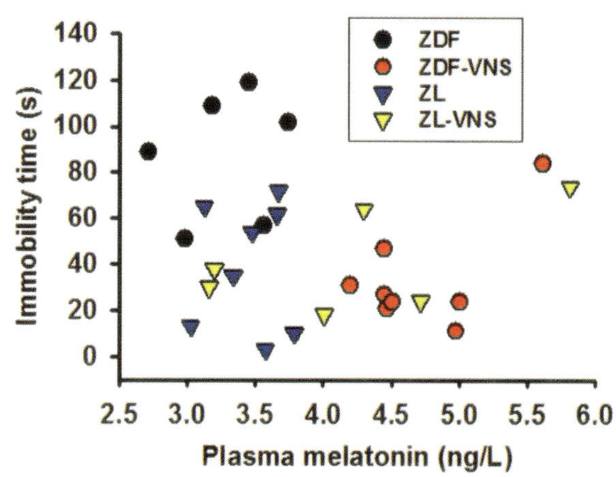

Figure 4. Correlation of melatonin concentration and immobility time in FST on day 35. Linear regression analysis found a strong negative correlation between the plasma melatonin concentration and the immobility time in forced swimming test in ZDF ($R = -0.544$) but not ZL rats ($R = 0.254$, also see Table 3).

Table 3. Correlations between plasma melatonin concentration and immobility time in FST.

Rat group	ZDF	ZL
Expected melatonin level from immobility time	$y = 4.832 - 0.0130x$ $R = -0.544$	$y = 3.465 + 0.00752x$ $R = 0.245$
Expected immobility time from melatonin level	$y = 152.57 - 22.766x$ $R = -0.544$	$y = 9.481 + 7.958x$ $R = 0.245$

defected interaction between NMDA receptor and melatoninergic system in the brain may play a role in depression. As for the ZDF rats, the depression condition may be worse because they are genetically deficient in leptin receptor and are resistant to leptin, which is an adipocyte-derived hormone with antidepressant-like properties [22].

Under physiological conditions, the main source of melatonin is pineal gland [23]. The pineal gland is innervated by both noradrenergic sympathetic and cholinergic parasympathetic fibers [24–26]. While light exposure would activate sympathetic system and reduce pineal melatonin production [25], other environmental factors that modulate the autonomic nervous system or cause epinephrine secretion from adrenal medulla (e.g., distress, insulin-induced hypoglycemia) can override the inhibitory effects of light and accelerate melatonin synthesis [24]. There is also direct evidence that acupuncture elevates melatonin level in pineal gland and subsequently in serum in an animal model of seizures [27].

The taVNS shows antidepressive efficacy even in pinealectomized rats, implying that acupuncture works through the modulation of extrapineal melatonin secretion. Beside the pineal gland, melatonin is also secreted from retina, digestive tract, born marrow, skin, kidneys, ovaries, testis, circulating leukocytes, and many other sources [28]. It should be noted that, these extrapineal melatonin sources not only have a huge total volume, some of them are also rich in melatonin, for example, the melatonin pool of gastrointestinal tract [29] and bone marrow [30]. The concentration of melatonin in both pools surpasses blood melatonin levels by 2 to 3 orders of magnitude and the gastrointestinal tract alone contains over 400× more melatonin than in the pineal gland [29]. A critical factor beneficial for the acupuncture to functionally release melatonin from these extra-pineal sources is that they are innervated by vegetative nervous system and the release of melatonin therefrom is out of the photoperiodical regulation [29,30].

Interestingly, taVNS had differential antidepressive function if compared between ZDF and ZL rats. While taVNS worked well in ZDF rats it had limited efficiency in ZL rats, a similar phenomenon to melatonin treated experimental animals [31]. This may be due to a reduced parasympathetic activity that impedes melatonin secretion in ZDF but not ZL rats.

It should be pointed out that, all the results to date about the vagal nerve stimulation and its triggering and enhancing function to melatonin secretion were reached from preclinical studies in which animals were anesthetized. Thus it is still not clear whether melatonin secretion can be enhanced in a conscious state. Further studies are needed to elucidate the vagal nerve stimulation and melatonin secretion in alert states.

Taken together, the taVNS will trigger a tidal release of melatonin and enhance its production, which in turn will be antidepressive by inhibiting the NMDA induced current and down-regulate the expression of NMDA receptors [4,32,33]. Since taVNS induced tidal melatonin release may be maintained for several hour period, it may be used clinically in melatonin deficient patients, such as patients with insomnia and depression.

Conclusion

Our results support conclusions that ZDF rats are a good depression rodent model and that taVNS is antidepressive by triggering tidal secretion of melatonin and simultaneously increase its production.

Acknowledgments

Many thanks to Dr. J. Mao (Massachusetts General Hospital, Harvard Medical School) for generous assistance and consultant. We also thank Dr. B. Zhu (Institute of Acupuncture and Moxibustion, China Academy of Chinese Medical Sciences), Drs. Z.K. Guo, W.C. Yang, and X.H. Cai (Xinxiang Medical Univ.) and members of their laboratories for generous assistance.

Author Contributions

Conceived and designed the experiments: SW. Performed the experiments: SL XZ JZ HB XW. Analyzed the data: SW. Contributed reagents/materials/analysis tools: SW. Wrote the paper: SW PR MFM.

References

1. Rong P, Fang J, Kong J, Wang L, Meng H, et al (2012) Trancutanous vagus nerve stimulation for the treatment of depression: a study protocol for a double blinded randomized clinical trails. BMC Complement Altern Med12: 255.
2. Liu RP, Fang JL, Rong P, Zhao Y, Meng H, et al (2013) Effects of electroacupuncture at auricular concha region on the depressive status of unpredictable chronic mild stress rat models. Evid Based Complement Alternat Med 2013: 789674.
3. Dubocovich ML, Delagrange P, Krause DN, Sugden D, Cardinali DP, et al (2010) International Union of Basic and Clinical Pharmacology. LXXV. Nomenclature, classification, and pharmacology of G protein-coupled melatonin receptors. Pharmacol Rev 62: 343–380
4. Wang S, Tian Y, Song L, Lim G, Tan Y, et al (2012) Exacerbated mechanical hyperalgesia in rats with genetically predisposed depressive behavior: Role of melatonin and NMDA receptors. Pain 153: 2448–2457.
5. Zeng Q, Wang S, Lim G, Yang L, Mao J, et al (2008) Exacerbated mechanical allodynia in rats with depression-like behavior. Brain Res 1200: 27–38.
6. Maurizi CP (1984) Disorder of the pineal gland associated with depression, peptic ulcers, and sexual dysfunction. South Med J 77: 1516–1518.
7. Cardinali DP, Srinivasan V, Brzezinski A, Brown GM (2012) Melatonin and its analogs in insomnia and depression. J Pineal Res 52: 365–375.
8. Nelson E, Panksepp J, Ikemoto S (1994) The effects of melatonin on isolation distress in chickens. Pharmacol Biochem Behav 49: 327–333.
9. Lee JH, Choi TY, Lee MS, Lee H, Shin BC, et al (2013) Acupuncture for acute low back pain: a systematic review. Clin J Pain 29: 172–185.
10. Lyons Z, van der Watt G, Shen Z, Janca A (2012) Acupuncture and Chinese herbs as treatments for depression: an Australian pilot study. Complement Ther Clin Pract 18: 216–220.
11. Mischoulon D, Brill CD, Ameral VE, Fava M, Yeung AS (2012) A pilot study of acupuncture monotherapy in patients with major depressive disorder. J Affect Disord 141: 469–473.
12. Yeung AS, Ameral VE, Chuzi SE, Fava M, Mischoulon D (2011) A pilot study of acupuncture augmentation therapy in antidepressant partial and non-responders with major depressive disorder. J Affect Disord 130: 285–289.
13. Zhang ZJ, Chen HY, Yip KC, Ng R, Wong VT (2010) The effectiveness and safety of acupuncture therapy in depressive disorders: systematic review and meta-analysis. J Affect Disord 124: 9–21.

14. La Marca R, Nedeljkovic M, Yuan L, Maercker A, Elhert U (2010) Effects of auricular electrical stimulation on vagal activity in healthy men: evidence from a three-armed randomized trial. Clin Sci (Lond) 118: 537–546.
15. Preiss K, Brennan L, Clarke D (2013) A systematic review of variables associated with the relationship between obesity and depression. Obes Rev 14: 906–918.
16. Huang F, Dong J, Kong J, Wang H, Meng H (2014) Effect of transcutaneous auricular vagus nerve stimulation on impaired glucose tolerance: a pilot randomized study. BMC Complement Altern Med 14: 203.
17. Maganhin CC, Simões RS, Fuchs LF, Oliveira-Filho RM, Simões Mde J, et al (2009) Rat pinealectomy: a modified direct visual approach. Acta Cir Bras 24: 321–324.
18. Bardgett ME, McCarthy JJ, Stocker SD (2010) Glutamatergic receptor activation in the rostral ventrolateral medulla mediates the sympathoexcitatory response to hyperinsulinemia. Hypertension 55: 284–290.
19. Ward KR, Bardgett JF, Wolfgang L, Stocker SD (2011) Sympathetic response to insulin is mediated by melanocortin 3/4 receptors in the hypothalamic paraventricular nucleus. Hypertension 57: 435–441.
20. Mathews DC, Henter ID, Zarate CA (2012) Targeting the glutamatergic system to treat major depressive disorder: rationale and progress to date. Drugs 72: 1313–1333.
21. Wang S, Zhang L, Lim G, Sung B, Tian Y, et al (2009) A combined effect of dextromethorphan and melatonin on neuropathic pain behavior in rats. Brain Res 1288: 42–49.
22. Guo M, Lu Y, Garza JC, Li Y, Chua SC, et al (2012) Forebrain glutamatergic neurons mediate leptin action on depression-like behaviors and synaptic depression. Transl Psychiatry 2: e83.
23. Brzezinski A (1997) Melatonin in humans. N Engl J Med 336: 186–195.
24. Spence DW, Kayumov L, Chen A, Lowe A, Jain U, et al (2004) Acupuncture increases nocturnal melatonin secretion and reduces insomnia and anxiety: a preliminary report. J Neuropsychiatry Clin Neurosci 16: 19–28.
25. Samuels N (2005) Integration of hypnosis with acupuncture: possible benefits and case examples. Am J Clin Hypn 47: 243–248.
26. DeBenedittis G, Cigada M, Bianchi A, Signorini MG, Cerutti S (1994) Autonomic changes during hypnosis: a heart rate variability power spectrum analysis as a marker of sympatho-vagal balance. Int J Clin Exp Hypn 42: 140–152.
27. Chao DM, Chen G, Cheng JS (2001) Melatonin might be one possible medium of electroacupuncture anti-seizures. Acupunct Electrother Res 26: 39–48.
28. Esposito E, Cuzzocrea S (2010) Antiinflammatory activity of melatonin in central nervous system. Curr Neuropharmacol 8: 228–242.
29. Bubenik GA (2002) Gastrointestinal melatonin: localization, function, and clinical relevance. Dig Dis Sci 47: 2336–2348.
30. Conti A, Conconi S, Hertens E, Skwarlo-Sonta K, Markowska M, et al (2000) Evidence for melatonin synthesis in mouse and human bone marrow cells. J Pineal Res 28: 193–202.
31. Paul P, Lahaye C, Delagrange P, Nicolas JP, Canet E, et al (1999) Characterization of 2-[125I]iodomelatonin binding sites in Syrian hamster peripheral organs. J Pharmacol Exp Ther 290: 334–340.
32. Kaster MP, Machado DG, Santos AR, Rodrigues AL (2012) Involvement of NMDA receptors in the antidepressant-like action of adenosine. Pharmacol Rep 64: 706–713.
33. Ghasemi M, Raza M, Dehpour AR (2010) NMDA receptor antagonists augment antidepressant-like effects of lithium in the mouse forced swimming test. J Psychopharmacol 24: 585–594.

Cost-Effectiveness of Collaborative Care for Depression in UK Primary Care: Economic Evaluation of a Randomised Controlled Trial (CADET)

Colin Green[1*], David A. Richards[1], Jacqueline J. Hill[2], Linda Gask[3], Karina Lovell[4], Carolyn Chew-Graham[5], Peter Bower[3], John Cape[6], Stephen Pilling[6], Ricardo Araya[7], David Kessler[7], J. Martin Bland[8], Simon Gilbody[9], Glyn Lewis[10], Chris Manning[11], Adwoa Hughes-Morley[3], Michael Barkham[12]

1 University of Exeter Medical School, University of Exeter, Exeter, United Kingdom, **2** Mood Disorders Centre, University of Exeter, Exeter, United Kingdom, **3** Centre for Primary Care at the Institute of Population Health, University of Manchester, Manchester, United Kingdom, **4** School of Nursing, Midwifery, and Social Work, University of Manchester, Manchester, United Kingdom, **5** Primary Care and Health Sciences, Keele University, Keele, United Kingdom, **6** Research Department of Clinical, Educational, and Health Psychology, University College London, London, United Kingdom, **7** School of Social and Community Medicine, University of Bristol, Bristol, United Kingdom, **8** Department of Health Sciences, University of York, York, United Kingdom, **9** Department of Health Sciences at Hull York Medical School, University of York, York, United Kingdom, **10** Mental Health Sciences Unit, University College London, London, United Kingdom, **11** Upstream Healthcare, Teddington, United Kingdom, **12** Department of Psychology, University of Sheffield, Sheffield, United Kingdom

Abstract

Background: Collaborative care is an effective treatment for the management of depression but evidence on its cost-effectiveness in the UK is lacking.

Aims: To assess the cost-effectiveness of collaborative care in a UK primary care setting.

Methods: An economic evaluation alongside a multi-centre cluster randomised controlled trial comparing collaborative care with usual primary care for adults with depression (n = 581). Costs, quality-adjusted life-years (QALYs), and incremental cost-effectiveness ratios (ICER) were calculated over a 12-month follow-up, from the perspective of the UK National Health Service and Personal Social Services (i.e. Third Party Payer). Sensitivity analyses are reported, and uncertainty is presented using the cost-effectiveness acceptability curve (CEAC) and the cost-effectiveness plane.

Results: The collaborative care intervention had a mean cost of £272.50 per participant. Health and social care service use, excluding collaborative care, indicated a similar profile of resource use between collaborative care and usual care participants. Collaborative care offered a mean incremental gain of 0.02 (95% CI: –0.02, 0.06) quality-adjusted life-years over 12 months, at a mean incremental cost of £270.72 (95% CI: –202.98, 886.04), and resulted in an estimated mean cost per QALY of £14,248. Where costs associated with informal care are considered in sensitivity analyses collaborative care is expected to be less costly and more effective, thereby dominating treatment as usual.

Conclusion: Collaborative care offers health gains at a relatively low cost, and is cost-effective compared with usual care against a decision-maker willingness to pay threshold of £20,000 per QALY gained. Results here support the commissioning of collaborative care in a UK primary care setting.

Editor: Andrea Icks, Heinrich-Heine University, Faculty of Medicine, Germany

Funding: This report is independent research funded by the UK Medical Research Council (MRC; reference G0701013, www.mrc.ac.uk), managed by the National Institute for Health Research (NIHR, www.nihr.ac.uk), on behalf of the MRC-NIHR partnership. Research was supported by NIHR Collaboration for Leadership in Applied Health Research and Care South West Peninsula at the Royal Devon and Exeter NHS Foundation Trust. The views expressed are those of the author(s) and not necessarily those of the NHS, the NIHR, or the Department of Health. The funders had no role in study design, data collection and analysis, decision to publish, or preparation of the manuscript.

Competing Interests: The authors have declared that no competing interests exist.

* Email: c.green@exeter.ac.uk

Introduction

Depression is a long term and disabling condition with well documented negative impacts on health status and on health care resources [1,2]. In most cases the responsibility for treatment of people with depression falls on primary care [3], but the organisation of care in this setting can face many challenges. These include barriers between generalist and specialist mental health professionals, poor patient adherence to pharmacological treatment [4], and a shortage of specialists to provide psychological therapies [5]. Against this backdrop there is a growing role for organisational interventions to support the management of depression, and collaborative care has been shown to be an effective intervention that supports the organisation of health care for depression [6]. Collaborative care is a complex intervention, developed in the United States, incorporating a multi-professional approach to patient care; a structured management plan; scheduled patient follow-ups; and enhanced inter-professional communication [7]. In practice this is achieved by the introduction of a care manager into primary care, responsible for delivering care to patients with depression under supervision from a specialist, and for liaising between primary care clinicians and mental health specialists. Systematic reviews, of studies mostly conducted in the United States, demonstrate that collaborative care improves depression outcomes [6,8], and a recent randomised control trial, the CADET Trial of collaborative care for depression in UK primary care, has shown it to be effective in the UK healthcare system [9]. Evidence indicates that collaborative care is cost-effective in the setting of the United States healthcare system [10,11], however, evidence on the cost effectiveness of collaborative care for depression in the UK has been lacking until now [10,11]. We report here the results of an economic evaluation of collaborative care versus usual care carried out in the UK alongside the CADET trial.

Methods

Study/Trial design

The aim of the CADET trial was to determine the effectiveness and cost-effectiveness of collaborative care when added to usual care compared to usual care alone in the management of patients with moderate to severe depression in UK primary care. The design of this multi-centre, two group cluster randomised controlled trial, and methods for the economic evaluation, are described in detail in the published protocol [12]. In brief, we recruited participants from electronic case records of general practices in three UK sites: Bristol, London and Greater Manchester. Recruitment included patients newly identified as depressed, with or without one or more previous depressive episodes, and those with an existing diagnosis of depression which was not responding to primary care management. Eligible participants were people aged 18+ who met ICD-10 criteria for a depressive episode on the revised Clinical Interview Schedule (CIS-R) [13]. Ethical approval for the trial on which this economic evaluation is based was given by the UK NHS Health Research Authority, NRES Committee South West (NRES/07/H1208/60). All participants gave written informed consent before taking part in the study. No minors/children were enrolled in the study. Written consent forms were co-signed by participant and the person taking consent, and were securely stored in both original form and electronically. The ethics approval included approval of both the procedure and the forms and documentation used for consent. We excluded those at high risk of suicide, psychosis, bi-polar disorder, those whose depression was associated with bereavement, people whose primary presenting problem was alcohol or drug abuse, and those receiving psychological treatment for their depression via mental health services. We randomly allocated practices into collaborative care or usual care, using a minimisation approach, to minimise imbalance between treatment groups, using site (Bristol, London. Manchester), Index of Multiple Deprivation (IMD) rank [14], number of GPs, and practice size.

Interventions

Participants allocated to the control condition, treatment as usual (TAU), received care from their general practitioner according to usual clinical practice for these patients, including treatment by antidepressants and referral for other treatments, including UK Improving Access to Psychological Therapies (IAPT) services.

The collaborative care intervention consisted of usual care from the GP, and additionally care managers were expected to provide between 6–12 contacts with participants over a period of 14 weeks: with these expected to comprise 30–40 minutes for one initial face to face appointment followed by 15–20 minute telephone contacts thereafter. Contacts included: education about depression; medication management; behavioural activation [15]; and relapse prevention instructions [16]. Care managers provided GPs with advice on medication and regular updates on patient progress including medication adherence.

Care managers had existing UK mental health qualifications (psychological wellbeing practitioners, counsellors or nurses) and were then trained specifically to deliver the intervention within the collaborative care framework. They received weekly supervision from a specialist mental health professional, a clinical psychologist, psychiatrist, an academic GP with special interest in mental health or a senior nurse psychotherapist. Individual patients were discussed in supervision at least monthly, facilitated through a bespoke computerised patient management system (PC-MIS-http://www.pc-mis.co.uk).

Outcome measures

Clinical effectiveness was assessed using depression severity as the primary outcome, measured by the Patient Health Questionnaire-9 (PHQ-9) [17]. The PHQ-9 is a nine-item questionnaire, which records the core symptoms of depression, with scores ranging from 0 to 27 where higher scores indicate a greater severity of depression. Secondary outcomes were quality of life using the SF-36 [18], worry and anxiety using the GAD-7 [19], patient satisfaction using the CSQ8 [20], health care service use using a patient questionnaire, and health state values (health-related quality-of-life) using the EQ-5D 3L [21,22]. All measures were collected at baseline, four months and 12 months post randomisation (except patient satisfaction, measured at four months only).

Cost-effectiveness analyses

In our economic evaluation we adopted the perspective of the UK NHS and Personal Social Services (Third Party Payer perspective), with a broader participant and carer perspective considered in sensitivity analyses. Our primary economic endpoint was the cost per quality-adjusted life-year at 12-month follow-up. To assess cost-effectiveness we estimated the additional cost for delivery of the collaborative care intervention, the costs associated with health and social care service use, and estimated quality-adjusted life-years (QALYs). QALYs are a commonly used summary measure of health-related quality-of-life, taking account of both quality and quantity of life, and are increasingly used to compare the cost-effectiveness of interventions across a broad range of health and related contexts [23]. We estimated QALYs over the 12-month trial follow-up, using the EQ-5D trial data, applying UK tariffs obtained from a UK general population survey to value the EQ-5D health states [24]. In addition, to inform sensitivity analyses, we used trial data from the SF-36 to estimate QALYs using the SF-6D, which presents tariffs obtained from a UK general population survey to value health states [25]. We derived QALY estimates using data from baseline, 4-month

Table 1. Unit costs for different types of health and social care resource items.

Resource item	Unit costs*	Source of cost data	Basis of estimate
GP (at surgery/practice)	£36.00	PSSRU 2011	GP appt/surgery; based on costing at 11.7 mins
GP (at home)	£121.00	PSSRU 2011	
Practice Nurse (surgery)	£15.00	PSSRU 2011	15.5 min/hourly patient-related cost
Practice Nurse (home)	£30.00	PSSRU 2011	25 min/hourly home visiting cost
Walk-in-centre (appt)	£41.00	PSSRU 2011	Walk-in-service (not admitted)
Counsellor	£60.00	PSSRU 2011	Per consultation
Mental health worker	£76.00	PSSRU 2011	MH Nurse, £76 per 1 hour contact (assumed 1 hr)
Social Worker/Care Manager	£212.00	PSSRU 2011	Per 1 hour contact (assumed 1 hr)
Home help/Care Worker	£18.00	PSSRU 2011	Per weekday hour
Occupational Therapist	£82.00	PSSRU 2011	Community based OT, per 1 hour of client contact (assumed 1 hr)
Voluntary Group (e.g. MIND/CRUISE)	£21.73	PSSRU 2010	Cost per user session, voluntary/non-profit organisation (£21 session/2010).
Acute psychiatric ward (bed day)	£312.00	PSSRU 2011	Cost per bed day
Long-stay ward (bed day)	£222.52	PSSRU 2010	Cost per bed day (£215/2010)
Gen Med ward (bed day)	£321.00	PSSRU 2011	weighted ave. All adult mental health inpatient days
A & E (contact)	£106.00	PSSRU 2011	Contact, not admitted
Day hospital (Attend/day)	£126.00	PSSRU 2011	Cost per day, weighted ave of all adult attendances
Psychiatrist (outpatient contact)	£161.38	NHS Ref Costs**	2008–09 per consult (code MHOPFUA2, £155)
Psychologist (outpatient contact)	£135.00	PSSRU 2011	Cost per contact hour (assumed 1 hr)
Psychiatric Nurse/Care Coordinator (outpatient contact)	£76.00	PSSRU 2011	MH Nurse, £76 per 1 hour contact (assumed 1 hr)
Other Outpatient contact	£143.00	PSSRU 2011	Outpatient consultant services, weighted average
Day care centre (comm. serv/social care)	£34.00	PSSRU 2011	Cost per user session
Drop in Club (comm. serv/social care)	£34.00	PSSRU 2011	Assume cost as day centre, cost per user session
Help from friends/relatives (hrs)	£18.00	PSSRU 2011	Use cost per hour, based on unit cost for home help/care worker (as above).
Lost work (day) (friends/relatives)	£99.6	ONS 2011	Based on median gross weekly earnings in 2011 for f/t employees at £498.
Travel cost per mile (patient own car)	£0.44		Assumed reclaim/expense rate (running cost per mile)

*Unit costs at 2011 prices/costs.
**Costs uprated/adjusted to 2011 prices using HCHS index reported in PSSRU Unit Costs of Health Care [27].
PSSRU Unit Costs of Health Care 2011 [27].
NHS Ref Costs 2008–09 - http://www.ons.gov.uk/ons/dcp171778_256900.pdf (Accessed 18/05/12).

and 12-month assessments, applying the area-under-the-curve approach, a recognised approach for assessing repeated measures data [26], as recommended by Brazier and colleagues [23].

We collected resource use associated with delivery of the collaborative care intervention within the trial, comprising care manager contact time, and supervision of care managers by specialists. We collected other health and social care resource use by participants over the 12-month follow-up and data on informal care from friends/relatives and patient costs using self-report, interviewer administered, questionnaires (at 4 and 12-months; covering the prior 4-month and prior 8-month time periods respectively). We collected this same data at the baseline assessment, with participants reporting resource use over the 6-month period prior to baseline assessment.

We combined data on resource use with published unit costs to estimate mean cost per participant by using healthcare resource values from unit costs in nationally available data sources, adjusted for inflation where necessary, in British pounds sterling (£) at 2011 costs, see Table 1. In estimates of the intervention cost for collaborative care, we based care manager costs on costs for UK NHS Agenda for Change (AfC) band 5 staff costs, using a unit cost of £65 per hour for patient contact time [27], equivalent to Mental Health Nurse. This unit cost includes all staff cost components, and an allowance of contact time to non-contact time of 1:0.89 (see [27], Table 10.2). We based supervision costs on a unit cost of £135 per hour for Clinical Supervisors, based on full costs for specialist mental health professionals at NHS AfC band 8a ([27], Table 9.5).

Statistical methods

We analysed data on an intention-to-treat basis, in accordance with an analysis plan drawn up prior to the analysis of data [12]. We undertook analyses in STATA, version 12. Our primary economic analyses estimated mean cost and mean QALY by treatment allocation, and estimated differences between groups over 12-months, adjusting for baseline measures, and using pre-specified covariates for age (individual level), and at the cluster level covariates for deprivation (IMD), site, and practice size. We used a multi-level regression model (STATA, xtmixed) for the primary analyses, to consider the hierarchical (clustered) nature of the data, presenting the intraclass correlation coefficient (ICC) for the main analyses. We undertook data analyses using generalised linear models (GLM), with appropriate family and link components, to account for the potentially non-normally distributed nature of cost data. GLM model results were not different to those using the multi-level model applied in the main analyses.

Table 2. Mean health and social care resource use (quantities) over 12 month follow-up.

Resource item	Usual Care		Collaborative Care	
	n=305		n=276	
	n	Mean (SD) [range]	n	Mean (SD) [range]
Primary/Community Care:				
GP (surgery/practice)	244	**8.21** (6.69) [0–56]	217	**7.77** (6.78) [0–45]
GP (at home)	247	**0.12** (0.80) [0–11]	218	**0.05** (0.27) [0–3]
Nurse (surgery/practice)	247	**1.77** (3.08) [0–24]	215	**1.68** (3.10) [0–32]
Nurse (at home)	247	**0.06** (0.46) [0–4]	218	**0.05** (0.45) [0–6]
Walk-in-centre (attendance)	247	**0.32** (0.87) [0–8]	217	**0.31** (0.86) [0–5]
Counsellor	246	**3.58** (11.26) [0–116]	212	**2.67** (7.21) [0–48]
Mental Health worker	247	**0.58** (3.51) [0–50]	215	**0.79** (3.72) [0–36]
Social worker	247	**0.34** (1.79) [0–14]	218	**0.58** (3.94) [0–33]
Home help/Care Worker	247	**4.35** (47.27) [0–722]	218	**1.24** (15.07) [0–220]
Occupational Therapist	247	**0.22** (0.98) [0–9]	218	**0.13** (0.61) [0–5]
Voluntary Group	247	**0.94** (5.80) [0–64]	218	**0.22** (1.39) [0–16]
Secondary Care:				
Hospital admissions, n+	247	34	218	28
Acute Psychiatric ward (days)	247	-	218	**0.46** (6.77) [0–100][1]
Psychiatric rehab ward	247	-	218	-
Long stay ward	247	**0.06** (0.94) [0–15]	218	-
Psychiatric ICU ward	247	-	218	-
General Medical ward (days)	247	**0.48** (2.02) [0–21]	217	**0.42** (1.67) [0–12]
Other hospital ward/stay	247	**0.28** (1.58) [0–17]	218	**0.39** (2.12) [0–24]
A & E (attendance)	247	**0.40** (0.93) [0–7]	218	**0.34** (0.76) [0–5]
Day hospital (attendance)	247	**0.60** (2.22) [0–24]	218	**0.36** (1.19) [0–12]
Outpatient appointment	247	**2.62** (5.60) [0–58]	217	**2.63** (5.63) [0–65]
Social care:				
Used day care services (%)+	247	**3%/2%**	218	**4%/3%**
Day care centre	247	**0.28** (4.54) [0–70]	218	**0.07** (1.08) [0–16]
Drop in club	247	**0.56** (5.26) [0–70]	218	**0.12** (1.40) [0–20]
Day care other	247	**0.39** (2.85) [0–28]	217	**0.65** (5.67) [0–74]
Informal care from friends/relatives:				
Had help/care from friends/relatives (%)+		**45%/48%**		**38%/35%**
Hours per week help from friends/relatives#	230	**6.11** (15.44) [0–112]	209	**3.95** (10.11) [0–104]
Report time off work for friends/relatives (%)+		**7%/9%**		**7%/10%**

Table 2. Cont.

Resource item	Usual Care		Collaborative Care	
	n = 305		n = 276	
	n	Mean (SD) [range]	n	Mean (SD) [range]
Days lost work by friends/relatives	246	**4.05** (29.14) [0–360]**	217	**1.65** (11.28) [0–144**]
Patient other costs:				
OTC medications (£)	246	**28.40** (57.90) [0–429]**	215	**40.31** (68.61) [0–507]**
Travel costs (£)	246	**10.98** (30.30) [0–320]	216	**14.33** (37.57) [0–202]
Own care travel (miles)	246	**26.12** (77.68) [0–600]	214	**31.53** (138.95) [0–1862]
Other 'one-off' costs (£)	246	**35.77** (144.35) [0–1569]	218	**51.58** (213.53) [0–1,998]

[1]includes one participant with 100 days in psychiatric ward/admission.
[+]Here this data refers to proportion with hospital stay [resource use] at 4 mths follow-up and at 12 months follow-up (mths 5–12) questionnaire.
[#]this is a weekly number of hours (weighted average of data reported at 4-mth and 12 mth follow-up), and requires×52 weeks for annual estimate of hours.
*****Kruskal-Wallis (non-parametric) test: no statistically significant differences between groups, other than for OTC cost, and cost for days lost work by friends/ relatives, which are statistically significant at $p \leq 0.05$.***

We conducted a number of sensitivity analyses for areas of uncertainty in the cost effectiveness analyses: 1) we considered the effect of missing data, estimated by multiple imputation (STATA MI command, with 25 replicated datasets), using all available data on the target variable together with covariates for individual and cluster variables used in the base case regression analyses [28]; 2) we undertook analyses using a broader analytical perspective, including estimated costs for informal care and participant out-of-pocket expenses; 3) we analysed data for a scenario using the SF-6D [25] as an alternative QALY outcome measure; 4) we considered uncertainty in the intervention costs; 5) we analysed a scenario where one participant, with an extremely high level of self-reported resource use, was excluded, as this potentially offers a more likely and policy-relevant estimate of cost-effectiveness.

We combined estimates of incremental cost and incremental benefit to present incremental cost effectiveness ratios (ICERs), allowing decision-makers to assess value for money using the cost per QALY estimates ($ICER = (Cost_{CC} - Cost_{TAU})/(QALY_{CC} - QALY_{TAU})$). We used the NICE threshold of £20,000 to £30,000 per QALY [29,30], i.e. the expected Payer willingness to pay per unit of additional outcome, to assess the cost-effectiveness of collaborative care, with ICERs below these values regarded as cost-effective. We used the non-parametric bootstrap approach [31], with 10,000 replications, to estimate 95% confidence intervals around estimated cost differences, and for QALY differences, in order to address uncertainty. To present the level of uncertainty on cost-effectiveness estimates we used the cost-effectiveness plane to present combinations of incremental cost and incremental QALY data from bootstrap replicates, and used the cost-effectiveness acceptability curve (CEAC), with the 'net benefit statistic' (net monetary benefit = (incremental QALY×willingness to pay per QALY) − incremental cost)) [32,33], to present the probability that the intervention is cost-effective (i.e. incremental net benefit statistic is >0), against a range of potential cost-effectiveness thresholds.

Results

We recruited a total of 581 participants to the CADET trial, from 49 practice clusters. The majority (55·6%) of participants fulfilled criteria for a moderately severe depressive episode with a further 29·9% meeting criteria for severe depression, 14.3% mild depression, and 72·6% having suffered from depression in the past. At baseline, 82% of participants had been prescribed antidepressant medication by their GP. The mean age was 44·8 years (SD 13·3), and 71·9% were women. A total of 276 participants were allocated to collaborative care and 305 allocated to usual care. Full trial results have been presented elsewhere [9]. In brief, however, we found that collaborative care improved depression immediately after treatment compared to usual care, with effects persisting to 12-month follow-up. After adjustment for baseline depression, the mean depression score was 1.33 PHQ-9 points lower (95% CI 0.35 to 2.31, p = 0.009) in collaborative care than in usual care at 4-months, and 1.36 lower (95% CI 0.07 to 2.64, p = 0.04) at 12 months. This difference equated to a standardised effect size of 0.26 (0.07 to 0.46). Patients receiving collaborative care had better outcomes than usual care in terms of depression recovery (odds ratio 1.67 (95% confidence interval 1.22 to 2.29); number needed to treat = 8.4) and response to treatment (odds ratio 1.77 (95% confidence interval 1.22 to 2.58); number needed to treat = 7.8).

Cost for Collaborative Care

Our estimated mean cost per participant for the delivery of the collaborative care intervention was £272.50. This cost estimate comprises care manager costs at £232, and clinical supervision costs of £40.50. We based care manager costs on data available from electronic participant level records on 235 participants receiving collaborative care, from 10 Care managers, reporting mean (SD) care manager time per participant of 214.15 (115) minutes. We based clinical supervision costs on data collected from supervision records (n = 220 records) reporting a mean supervision time for care managers, in weekly sessions, at 35 minutes, with six participants discussed on average per session (based on data from

Table 3. Estimated mean cost (£'s) for health, social care, and other resource use, over 12 month follow-up.

Resource item	12-mth Follow-up			
	Usual Care		Collaborative Care	
	n	£ Mean (SD)	n	£ Mean (SD)
Primary/Community:				
GP (surgery/practice)	244	295.52 (241)	217	279.76 (243)
GP (at home)	247	14.21 (97)	218	5.55 (32)
Nurse (surgery/practice)	247	26.54 (46)	215	25.19 (46)
Nurse (at home)	247	1.94 (14)	218	1.38 (13)
Walk-in-centre (attendance)	247	13.28 (35)	217	12.66 (35)
Counsellor	246	214.63 (676)	212	160.47 (433)
Mental Health worker	247	44 (267)	215	59.74 (283)
Social worker	247	72.10 (379)	218	122.53 (835)
Home help/Care Worker	247	78.27 (851)	218	22.38 (271)
Occupational Therapist	247	18.26 (80)	218	10.53 (50)
Voluntary Group	247	20.50 (126)	218	4.88 (30)
Secondary Care:				
Acute Psychiatric ward	247	0	218	143.12 (2,113)
Psychiatric rehab ward	247	0	218	0
Long stay ward	247	13.51 (212)	218	0
Psychiatric ICU ward	247	0	218	0
General Med ward	247	154.65 (649)	217	134.61 (535)
Other hosp ward/stay	247	90.97 (507)	218	123.69 (682)
A & E	247	43.06 (99)	218	36.47 (81)
Day hospital	247	74.99 (280)	218	45.08 (150)
Out Patient Appt, Psychiatrist	247	26.79 (148)	217	43.88 (170)
Out Patient Appt, Psychologist	247	25.14 (313)	217	25.51 (296)
Out Patient Appt, Psychiatric Nurse	247	8.92 (67)	217	12.61 (166)
Out Patient Appt, Other	246	306.93 (588)	215	285.34 (498)
Social care:				
Day care centre	247	9.64 (151)	218	2.50 (37)
Drop in club	247	19.13 (179)	218	4.06 (48)
Day care other	247	13.35 (97)	217	22.09 (193)
Informal care from friends/relatives:				
help from friends/relatives	230	5,714.73 (14,455)	209	3,698.50 (9,462)
Days lost work by friends/relatives	246	403.26 (2,902)	217	164.78 (1,123)
Patient other costs:				
OTC medications	246	28.40 (58)	215	40.31 (69)
Travel costs	246	10.98 (30)	216	14.33 (38)
Own car travel	246	11.75 (35)	214	14.19 (63)
'one-off' costs	246	35.77 (144)	218	51.58 (213)

Kruskal-Wallis (non-parametric) test: no statistically significant differences between groups, other than for OTC cost, and cost for days lost work by friends/ relatives, which are statistically significant at $p \leq 0.05$.
(Appt = appointment; OTC = over the counter).

164 records). We assumed from this data that participants were discussed in three supervisory sessions (over the course of the intervention), at six minutes per participant per session.

Probabilistic analyses used to explore uncertainty around the main cost component, drawing from the distribution of contact time for care managers (mean 214.5 mins, SD 115 mins), showed that in 95% of simulations (cost estimates) the estimated cost of collaborative care was between £101 and £592 per participant (median £249).

NHS and Social Care Resource Use and Costs

We found no statistically significant differences between treatment groups in use of resources during the six months prior to baseline assessment (see Table S1). Table 2 presents resource

Table 4. Estimated costs, and cost differences (adjusted, unadjusted), over 12-month follow-up, by group.

Resource item	Usual Care n = 305		Collaborative Care n = 276		Difference (no adjustment)	Difference, adjusted for baseline and participant/cluster covariates*
	n	Mean (SD) £	n	Mean (SD) £	£	Mean (95% CI)** £
Primary and community services/care	243	801.49 (1,476.98)	208	715.86 (1,220.06)	–85.63	–116.48 (–341.06, 110.91)
Secondary care: hospital stay	247	259.14 (835.40)	217	402.65 (2,282.88)	143.51	160.92 (–70.81, 481.70)
Secondary care: outpatient care	246	368.03 (781.43)	215	368.09 (692.60)	0.06	–30.68 (–148.85, 111.70)
Secondary care: day hospital	247	74.99 (280.31)	218	45.08 (149.65)	–29.91	–14.52 (–50–13, 17.94)
A & E	247	42.06 (98.66)	218	36.47 (80.51)	–5.59	–5.87 (–22.39, 9.99)
Day services and care	247	42.12 (334.85)	217	28.67 (203.43)	–13.45	1.83 (–38.51, 41.01)
Total NHS and personal social services (excl Collab Care)	242	1,570.70 (2,441.55)	205	1,614.32 (3,714.49)	43.62	1.78 (–454.82, 640.81)
CADET collaborative care		-		272.50	272.50	-
Total NHS and personal social services	242	**1,570.70** (2,441.55)	205	**1,886.82** (3,714.49)	**316.12**	**270.72 (–202.98, 886.04)**[#1]
Patient personal costs (OTC/meds, travel costs, plus patient 'one-off' costs)	244	86.64 (175.50)	211	120.79 (260.37)	34.15	24.95 (–12.41, 65.61)
Informal care costs	230	5,714.73 (14,455.18)	209	3,698.50 (9,642.61)	–2,016.23	–1,114.13 (–3,366.09, 1,117.32)
TOTAL costs (NHS and patient/related costs)	223	**7,010.59** (13,492.42)	195	**5,764.48** (10,796.40)	**–1,246.11**	**–312.83 (–2,339.92, 2,035.27)**[#2]

*regression analyses using multilevel model ('xtmixed' STATA), with baseline value as covariate, age, and cluster level covariates.
**95% Confidence intervals estimated using non-parametric bootstrap method.
[#1]ICC = 0.0000 (95% CI 0.0000, 0.0000).
[#2]ICC = 0.0000 (95% CI 0.0000, 0.0000).
On cost estimates for individual items/categories, ANOVA showed no statistically significant differences between groups; [note: informal care cost difference at p = 0.088].

use over the 12-month follow-up, and Table 3 presents the costs associated with resource use over 12-month follow-up. Table 4 presents cost data by category with comparison by category by treatment group. We found a broadly similar pattern of resource use across groups, with estimated mean costs for NHS and social care (Third Party Payer perspective), excluding the collaborative care intervention, at £1,571 and £1,614 respectively for usual care and collaborative care participants. After adjustment for baseline cost and individual and cluster covariates the cost difference was not statistically significant, with wide confidence intervals. When including the cost for the collaborative care intervention, the mean total NHS and social care costs were £1,571 and £1,887 for usual care and collaborative care participants respectively, but similarly, after adjustment the cost difference of £271 was not statistically significant. Excluding the intervention cost, the one area of substantial cost difference between groups was on hospital stay, with a mean cost difference of £161 (regression adjusted estimate). This estimated difference in hospital cost was driven by one participant in the collaborative care group, who reported an acute psychiatric hospital stay of 100 days. When we excluded that one participant from analyses, the cost difference for hospital stay was adjusted to £34 (–119 to 189), and the related differences in NHS and social care, without collaborative care costs and with collaborative care costs, were adjusted to –£209 (less cost for collaborative care), and £63 (additional cost for collaborative care) respectively.

Broader Participant Level and Social Costs

Tables 2 and 3 report resource use and cost estimates associated with informal care from friends and/or relatives, and other patient out-of-pocket expenses. Our findings show that informal care costs, when estimated using a shadow price for informal care (an estimate of £18 per hour, see Table 1), represented the largest resource and cost burden associated with participants' depression. Participants in the treatment as usual group reported a high use of informal care, which resulted in a higher mean (SD) cost estimate, over 12-months, at £5,715 (£14,455) compared to £3,699 (£9,462) in the collaborative care group. However there is wide variation in the self-report data as shown by the large standard deviations. When adjusting for baseline costs and other covariates the difference in estimated cost for informal care was –£1,114 (95% CI –£3,366 to £1,117), with lower costs for the collaborative care group, and, therefore, lower total costs in the collaborative care group (Table 4).

Quality-Adjusted Life-Years

Table 5 reports data on health state values for the EQ-5D and the SF-6D, and the estimated QALY values over 12-months. When adjusted for baseline and for individual and cluster covariates we found a difference of 0.02 (95% CI –0.02 to 0.06) in the QALY over 12 months for the EQ-5D, and 0.017 (95% CI 0.000 to 0.032) for the SF-6D. Both measures showed a QALY

Table 5. Health State Values and QALY comparisons (adjusted, unadjusted), over 12-month follow-up, by group.

Measure (time-point)	Usual Care n = 305		Collaborative Care n = 276		Difference (no adjustment)	Difference, adjusted for baseline and participant/cluster covariates*
	n	Mean (SD) [range]	n	Mean (SD) [range]		Mean (95% CI)**
EQ-5D: Baseline	305	0.464 (0.313) [−0.29, 1.00]	276	0.504 (0.288) [−0.349, 1.00]	0.040	
EQ-5D: 4-month	273	0.557 (0.331) [−0.239, 1.00]	228	0.599 (0.341) [−0.484, 1.00]	0.042	
EQ-5D: 12-month	254	0.593 (0.338) [−0.349, 1.00])	227	0.650 (0.317) [−0.484, 1.00])	0.057	
EQ-5D: QALY (12-month)	**248**	**0.554 (0.286) [−0.27, 0.97]**	**218**	**0.605 (0.261) [−0.29, 0.97]**	0.051*	**0.019 (−0.019, 0.06)**#
SF-6D: Baseline	303	0.538 (0.86) [0.30, 0.77]	274	0.540 (0.83) [0.30, 0.82]	0.002	
SF-6D: 4-month	269	0.597 (0.126) [0.30, 1.00]	227	0.614 (0.140) [0.32, 1.00]	0.017	
SF-6D: 12-month	250	0.605 (0.131) [0.30, 1.00])	223	0.634 (0.144) [0.30, 1.00])	0.029*	
SF-6D: QALY (12-month)	241	**0.591 (0.109) [0.30, 0.90]**	211	**0.609 (0.114) [0.35, 0.91]**	0.018	**0.0168 (0.000, 0.032)**

#ICC = 0.0000 (95% CI 0.0000, 0.0000).
*ANOVA, p≤0.05.
**regression analyses using multilevel model ('xtmixed' STATA), with baseline.

gain for collaborative care, although the EQ-5D difference is not statistically significant.

Cost-Effectiveness Analyses

Table 6 presents data used to estimate cost per QALY, and the cost per QALY estimates, based on participants with data on costs and outcomes at follow-up. The base case cost per QALY for collaborative care was £14,248, adopting a NHS and social care perspective, with uncertainty around this estimated illustrated in Figure 1 (cost-effectiveness plane), and Figure 2 (CEAC). The probability that collaborative care is cost effective, compared to treatment as usual, is 0.58 at a willingness to pay of £20,000 per QALY, and 0.65 at a willingness to pay of £30,000 per QALY.

Sensitivity Analyses

Table 6 presents the results of our sensitivity analyses, where we estimated incremental costs and QALYs, and cost per QALY using alternative assumptions. In base case analyses 23% of cost data are missing at 12-month follow-up (21% in control; 25% in collaborative care), and 20% of QALY (EQ-5D) data are missing at the 12-month follow-up (19% in control; 21% missing in collaborative care). Imputation of missing data resulted in an estimated incremental cost of £292 and an incremental EQ-5D QALY gain of 0.017, with a cost per QALY of £17,490. Where we adopted a broader analytical perspective, including all participants with data on cost and outcome at follow-up, we estimated a mean cost saving of £313 with collaborative care, alongside the estimated incremental gain in QALYs (0.02). This, therefore, represents a position of dominance for the collaborative care intervention compared to treatment as usual. Using the SF-6D QALY estimate the cost per QALY increased to £16,114, with a 0.57 and 0.72 probability of being cost-effective at a willingness to pay of £20,000 and £30,000 per QALY respectively. When we analysed CEA using an alternative cost for the collaborative care intervention, assuming a cost of £338.80 per participant (compared to base case of £272.50) to allow for additional clinical supervision time to the care manager, and therefore per participant, and for supervision from a psychiatrist (unit cost per hour, £267, [27]) the base case cost per QALY estimate increased to £17,738. When we undertook a scenario the same as the base case but with one participant, with extremely high resource use, excluded from analyses the cost per QALY was reduced to an estimate of £3,334 with a 0.76 and 0.79 probability of being cost-effective at a willingness to pay of £20,000 and £30,000 per QALY respectively.

Discussion

Our results show that collaborative care is cost-effective, compared to usual care, in treating people with depression in a UK primary care setting, where providers are willing to pay up to £20,000 per QALY gained. When taking a broader analytical perspective, and including costs associated with informal care, results show that collaborative care is expected to be cost saving, with expected health gains, and therefore dominates the usual care comparator. Previous reviews [10,34] have reported on economic analyses related to collaborative care, across a range of settings, including care for depression. These reviews have identified evidence from cost-utility (cost per QALY) studies to support the economic value of collaborative care for depression in the United States healthcare system, and have also highlighted an absence of evidence for the UK. Results presented here for the CADET trial represent the first study to estimate the cost-effectiveness of collaborative care in a UK primary care setting.

Our cost-effectiveness analyses report an expected modest mean QALY gain at a relatively low cost. The relative effectiveness of collaborative care versus usual care reported in the CADET trial [9] is regarded as clinically meaningful in terms of recovery (defined as a follow up score of less than or equal to 9 on PHQ-9)

Table 6. Cost Effectiveness Analyses.

Scenario/Analyses	Difference, adjusted for baseline and participant/cluster covariates* Mean (95% CI)	ICER, Cost (£) per QALY	Probability Cost-effective at WTP‡ per QALY gained: £20,000 per QALY	£30,000 per QALY
Base Case:				
Total NHS and personal social services	£270.72 (−202.98, 886.04)			
EQ-5D: QALY (12-month)	0.019 (−0.019, 0.06)	**£14,248**	0.58	0.65
Sensitivity Analyses:				
(1) Base Case CEA, with multiple imputation of missing data				
Total NHS and personal social services	£292.08 (−216.88, 801.04)			
EQ-5D: QALY (12-month)	0.017 (−0.020, 0.054)	£17.490	N/A	N/A
(2) CEA Using SF6D QALY data				
SF6D: QALY (12-month)	0.0168 (0.000, 0.032)	£16,114	0.57	0.72
(3) CEA when excluding one high cost participant				
Total NHS and personal social services	£63.34 (−295.98, 422.67)			
EQ-5D: QALY (12-month)	0.019 (−0.018, 0.06)	£3,334	0.76	0.79
(4) CEA using higher cost estimate for Collaborative Care, at mean cost of £338.80				
Total NHS and personal social services	£337.02 (−136.67, 952.34)	£17,738	0.54	0.62
(5) CEA using a broader perspective, including patient costs and informal care costs	−£312.83 (−2,339.93, 2,035.27)	Collaborative Care is dominant**	N/A	N/A

*Adjusting for baseline measures, and pre-specified covariates for age (individual level), and (at the cluster level) deprivation (IMD), site, and practice size.
**Dominance: lower expected costs, with greater expected QALY gain.
‡WTP = willingness to pay; based in the assessment of incremental net benefit statistic, and WTP thresholds commonly applied in the UK NHS (NICE, 2013).

and treatment response (defined as a 50% reduction or greater at follow up compared to baseline PHQ-9). Although, as seen in the QALY data, the average individual treatment response was modest, at 12 months 56% of patients receiving collaborative care were 'recovered', 15% more than in usual care, and 49% responded to treatment, 13% more than in usual care. Whilst the mean QALY gains are modest, they are comparable, and favourable, to those recently reported for evaluation of a UK Improving Access to Psychological Therapies (IAPT) service [35], which estimated a mean EQ-5D QALY gain of 0.014 (SF6D gain of 0.008). In the IAPT evaluation, the SF6D values at baseline and follow-up are a little higher than those for CADET, probably reflecting the fact that the patient group had a lower mean PHQ-9 score compared to CADET participants. Our estimated costs for health and social care in CADET are similar to those reported in the IAPT service evaluation, for IAPT service or comparator mental healthcare services [35]. QALY gains from the collaborative care intervention are in a similar range to those reported for evaluation of therapist-delivered CBT for depression [36], where a mean (95% CI) incremental QALY benefit is reported at 0.027 (−0.012 to 0.066).

Our base case difference in health and social care (NHS and PSS) costs, over 12 months (£271), and the subsequent cost per QALY estimate, of £14,248 are heavily influenced by one participant who reported extremely high levels of service use for specialist care, including a 100-day stay in an acute psychiatric hospital. This participant, in the collaborative care group, had an estimated service use cost of £48,522, compared to a mean cost of £1,637 for all other trial participants with cost data over 12-months (n = 446); 94% of participants have cost estimates at less than £5,000; all but four participants have costs at less than £10,000; three participants have costs estimated between £10,000 and £24,000. When we excluded this one participant from analyses, the difference in NHS and PSS costs, when including cost for collaborative care, was £63, between collaborative care and usual care, with an estimated cost per QALY of £3,334. For

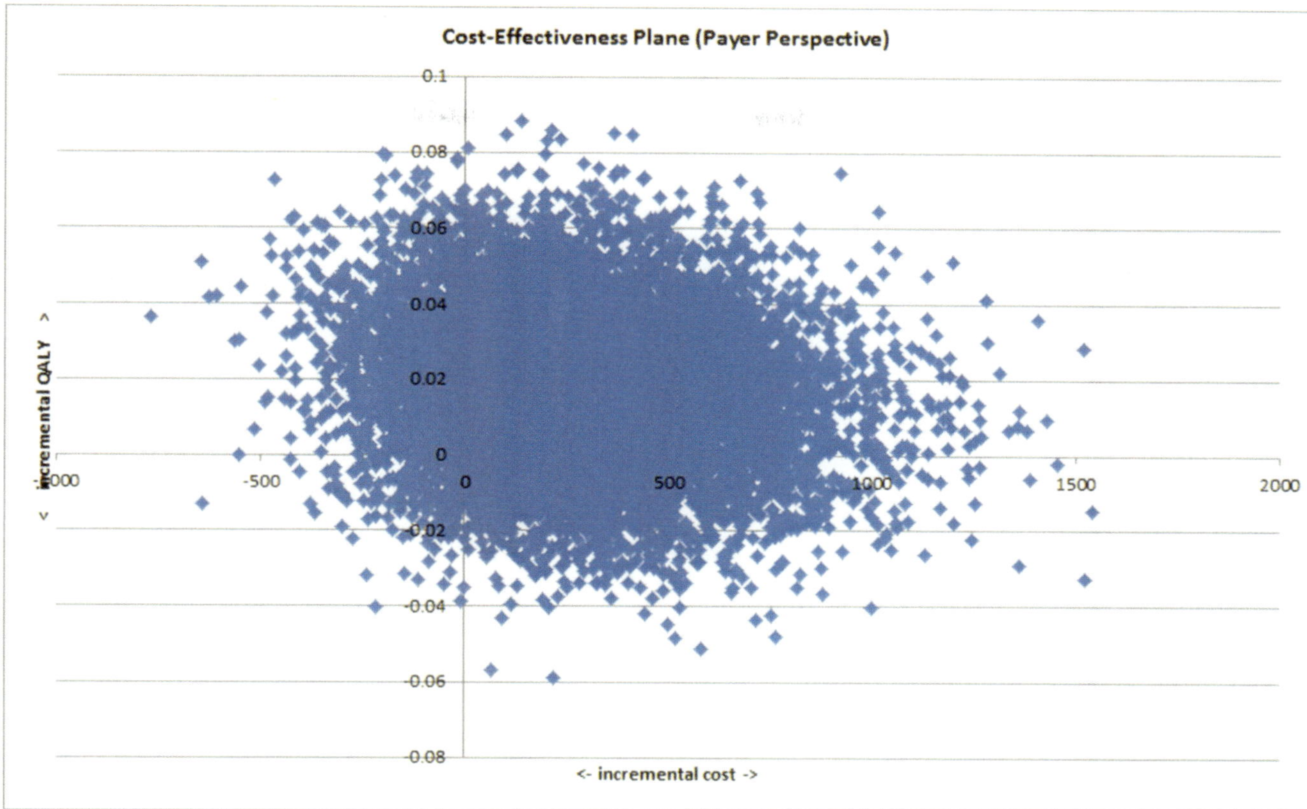

Figure 1. Cost-effectiveness plane (Payer perspective).

our primary analysis we retained the intent to treat principle, and this one participant is included in the base case analyses, but we would suggest that the likely cost-effectiveness of collaborative care in practice might be closer to the estimate in the sensitivity analyses with this one participant excluded.

Although there is uncertainty in the cost and QALY data, our probabilistic analyses indicate that collaborative care has a 58% or 65% probability of being cost-effective, at commonly assumed UK NHS willingness to pay of £20,000 or £30,000 per QALY. Where we considered uncertainty around the CEA estimate that excludes one participant with high service use and costs (£3,334 per QALY), the probability of being cost effective at these cost per QALY thresholds is above 75%. Given the wide variation in the costs reported for general health and social care resource use, and the uncertainty in the profile of resource use, a simplistic view would be to have an expectation that the introduction of collaborative care will involve an additional cost of £272.50 per participant for the UK NHS, and this potential cost alongside estimated EQ-5D QALY gains, results in an expected cost per QALY gain of £14,342, which is similar to the base case analyses presented here and represents a cost effective use of NHS resources.

Strengths and Limitations

The CADET trial was a high quality RCT with an integrated economic evaluation, reported here. The analyses follow good practice for economic evaluation, and our within-trial analysis demonstrates cost-effectiveness at the willingness to pay threshold of £20,000 per QALY, without the need to extrapolate potential benefits over the longer term. Our analyses use data collected within trial to estimate resource use and cost associated with delivery of the intervention, but rely on self-report data, from interviewer administered questionnaires, to estimate health and social care service use, and to estimate broader resource impacts. There is no consensus in the economic evaluation literature on the relative merits of different methods for collection of resource use data [37–39], but routinely collected service use data may have provided a more rigorous estimate of service use, particularly for primary care contacts [40]. However, there are difficulties and costs related to collection of service use data from 42 general practices, and from other necessary routine data collection for aspects of care not recorded in GP records, therefore we chose to use participant self-report data. Difficulties collecting detailed data via self-report on medications, related to potential for variation in medication names, dose, the potential for people to be on medications for a wide range of co-morbid conditions, and other factors, can lead to errors in self-reporting. These issues led to the exclusion of medication costs from the economic analysis plan [12], and this may be a limitation in the results presented here, as medication adherence has been shown to be one of the potential benefits from collaborative care [8]. However, most participants in both collaborative care and the usual care groups remained on antidepressant prescriptions (74.8% v 73.8% at four months; 69.7% v 69.2% at 12 months).

The perspective on the analyses do not extend to the broad welfare and economic impacts of depression, including impact on productivity costs, as such costs are not included in the reference case analyses suggested by NICE [29] for UK analyses. However, data collection did cover aspects of care and support, and patient costs that have extended the primary perspective (of NHS and PSS costs) to a broader patient and societal orientated perspective. We

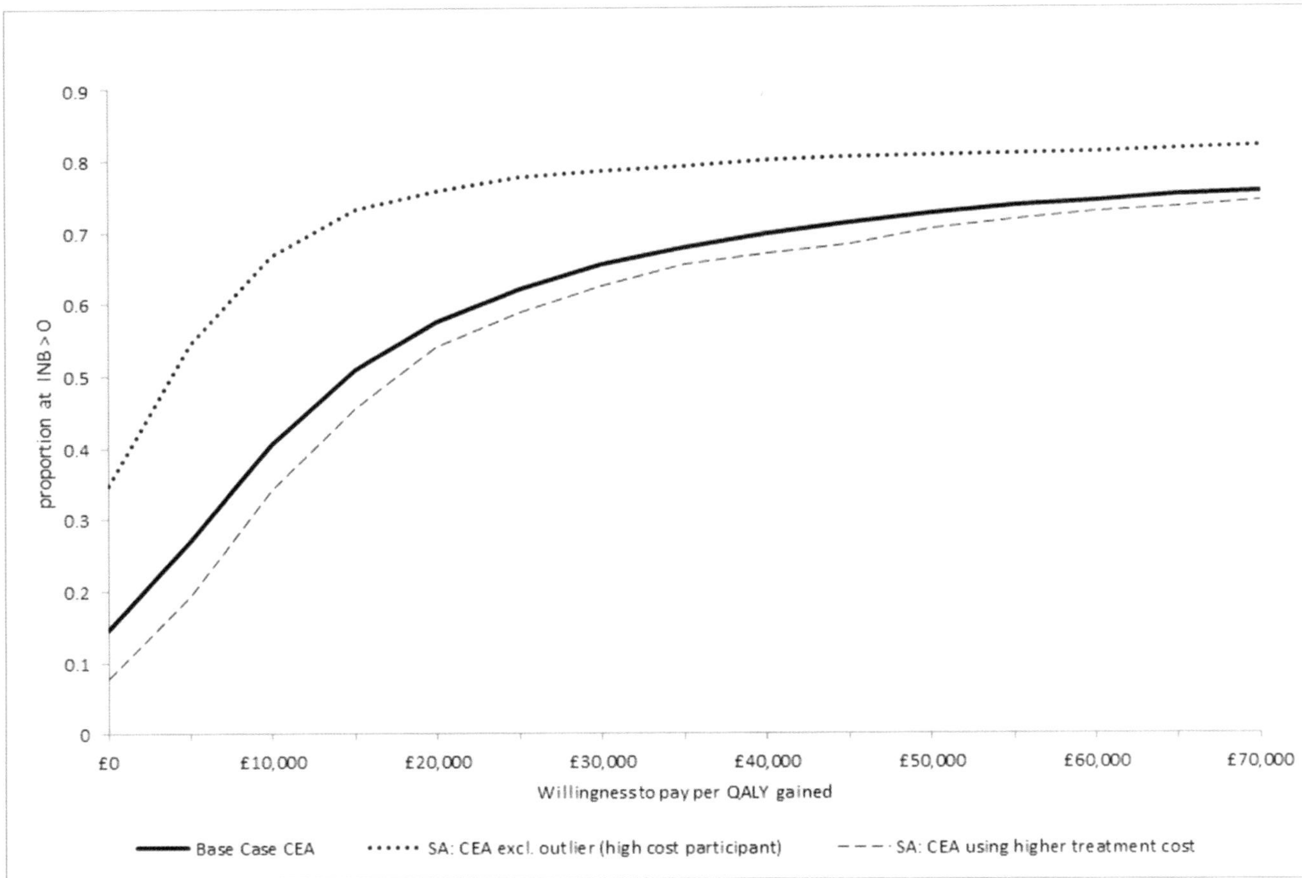

Figure 2. Cost-effectiveness acceptability curves.

accept that the use of a relatively small number of categories for these broader considerations may be a limitation in the analyses. However, as in other studies (e.g. [41]) we found that resources, and estimated costs, associated with informal care were a dominant aspect of care and costs, when taking a wider perspective, and provided clear guidance on the magnitude of costs at a wider perspective.

As discussed above, our estimated differences in costs, and in EQ-5D QALYs, did not reach statistical significance, introducing some uncertainty. However, the methods used in cost-effectiveness analyses account for uncertainty through replication of the estimates of incremental costs and QALYs, using the non-parametric bootstrap approach. The presentation of uncertainty using the CEAC, allows decision makers to consider the likelihood of collaborative care providing a cost-effective use of resources.

Implications

The CADET trial has shown that collaborative care improves depression immediately after treatment compared to usual care, it also has effects that persist to 12 month follow-up and is preferred by patients over usual care, and here our economic analysis of collaborative care also shows that it is cost effective in the UK. We have therefore, responded to the evidence needs, and answered the specific request for evidence required by NICE [11], on the clinical and cost effectiveness of collaborative care, in that our positive findings on the cost-effectiveness of collaborative care adds to the evidence for its sustained clinical effectiveness.

Given that collaborative care is more effective over a sustained period of time than usual care and represents value for money against commonly used thresholds for cost per QALY, we suggest that commissioners of healthcare in the UK and elsewhere organise their depression management services using a collaborative care model. Evidence here indicates that services should be commissioned to support the management of patients with depression in UK primary care using a collaborative care model, as it would be both effective and cost effective to do so. Although the introduction of collaborative care will involve additional resources for the delivery of the intervention, there is reasonable potential for cost saving against other areas of health and social care over time.

Where we have included informal care costs in our analyses, the finding that collaborative care is the dominant intervention, compared to care as usual, is an important issue. Family members and others involved in informal care are contributing to the care of depression in a substantial manner. As Richard Layard and others have often asserted [42], the implications of these care costs on productivity is a significant burden on the economic activity of a nation. The introduction of collaborative care has the potential to relieve some of the significant burden that falls on informal carers, and can reduce this economic load.

Supporting Information

Table S1 Estimated mean baseline cost (£'s) for health, social care, and other resource use.

Acknowledgments

We thank Leala Watson for assistance with the revision of this manuscript.

Author Contributions

Conceived and designed the experiments: CG DAR JJH LG KL CC-G PB JC SP RA DK JMB SG GL CM AH-M MB. Performed the experiments: DAR LG KL CC-G PB JC SP RA DK SG GL MB. Analyzed the data: CG JMB. Contributed to the writing of the manuscript: CG DAR JJH LG KL CC-G PB JC SP RA DK JMB SG GL CM AH-M MB.

References

1. Mann R, Gilbody S, Richards D (2009) Putting the 'Q' in depression QALYs: a comparison of utility measurement using EQ-5D and SF-6D health related quality of life measures. Soc Psychiatry Psychiatr Epidemiol 44: 569–578.
2. McCrone P, Dhanasiri S, Patel A, Knapp M, Lawton-Smith S (2008) Paying the Price. The Cost of Mental Health Care in England to 2006. King's Fund.
3. Meltzer H, Gill B, Petticrew M, Hinds K (1995) OPCS Surveys of Psychiatric Morbidity in Great Britain, Report 2: Physical complaints, service use and treatment of adults with psychiatric disorders. London: HMSO.
4. Simon G, Ludman E, Tutty S, Operskalski B, Von Korff M (2004) Telephone psychotherapy and telephone care management for primary care patients starting antidepressant treatment: a randomized controlled trial. Journal of the American Medical Association 292: 935–942.
5. Gask L (2005) Overt and covert barriers to the integration of primary and specialist mental health care. Social Science and Medicine 61: 1785–1794.
6. Gilbody S, Bower P, Fletcher J, Richards D, Sutton AJ (2006) Collaborative care for depression: a cumulative meta-analysis and review of longer-term outcomes. Arch Intern Med 166: 2314–2321.
7. Gunn J, Diggens J, Hegarty K, Blashki G (2006) A systematic review of complex system interventions designed to increase recovery from depression in primary care. BMC Health Services Research 6.
8. Archer J, Bower P, Gilbody S, Lovell K, Richards D, et al. (2012) Collaborative care for depression and anxiety problems. The Cochrane Database of Systematic Reviews 10: CD006525.
9. Richards DA, Hill JJ, Gask L, Lovell K, Chew-Graham C, et al. (2013) Clinical effectiveness of collaborative care for depression in UK primary care (CADET): cluster randomised controlled trial. Bmj 347: f4913.
10. Gilbody S, Bower P, Whitty P (2006) Costs and consequences of enhanced primary care for depression: systematic review of randomised economic evaluations. Br J Psychiatry 189: 297–308.
11. National Institute for Health and Clinical Excellence (2009) Depression: the Treatment and Management of Depression in Adults.: NICE clinical guideline 90 (CG90). Available: www.nice.org.uk/CG90.
12. Richards DA, Hughes-Morley A, Hayes RA, Araya R, Barkham M, et al. (2009) Collaborative Depression Trial (CADET): multi-centre randomised controlled trial of collaborative care for depression–study protocol. BMC Health Serv Res 9: 188.
13. Lewis G, Pelosi AJ, Araya R, Dunn G (1992) Measuring psychiatric disorder in the community: a standardized assessment for use by lay interviewers. Psychol Med 22: 465–486.
14. Department for Communities and Local Government (2008) The English Indices of Multiple Deprivation 2007. London: HMSO.
15. Ekers D, Richards D, Gilbody S (2008) A meta-analysis of randomized trials of behavioural treatment of depression. Psychol Med 38: 611–623.
16. Irvin JE, Bowers CA, Dunn ME, Wang MC (1999) Efficacy of relapse prevention: a meta-analytic review. J Consult Clin Psychol 67: 563–570.
17. Kroenke K, Spitzer RL, Williams JB (2001) The PHQ-9: validity of a brief depression severity measure. J Gen Intern Med 16: 606–613.
18. Ware J, Sknow K, Kosinski M, Gandek B (1993) SF-36 Health Survey: Manual and Interpretation Guide. Boston, MA: The Health Institute, New England Medical Centre.
19. Spitzer RL, Kroenke K, Williams JB, Lowe B (2006) A brief measure for assessing generalized anxiety disorder: the GAD-7. Arch Intern Med 166: 1092–1097.
20. Attkisson CC, Zwick R (1982) The client satisfaction questionnaire. Psychometric properties and correlations with service utilization and psychotherapy outcome. Eval Program Plann 5: 233–237.
21. EuroQol Group (1990) EuroQol–a new facility for the measurement of health-related quality of life. Health Policy 16: 199–208.
22. EuroQol Group (1996) EQ-5D user guide. Rotterdam. Netherlands: The EuroQol Group.
23. Brazier J, Ratcliffe J, Salomon J, Tsuchiya A (2007) Measuring and Valuing Health Benefits for Economic Evaluation. Oxford: Oxford University Press.
24. Dolan P (1997) Modeling valuations for EuroQol health states. Med Care 35: 1095–1108.
25. Brazier J, Roberts J, Deverill M (2002) The estimation of a preference-based single index measure for health from the SF-36. Journal of Health Economics 21: 271–292.
26. Matthews JN, Altman DG, Campbell MJ, Royston P (1990) Analysis of serial measurements in medical research. Bmj 300: 230–235.
27. Curtis L (2011) Unit Costs of Health & Social Care. Canterbury: Personal Social Services Research Unit.
28. Royston P (2004) Multiple imputation of missing values. Stata Journal 4: 227–241.
29. National Institute for Health and Care Excellence (2013) Guide to the methods of technology appraisal. London: National Institute for Health and Care Excellence.
30. National Institute for Health and Clinical Excellence (2008) Guide to the methods of technology appraisal. London: National Institute for Health and Clinical Excellence.
31. Briggs A, Schulpher M, Claxton K (2006) Decision modelling for health economic evaluation. Oxford: Oxford University Press.
32. Fenwick E, Byford S (2005) A guide to cost-effectiveness acceptability curves. Br J Psychiatry 187: 106–108.
33. Drummond M, Schulpher M, Torrance G, O'Brien B, Stoddart G (2005) Methods for the Economic Evaluation of Health Care Programmes. 3rd Edition. Oxford: Oxford University Press.
34. Jacob V, Chattopadhyay SK, Sipe TA, Thota AB, Byard GJ, et al. (2012) Economics of collaborative care for management of depressive disorders: a community guide systematic review. Am J Prev Med 42: 539–549.
35. Mukuria C, Brazier J, Barkham M, Connell J, Hardy G, et al. (2013) Cost-effectiveness of an improving access to psychological therapies service. Br J Psychiatry 202: 220–227.
36. Hollinghurst S, Peters TJ, Kaur S, Wiles N, Lewis G, et al. (2010) Cost-effectiveness of therapist-delivered online cognitive-behavioural therapy for depression: randomised controlled trial. Br J Psychiatry 197: 297–304.
37. Byford S, Leese M, Knapp M, Seivewright H, Cameron S, et al. (2007) Comparison of alternative methods of collection of service use data for the economic evaluation of health care interventions. Health Econ 16: 531–536.
38. Lairson DR, Basu R, Begley CE, Reynolds T (2009) Concordance of survey and billing data in a study of outpatient healthcare cost and utilization among epilepsy patients. Epilepsy Res 87: 59–69.
39. Wolinsky FD, Miller TR, An H, Geweke JF, Wallace RB, et al. (2007) Hospital episodes and physician visits: the concordance between self-reports and medicare claims. Med Care 45: 300–307.
40. Petrou S, Murray L, Cooper P, Davidson LL (2002) The accuracy of self-reported healthcare resource utilization in health economic studies. Int J Technol Assess Health Care 18: 705–710.
41. Romeo R, Knapp M, Hellier J, Dewey M, Ballard C, et al. (2013) Cost-effectiveness analyses for mirtazapine and sertraline in dementia: randomised controlled trial. Br J Psychiatry 202: 121–128.
42. Layard R (2006) The depression report: a new deal for depression and anxiety disorders: London School of Economics.

Risk of Developing Depressive Disorders following Rheumatoid Arthritis: A Nationwide Population-Based Study

Shu-Li Wang[2], **Cheng-Ho Chang[1]**, **Li-Yu Hu[1]**, **Shih-Jen Tsai[3,4]**, **Albert C. Yang[3,4,5]**, **Zi-Hong You[6,7]***

1 Department of Psychiatry, Kaohsiung Veterans General Hospital, Kaohsiung, Taiwan, **2** Department of Dental Laboratory Technology, Central Taiwan University of Science and Technology, Taichung, Taiwan, **3** Department of Psychiatry, Taipei Veterans General Hospital, Taipei, Taiwan, **4** School of Medicine, National Yang-Ming University, Taipei, Taiwan, **5** Center for Dynamical Biomarkers and Translational Medicine, National Central University, Chungli, Taiwan, **6** Division of Nephrology, Department of Internal Medicine, Taichung Veterans General Hospital, Chia-Yi Branch, Chia-Yi, Taiwan, **7** Institute of Medicine, Chung Shan Medical University, Taichung, Taiwan

Abstract

Background & Aims: To evaluate the risk of depressive disorders among rheumatoid arthritis (RA) by using the Taiwan National Health Insurance Research Database (NHIRD).

Methods: We conducted a retrospective study of a matched cohort of 18 285 participants (3 657 RA patients and 14 628 control patients) who were selected from the NHIRD. Patients were observed for a maximum of 10 years to determine the rates of newly diagnosed depressive disorders, and Cox regression was used to identify the risk factors associated with depressive disorders in RA patients.

Results: During the 10-year follow-up period, 205 (11.2 per 1000 person-years) RA patients and 384 (5.1 per 1000 person-years) control patients were diagnosed with depressive disorders. In RA patients, most depressive disorders (n = 163, 80%) developed with five years of being diagnosed with RA. The incidence risk ratio of depressive disorders between RA patients and control patients was 2.20 (95% confidence interval [CI], 1.84–2.61, $P<.001$). After adjusting for age, sex, and comorbidities, RA patients were 2.06 times more likely to develop depressive disorders (95% CI, 1.73–2.44, $P<.001$) compared with the control patients. Hyperthyroidism (HR = 1.67) was an independent risk factor for depressive disorders in patients with RA.

Conclusions: The likelihood of developing depressive disorders is greater among RA patients than among patients without RA. Symptoms of depression should be sought in patients with RA.

Editor: Melvin G. McInnis, University of Michigan, United States of America

Funding: This study was supported by a grant from the Taipei Veterans General Hospital (V101D-001-2) and SJT received the funding. The funder had no role in study design, data collection and analysis, decision to publish, or preparation of the manuscript.

Competing Interests: The authors have declared that no competing interests exist.

* Email: zihongyou@gmail.com

These authors contributed equally to this work.

Introduction

Rheumatoid arthritis (RA) is a systemic chronic autoimmune disorder affecting primarily cartilage and bone. In addition, several organs such as lung, vessels, and kidney may be involved. In general, RA affects 0.5–1% of the population [1]. Despite of substantial advances in medical treatment, chronic pain, fatigue, and functional disability causes much psychosocial burden for these patients with RA [2,3].

Therefore, interest in the psychiatric aspects of rheumatoid arthritis has grown. Several studies have reported a high depression prevalence rate in patients with RA [4–12], and a significant correlation was observed among depression and increased pain levels in patients with RA [13]. Comorbid depression has been also shown to independently increase disability and a low quality of life in patients with RA [14–18]. In addition, depression has been demonstrated to be an independent risk factor for non-suicide mortality in patients with RA [19]. Hence, the depression symptoms should be examined in patients with RA because depression is a modifiable illness that is amenable to treatment.

However, in previous studies focusing on depression among patients with RA, depression was often evaluated by using rating scales, such as the Beck Depression Inventory or the Epidemiological Studies Depression Scale, rather than diagnosis by a psychiatrist [5–12]. The real prevalence rate of clinical depressive disorders in patients with RA remains unknown. In addition, the design of former studies prevented the temporal causal relationship between RA and depressive disorders from being clarified because the designs of these studies were almost cross-sectional studies [4–12]. Furthermore, whether there is an independent risk factor for newly diagnosed depressive disorders in patients with RA has never been studied.

We performed a population-based retrospective cohort study using data derived from the National Health Insurance (NHI) system in Taiwan. The purpose of our study was to determine whether RA was associated with an increased risk of clinical depressive disorders. Independent risk factors for newly diagnosed depressive disorders among the patients with RA were also identified.

Materials and Methods

Data Sources

Instituted in 1995, the NHI program is a mandatory health insurance program that offers comprehensive medical care coverage, including outpatient, inpatient, emergency, and traditional Chinese medicine, to all residents of Taiwan; the coverage rate is as high as 99% [20]. The NHI research database (NHIRD) contains comprehensive information regarding clinical visits, including prescription details and diagnostic codes based on the International Classification of Diseases, ninth revision, Clinical Modification (ICD-9-CM). The NHIRD is managed by the National Health Research Institutes (NHRI) and confidentiality is maintained according to the directives of the Bureau of the NHI. The data source for our study was the Longitudinal Health Insurance Database 2005 (LHID 2005), which is a dataset of NHIRD. Data for the LHID was collected by systematically and randomly sampling from the NHIRD; the database included the data of one million individuals. The NHRI of Taiwan reports that there were no significant differences in gender distribution, age distribution, or average insured payroll-related amount between the patients in the LHID and those in the original NHIRD [21]. Detailed information about the data source is provided on the NHRI website (http://nhird.nhri.org.tw). Comments, problems or requests about the data application could be sent to e-mail address at the NHRI (e-mail: nhird@nhri.org.tw).

Ethics Statement

The Institutional Review Board of the Taipei Veterans General Hospital approved this study (2013-03-035AC). Written consent from study patients was not obtained because the NHI dataset consists of de-identified secondary data for research purposes, and the Institutional Review Board of Taipei Veterans General Hospital issued a formal written waiver for the need for consent.

Study Population

Using data extracted from the LHID 2005, we conducted a retrospective cohort study of patients aged 20 years and older who were newly diagnosed with RA by a rheumatologist between January 1, 2000 and December 31, 2008. RA was defined as ICD-9-CM code: 714. We excluded patients who were diagnosed with depressive disorders (ICD-9-CM code: 296.2X-296.3X, 300.4, and 311.X) before enrollment. Insurance premiums, calculated according to the beneficiary's total income, were used to estimate monthly income. Monthly income was grouped into low income (monthly income <20,000 New Taiwan Dollar [NTD]), median income (20,000 NTD≤monthly income <40,000 NTD), and high income (monthly income ≥40,000 NTD). Urbanization was divided into three groups: urban, suburban, and rural. Urbanization and monthly income levels were used to represent socioeconomic status. For each cirrhotic patient included in the final cohort, 4 age-, sex-, and enrolment-date-matched control patients who were not diagnosed with rheumatoid arthritis or depressive disorder were randomly selected from the LHID 2005. All RA and control patients were observed until diagnosed with a depressive disorder by a psychiatrist, death, withdrawal from the NHI system, or December 31, 2009. The primary clinical outcome assessed was psychiatrist-diagnosed depressive disorder.

Statistical Analyses

The incidence of newly diagnosed depressive disorders in the RA and control patients, stratified by gender and age (equal or older than 60 years old or younger than 60 years old) was calculated. Independent *t*-tests and chi-squared tests were used to examine the differences in the demographic characteristics between the RA and control patients.

A Cox proportional-hazards regression model was used to identify variables that predicted depressive disorder in the RA and control patients, and in the RA patients only. Control variables, such as age; sex; common comorbidities, including hypertension, diabetes mellitus, dyslipidemia, coronary artery disease, congestive heart failure, cirrhosis, hyperthyroidism, hypothyroidism, cerebrovascular disease, and malignancy; urbanization; and monthly income were included as covariates in the univariate model. Factors that demonstrated a moderately significant statistical relationship in the univariate analysis ($P<.1$) were entered by forward selection in a multivariate Cox proportional-hazards regression model [22].

The Perl programming language (version 5.12.2) was used to extract and compute data. The Microsoft SQL Server 2005 (Microsoft Corp., Redmond, WA, USA) was used for data linkage, processing, and control sampling. IBM SPSS (version 19.0 for Windows; IBM Corp., New York, NY, USA) and SAS statistical software (version 9.2; SAS Institute Inc., Cary, NC, USA) were used to perform all statistical analyses. The comparisons resulting in a *P*-value of less than .05 were considered to indicate a statistically significant relationship.

Results

Participant Selection (Figure 1)

The sample comprised 3657 RA patients and 14 628 control patients without depression, among whom 72.8% were female. The median age at enrollment was 51 years (interquartile range [IQR], 41–61 years), and the median follow-up period was 4.72 years (IQR, 2.59–7.42 years) for RA patients and 4.92 years (IQR, 2.69.21–7.55 years) for control patients. The comorbidities, including hypertension, diabetes mellitus, dyslipidemia, congestive heart failure, hyperthyroidism, hypothyroidism, and cerebrovascular disease were more common in RA patients than control patients. The comparisons of the demographic and clinical variables between the RA and control patients are presented in Table 1.

Incidence Rate of Depressive Disorders

During the study period, 205 (11.2 per 1000 person-years) RA patients and 384 (5.1 per 1000 person-years) control patients were diagnosed with depressive disorders. The incidence risk ratio (IRR)

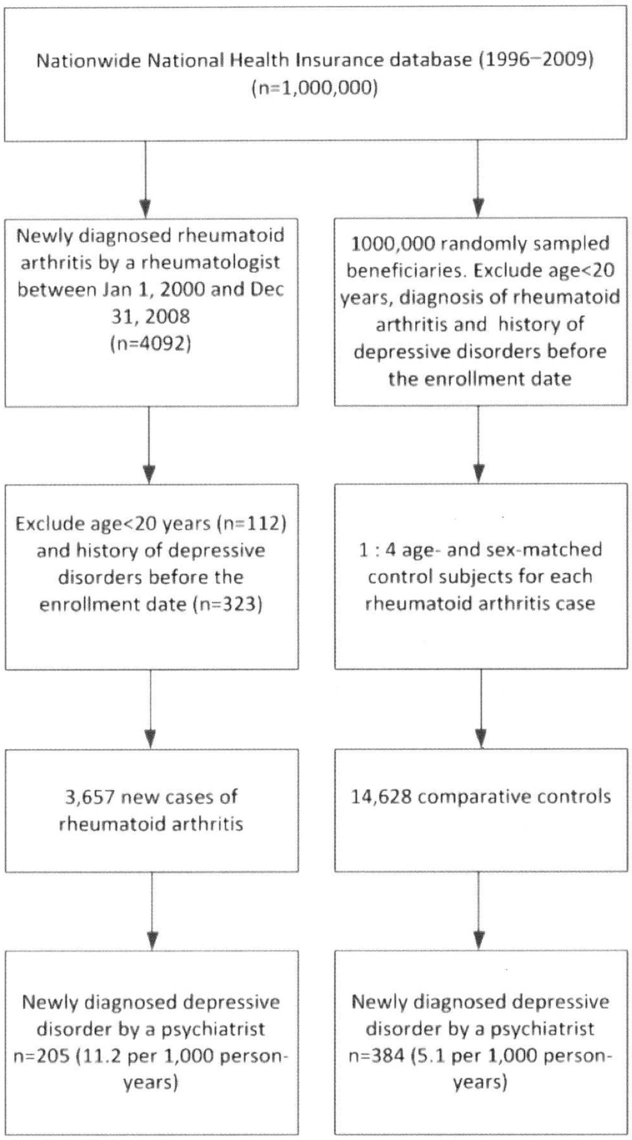

Figure 1. Flow chart of sample selection criteria.

of depressive disorders between RA patients and control patients was 2.20 (95% CI, 1.84–2.61, $P<.001$). When stratified by gender and age, the IRR of depressive disorders was still higher in the RA patients than in the control patients. The results are shown in Table 2. In RA patients, most depressive disorders (n = 163, 80%) developed with five years of being diagnosed with RA.

Rheumatoid arthritis on Risks of Clinical Depression

After adjusting for age, sex, comorbidities, urbanization, and monthly income, the hazard ratio (HR) for developing depressive disorders during the follow-up period was 2.06 times (95% CI, 1.73–2.44, $P<.001$) greater for the RA patients than for the control patients (Table 3 and figure 2).

Risks Factors for Depression in Rheumatoid arthritis Patients

In Table 4, we applied univariate analysis to predict the development of depressive disorders in the RA cohort, and the results demonstrated that the female sex (HR = 1.37, 95% CI, 0.98–1.90, $P = .063$), diabetes mellitus (HR = 1.39, 95% CI, 1.00–1.94, $P = .051$), hyperthyroidism (HR = 1.79, 95% CI, 1.09–2.94, $P = .022$), cerebrovascular disease (HR = 1.55, 95% CI, 0.99–2.41, $P = .054$) and high income (HR = 0.56, 95% CI, 0.34–0.94, $P = .028$) are significant prognostic factors. The multivariate analysis confirmed that hyperthyroidism (HR = 1.67, 95% CI, 1.01–2.76, $P = .045$) was an independent risk factor for depressive disorder in the patients with RA.

Discussion

The key findings of our study are that (1) the incidence rate of depressive disorders in patients with RA was 11.2 per 1000 person-year; (2) the risk of clinical depressive disorders was higher when patients with RA (HR = 2.06) and most depressive disorders (n = 163, 80%) developed within five years of being diagnosed with RA; (3) hyperthyroidism (HR = 1.67) might be an independent risk factor for depressive disorders among patients with RA.

The strengths of this study are the large sample size, the long follow-up period, and the diagnosis of clinical depressive disorders and rheumatoid arthritis by specialists. In addition, our study design involved an unbiased participant selection process. Because participation in the NHI is mandatory and all residents of Taiwan can access low-cost health care, referral bias is low and follow-up compliance is high.

Consistent with the results of previous studies [4–11], we found that the risk of depression in RA patients was higher than that in the non-RA control patients. Chronic inflammation is one of the possible causes. RA is a chronic inflammatory disease, and accumulating evidence implicates inflammation as a critical mediator in the pathophysiology of depressive disorders [23–26]. In the Cardiovascular Health Study of 4 268 patients, a significant association was noted between high levels of C-reactive protein and depression symptoms, even after adjusting for confounding factors [27]. Administration of cytokines including tumor necrosis factor-α in animal and human studies has been shown to induce depressive symptoms, including sleep disturbance, anorexia, loss of interest and mood disturbances [28]. Potential involved mechanisms include direct effects of pro-inflammatory cytokines on monoamine, dysregulation of the hypothalamic-pituitary-adrenal axis, impaired neuroplasticity and structural and functional brain changes [29].

The symptoms of RA such as pain and fatigue may be another possible cause for higher risk of depression in RA patients than that in the non-RA control patients. Symptoms of RA such as pain and fatigue may impair patients' function and quality of life and influence patients' perception of health status, and make the patients more prone to develop depressive symptoms [12,30]. RA patients often suffered pain and pain intensity was more clearly related to disability in RA patients [31]. Several studies have shown that chronic pain was an important risk factor for depression and suicidal behavior [32–34]. Previous study has shown that the degree of depression in RA patients varies in proportion to the level of pain [31].

Furthermore, physical comorbidities might be another possible cause for a higher prevalence of depressive disorder in RA patients. Our findings are consistent with the results of previous studies that found that a higher percentage of many physical comorbidities in RA patients, such as hypertension [35], diabetes mellitus [36], congestive heart failure [37], hypothyroidism [38], and cerebrovascular disease [39]. All of above diseases had been proposed to be related with increased the risk of depression [40–43].

Table 1. Baseline Characteristics of Patients with and without Rheumatoid Arthritis.

Demographic data	Patients with rheumatoid arthritis		Patients without rheumatoid arthritis		P-value
	n=3,657		n=14,628		
	n	%	n	%	
Age (years) (interquartile range)	51 (41–61)		51 (41–61)		
≥60	961	26.3	3,851	26.3	.966
<60	2,696	73.7	10,777	73.7	.
Sex					
Male	993	27.2	3972	27.2	.999
Female	2,664	72.8	10,656	72.8	.
Comorbidities					
Hypertension	1,186	32.4	4,032	27.6	<.001
Diabetes mellitus	687	18.8	2,305	15.8	<.001
Dyslipidemia	1,098	30.0	3,002	20.5	<.001
Coronary artery disease	45	1.2	168	1.1	.673
Congestive heart failure	172	4.7	533	3.6	.004
Cirrhosis	62	1.0	198	1.4	.117
Hyperthyroidism	219	6.0	477	3.3	<.001
Hypothyroidism	107	2.9	178	1.2	<.001
Cerebrovascular disease	316	8.6	929	6.4	<.001
Malignant neoplasms	96	2.6	338	2.3	.274
Degree of urbanization					
urban	2,238	61.2	8,787	60.1	.435
suburban	1,040	28.4	4,268	29.2	
rural	326	8.9	1,362	9.3	
Income group					
low income	1,731	47.3	7,151	48.9	.001
median income	1,430	39.1	5,820	39.8	
high income	496	13.6	1,657	11.3	
Follow-up years (median)	4.72 (2.59–7.42)		4.92 (2.69–7.55)		.004

Finally, long-term drug use in RA patients and inevitable side effects of various medications might also impaired quality of life in RA patients and increased the risk of depression in RA patients [44,45]. Previous study showed that disease-modifying drugs used for RA patients had been related to higher rates of depression, and suicidal ideation among RA patients, serving as an alert to the importance of considering also this factors in therapeutic decisions [46].

Table 2. Incidence of Depressive Disorders in Patients with and without Rheumatoid Arthritis.

	Patients with rheumatoid arthritis		Patients without rheumatoid arthritis		Risk ratio (95% CI)	P value
	No. of Depressive disorders	Per 1 000 person-years	No. of Depressive disorders	Per 1 000 person-years		
Total	205	11.2	384	5.1	2.20 (1.84–2.61)	<.001
Age						
≥60	49	2.8	109	1.4	1.85 (1.29–2.61)	<.001
<60	156	8.5	275	3.7	2.33 (1.91–2.85)	<.001
Sex						
Male	45	2.5	88	1.2	2.10 (1.44–3.05)	<.001
Female	160	8.7	296	3.9	2.22 (1.82–2.70)	<.001

CI indicates confidence interval.

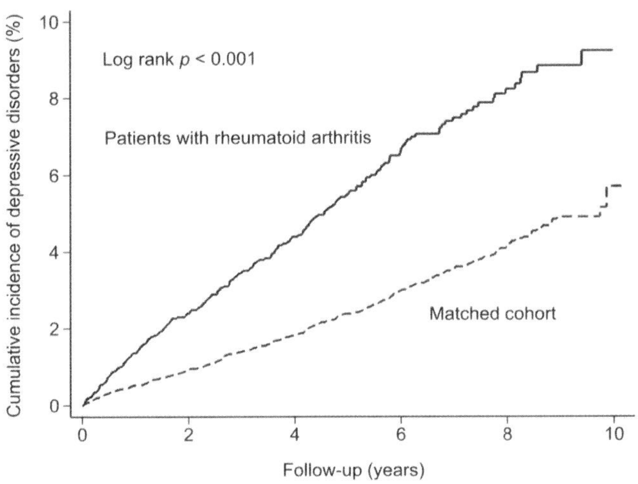

Figure 2. Cumulative incidence of depressive disorders in patients with rheumatoid arthritis (RA) and matched cohort.

According to previous studies, conservative estimates of the prevalence of depressive disorder among patients with RA ranged between 13 and 20% [13,45,47]. This prevalence rate was much higher than the rate calculated in this study. The possible reason for these two discrete findings might be partly due to difference in the methods of assessing depression [13]. In the most previous studies regarding RA and depression [5–12], rating scales, such as the Beck depression inventory, rather than diagnosis by a psychiatrist, were used for evaluation of depression in those studies. People who were recorded as depressed on rating scales may not meet the diagnostic criteria for clinical depressive disorders. However, depressive disorders in RA patients may be underdiagnosed in our study because symptoms of depressive disorders may mimic symptoms of RA, such as easily fatigue, sleep disturbance, and loss of interests with multiple somatic complaints. Physicians may have viewed RA patients' depressive symptoms as physical discomforts caused by RA and overlooked these symptoms, rather than viewing these symptoms as warning signs of depressive disorder.

There has been some discussion in the literature regarding the factors that influence the development of depression in patients with RA [48–50]. However, whether there is certain physical comorbidity as an independent risk factor for new-onset depressive disorders following a RA diagnosis has never been studied. In our study, we found that hyperthyroidism was an independent risk factor for depressive disorders in patients with RA. Studies have shown that mood disturbance, especially depressive disorders, often accompanies hyperthyroidism patients [51–54]. Alterations in components of the hypothalamic-pituitary-thyroid axis have been documented for the development of depressive disorder among patients with hyperthyroidism [53]. In addition, functional impairment caused by hyperthyroidism might play a vital role in causing psychological distresses including depressive disorders among patients with hyperthyroidism [55].

Table 3. Analyses of Risk Factors for Depressive Disorders in Patients with and without Rheumatoid Arthritis.

Predictive variables	Univariate analysis		Multivariate analysis	
	HR (95% CI)	***P* value**	**HR (95% CI)**	***P* value**
Rheumatoid arthritis	2.20 (1.86–2.60)	<.001	2.06 (1.73–2.44)	<.001
Age (<60 = 1, ≥60 = 0)	0.91 (0.76–1.10)	.327		
Sex (female = 1, male = 0)	1.34 (1.10–1.62)	.003	1.29 (1.06–1.57)	.011
Comorbidities				
Hypertension	1.39 (1.17–1.65)	<.001	1.00 (0.82–1.21)	.957
Diabetes mellitus	1.63 (1.34–1.99)	<.001	1.20 (0.96–1.50)	.116
Dyslipidemia	1.77 (1.48–2.12)	<.001	1.39 (1.14–1.71)	.001
Coronary artery disease	1.32 (0.62–2.77)	<.001	1.00 (0.47–2.13)	.995
Congestive heart failure	1.16 (0.75–1.79)	.505		
Cirrhosis	2.33 (1.39–3.89)	.001	1.91 (1.14–3.20)	.014
Hyperthyroidism	2.24 (1.61–3.12)	<.001	1.79 (1.27–2.52)	.001
Hypothyroidism	1.75 (1.01–1.76)	<.001	1.01 (0.57–1.78)	.973
Cerebrovascular disease	2.13 (1.65–2.76)	<.001	1.78 (1.36–2.33)	<.001
Malignant neoplasms	1.16 (0.65–2.05)	.622		
Degree of urbanization				
urban	Reference			
suburban	0.91 (0.76–1.10)	.319		
rural	0.85 (0.63–1.14)	.286		
Income group				
low income	Reference		Reference	
median income	0.94 (0.79–1.12)	.484	0.98 (0.83–1.17)	.847
high income	0.69 (0.51–0.92)	.013	0.75 (0.56–1.02)	.063

HR indicates hazard ratio; CI indicates confidence interval.

Table 4. Analyses of Risk factors for Depressive Disorders in Rheumatoid Arthritis Patients.

Predictive variables	Univariate analysis		Multivariate analysis	
	HR (95% CI)	*P* value	HR (95% CI)	*P* value
Age (<60 = 1, ≥60 = 0)	1.07 (0.77–1.47)	.701		
Sex (female = 1, male = 0)	1.37 (0.98–1.90)	.063	1.28 (0.92–1.79)	.146
Comorbidities				
Hypertension	1.13 (0.84–1.51)	.429		
Diabetes mellitus	1.39 (1.00–1.94)	.051	1.27 (0.90–1.78)	.171
Dyslipidemia	1.23 (0.91–1.66)	.174		
Coronary artery disease	0.97 (0.24–3.92)	.968		
Congestive heart failure	1.11 (0.57–2.16)	.766		
Cirrhosis	1.90 (0.85–4.29)	.120		
Hyperthyroidism	1.79 (1.09–2.94)	.022	1.67 (1.01–2.76)	.045
Hypothyroidism	1.34 (0.63–2.84)	.452		
Cerebrovascular disease	1.55 (0.99–2.41)	.054	1.46 (0.93–2.29)	.098
Malignant neoplasms	1.04 (0.43–2.54)	.925		
Degree of urbanization				
urban	Reference			
suburban	0.96 (0.71–1.31)	.793		
rural	0.78 (0.46–1.33)	.365		
Income group				
low income	reference		reference	
median income	1.04 (0.78–1.38)	.808	1.08 (0.81–1.44)	.603
high income	0.56 (0.34–0.94)	.028	0.62 (0.37–1.04)	.068

HR indicates hazard ratio; CI indicates confidence interval.

Our findings have certain limitations. Information regarding the family history of psychiatric disorders [56,57], lifestyle factors [58], self-perceived health, disability [59], and environmental factors (life stresses, such as recent major life event, domestic violence, childhood trauma, and social support) [60–63] are not included in the NHIRD, and all of which might be associated with the risk of development of depressive disorders. In addition, the severity of RA could not be ascertained. Whether the severity of RA influences the risk of developing depressive disorders warrants further study, despite previous studies indicating that disease activity of RA alone does not equate with depressive symptoms in RA patients reliably [47]. Furthermore, physicians may view RA patients' depressive symptoms as physical discomforts caused by RA and overlook these symptoms. Therefore, in our study, the incidence of clinical depressive disorders may be underestimated.

This population-based retrospective cohort study demonstrated that the risk of developing depressive disorders is higher among RA patients than those without RA, and that RA is an independent risk factor for depressive disorders. Hyperthyroidism is an independent risk factor for developing depressive disorders among patients with RA. Because depression was related to impairing the quality of life of RA patients, and depressive disorder is modifiable illness that is amenable to treatment, symptoms of depression should be sought in patients with RA. Future population-based prospective studies are needed to further investigate the association between RA and the risk of developing depressive disorders.

Acknowledgments

We thank Stephen Chow, Huei-Sing Chang, Cheng-Fang Hong, Chun-Hsin Hu, and Ai-Ling Hu for technical assistance. The study is based in part on data from the National Health Insurance Research Database, provided by the Bureau of National Health Insurance, Department of Health and managed by National Health Research Institutes. The interpretation and conclusions contained herein do not represent those of the Bureau of National Health Insurance, Department of Health or National Health Research Institutes.

Author Contributions

Conceived and designed the experiments: SLW LYH ZHY. Performed the experiments: SLW LYH SJT ACY. Analyzed the data: SLW LYH CHC. Contributed reagents/materials/analysis tools: SJT ACY. Contributed to the writing of the manuscript: SLW LYH ZHY.

References

1. Scott DL, Wolfe F, Huizinga TW (2010) Rheumatoid arthritis. Lancet 376: 1094–1108.
2. Rezvani A, Ayture L, Arslan M, Kurt E, Eroglu Demir S, et al. (2014) Affective temperaments in patients with rheumatoid arthritis. Int J Rheum Dis 17: 34–38.
3. Cross M, Smith E, Hoy D, Carmona L, Wolfe F, et al. (2014) The global burden of rheumatoid arthritis: estimates from the Global Burden of Disease 2010 study. Ann Rheum Dis.
4. Ahles TA, Khan SA, Yunus MB, Spiegel DA, Masi AT (1991) Psychiatric status of patients with primary fibromyalgia, patients with rheumatoid arthritis, and

subjects without pain: a blind comparison of DSM-III diagnoses. Am J Psychiatry 148: 1721–1726.
5. Callahan LF, Kaplan MR, Pincus T (1991) The Beck Depression Inventory, Center for Epidemiological Studies Depression Scale (CES-D), and General Well-Being Schedule depression subscale in rheumatoid arthritis. Criterion contamination of responses. Arthritis Care Res 4: 3–11.
6. Belza BL (1995) Comparison of self-reported fatigue in rheumatoid arthritis and controls. J Rheumatol 22: 639–643.
7. Serbo B, Jajic I (1991) Relationship of the functional status, duration of the disease and pain intensity and some psychological variables in patients with rheumatoid arthritis. Clin Rheumatol 10: 419–422.
8. Kasl SV, Cobb S (1969) The intrafamilial transmission of rheumatoid arthritis. V. Differences between rheumatoid arthritics and controls on selected personality variables. J Chronic Dis 22: 239–258.
9. Scheidt CE, Mueller-Becsangele J, Hiller K, Hartmann A, Goldacker S, et al. (2014) Self-reported symptoms of pain and depression in primary fibromyalgia syndrome and rheumatoid arthritis. Nord J Psychiatry 68: 88–92.
10. Allaire SH, Meenan RF, Anderson JJ (1991) The impact of rheumatoid arthritis on the household work performance of women. Arthritis Rheum 34: 669–678.
11. Lisitsyna TA, Zeltyn AE, Vel'tishchev D, Kovalevskaia OB, Seravina OF, et al. (2012) [Cognitive impairment and anxiety-depressive disorders in patients with rheumatoid arthritis]. Zh Nevrol Psikhiatr Im S S Korsakova 112: 96–103.
12. Coskun B, Coskun BN, Atis G, Ergenekon E, Dilek K (2014) Evaluation of sexual function in women with rheumatoid arthritis. Urol J 10: 1081–1087.
13. Dickens C, McGowan L, Clark-Carter D, Creed F (2002) Depression in rheumatoid arthritis: a systematic review of the literature with meta-analysis. Psychosom Med 64: 52–60.
14. Lowe B, Willand L, Eich W, Zipfel S, Ho AD, et al. (2004) Psychiatric comorbidity and work disability in patients with inflammatory rheumatic diseases. Psychosom Med 66: 395–402.
15. Lisitsyna TA, Veltishchev DY, Gerasimov AN, Seravina OF, Kovalevskaya OB, et al. (2013) [The magnitude of fatigue and its association with depression, pain, and inflammatory activity in rheumatoid arthritis]. Ter Arkh 85: 8–15.
16. van den Hoek J, Roorda LD, Boshuizen HC, van Hees J, Rupp I, et al. (2013) Long-term physical functioning and its association with somatic comorbidity and comorbid depression in patients with established rheumatoid arthritis: a longitudinal study. Arthritis Care Res (Hoboken) 65: 1157–1165.
17. Katz PP, Yelin EH (1994) Life activities of persons with rheumatoid arthritis with and without depressive symptoms. Arthritis Care Res 7: 69–77.
18. Wolfe F, Hawley DJ (1993) The relationship between clinical activity and depression in rheumatoid arthritis. J Rheumatol 20: 2032–2037.
19. Ang DC, Choi H, Kroenke K, Wolfe F (2005) Comorbid depression is an independent risk factor for mortality in patients with rheumatoid arthritis. J Rheumatol 32: 1013–1019.
20. Wu CY, Chen YJ, Ho HJ, Hsu YC, Kuo KN, et al. (2012) Association between nucleoside analogues and risk of hepatitis B virus-related hepatocellular carcinoma recurrence following liver resection. JAMA 308: 1906–1914.
21. Database. NHIR National Health Research Institutes.
22. Bednarek PH, Creinin MD, Reeves MF, Cwiak C, Espey E, et al. (2011) Immediate versus delayed IUD insertion after uterine aspiration. N Engl J Med 364: 2208–2217.
23. Lu Y, Feng L, Feng L, Nyunt MS, Yap KB, et al. (2013) Systemic inflammation, depression and obstructive pulmonary function: a population-based study. Respir Res 14: 53.
24. Pasco JA, Nicholson GC, Williams LJ, Jacka FN, Henry MJ, et al. (2010) Association of high-sensitivity C-reactive protein with de novo major depression. Br J Psychiatry 197: 372–377.
25. D'Mello C, Swain MG (2011) Liver-brain inflammation axis. Am J Physiol Gastrointest Liver Physiol 301: G749–761.
26. Madeeh Hashmi A, Awais Aftab M, Mazhar N, Umair M, Butt Z (2013) The fiery landscape of depression: A review of the inflammatory hypothesis. Pak J Med Sci 29: 877–884.
27. Kop WJ, Gottdiener JS, Tangen CM, Fried LP, McBurnie MA, et al. (2002) Inflammation and coagulation factors in persons >65 years of age with symptoms of depression but without evidence of myocardial ischemia. Am J Cardiol 89: 419–424.
28. Shimbo D, Chaplin W, Crossman D, Haas D, Davidson KW (2005) Role of depression and inflammation in incident coronary heart disease events. Am J Cardiol 96: 1016–1021.
29. Rosenblat JD, Cha DS, Mansur RB, McIntyre RS (2014) Inflamed moods: A review of the interactions between inflammation and mood disorders. Prog Neuropsychopharmacol Biol Psychiatry.
30. Katz PP, Yelin EH (2001) Activity loss and the onset of depressive symptoms: do some activities matter more than others? Arthritis Rheum 44: 1194–1202.
31. Peck JR, Smith TW, Ward JR, Milano R (1989) Disability and depression in rheumatoid arthritis. A multi-trait, multi-method investigation. Arthritis Rheum 32: 1100–1106.
32. Hassett AL, Aquino JK, Ilgen MA (2014) The risk of suicide mortality in chronic pain patients. Curr Pain Headache Rep 18: 436.
33. Hooley JM, Franklin JC, Nock MK (2014) Chronic pain and suicide: understanding the association. Curr Pain Headache Rep 18: 435.
34. Li JX (2014) Pain and depression comorbidity: A preclinical perspective. Behav Brain Res.
35. Manavathongchai S, Bian A, Rho YH, Oeser A, Solus JF, et al. (2013) Inflammation and hypertension in rheumatoid arthritis. J Rheumatol 40: 1806–1811.
36. Su CC, Chen Ie C, Young FN, Lian Ie B (2013) Risk of diabetes in patients with rheumatoid arthritis: a 12-year retrospective cohort study. J Rheumatol 40: 1513–1518.
37. Nicola PJ, Maradit-Kremers H, Roger VL, Jacobsen SJ, Crowson CS, et al. (2005) The risk of congestive heart failure in rheumatoid arthritis: a population-based study over 46 years. Arthritis Rheum 52: 412–420.
38. Raterman HG, van Halm VP, Voskuyl AE, Simsek S, Dijkmans BA, et al. (2008) Rheumatoid arthritis is associated with a high prevalence of hypothyroidism that amplifies its cardiovascular risk. Ann Rheum Dis 67: 229–232.
39. Wolfe F, Freundlich B, Straus WL (2003) Increase in cardiovascular and cerebrovascular disease prevalence in rheumatoid arthritis. J Rheumatol 30: 36–40.
40. Johansen A, Holmen J, Stewart R, Bjerkeset O (2012) Anxiety and depression symptoms in arterial hypertension: the influence of antihypertensive treatment. the HUNT study, Norway. Eur J Epidemiol 27: 63–72.
41. Freedland KE, Rich MW, Skala JA, Carney RM, Davila-Roman VG, et al. (2003) Prevalence of depression in hospitalized patients with congestive heart failure. Psychosom Med 65: 119–128.
42. Gothe F, Enache D, Wahlund LO, Winblad B, Crisby M, et al. (2012) Cerebrovascular diseases and depression: epidemiology, mechanisms and treatment. Panminerva Med 54: 161–170.
43. Guimaraes JM, de Souza Lopes C, Baima J, Sichieri R (2009) Depression symptoms and hypothyroidism in a population-based study of middle-aged Brazilian women. J Affect Disord 117: 120–123.
44. Pollard L, Choy EH, Scott DL (2005) The consequences of rheumatoid arthritis: quality of life measures in the individual patient. Clin Exp Rheumatol 23: S43–52.
45. Sheehy C, Murphy E, Barry M (2006) Depression in rheumatoid arthritis–underscoring the problem. Rheumatology (Oxford) 45: 1325–1327.
46. Pinho de Oliveira Ribeiro N, Rafael de Mello Schier A, Ornelas AC, Pinho de Oliveira CM, Nardi AE, et al. (2013) Anxiety, depression and suicidal ideation in patients with rheumatoid arthritis in use of methotrexate, hydroxychloroquine, leflunomide and biological drugs. Compr Psychiatry 54: 1185–1189.
47. Dickens C, Creed F (2001) The burden of depression in patients with rheumatoid arthritis. Rheumatology (Oxford) 40: 1327–1330.
48. Ramjeet J, Koutantji M, Barrett EM, Scott DG (2005) Coping and psychological adjustment in recent-onset inflammatory polyarthritis: the role of gender and age. Rheumatology (Oxford) 44: 1166–1168.
49. Covic T, Adamson B, Spencer D, Howe G (2003) A biopsychosocial model of pain and depression in rheumatoid arthritis: a 12-month longitudinal study. Rheumatology (Oxford) 42: 1287–1294.
50. Curtis R, Groarke A, Coughlan R, Gsel A (2005) Psychological stress as a predictor of psychological adjustment and health status in patients with rheumatoid arthritis. Patient Educ Couns 59: 192–198.
51. Placidi GP, Boldrini M, Patronelli A, Fiore E, Chiovato L, et al. (1998) Prevalence of psychiatric disorders in thyroid diseased patients. Neuropsychobiology 38: 222–225.
52. Kathol RG, Turner R, Delahunt J (1986) Depression and anxiety associated with hyperthyroidism: response to antithyroid therapy. Psychosomatics 27: 501–505.
53. Musselman DL, Nemeroff CB (1996) Depression and endocrine disorders: focus on the thyroid and adrenal system. Br J Psychiatry Suppl: 123–128.
54. Demet MM, Ozmen B, Deveci A, Boyvada S, Adiguzel H, et al. (2002) Depression and anxiety in hyperthyroidism. Arch Med Res 33: 552–556.
55. Lee H, Roh HS, Yoon JS, Lee SY (2010) Assessment of quality of life and depression in Korean patients with Graves' ophthalmopathy. Korean J Ophthalmol 24: 65–72.
56. Kaur G, Tee GH, Ariaratnam S, Krishnapillai AS, China K (2013) Depression, anxiety and stress symptoms among diabetics in Malaysia: a cross sectional study in an urban primary care setting. BMC Fam Pract 14: 69.
57. Tenev VT, Robinson RG, Jorge RE (2009) Is family history of depression a risk factor for poststroke depression? Meta-analysis. Am J Geriatr Psychiatry 17: 276–280.
58. Psaltopoulou T, Sergentanis TN, Panagiotakos DB, Sergentanis IN, Kosti R, et al. (2013) Mediterranean diet and stroke, cognitive impairment, depression: A meta-analysis. Ann Neurol.
59. Becofsky K, Baruth M, Wilcox S (2013) Physical functioning, perceived disability, and depressive symptoms in adults with arthritis. Arthritis 2013: 525761.
60. Monroe SM, Slavich GM, Gotlib IH (2013) Life stress and family history for depression: The moderating role of past depressive episodes. J Psychiatr Res.
61. Chuang CH, Cattoi AL, McCall-Hosenfeld JS, Camacho F, Dyer AM, et al. (2012) Longitudinal association of intimate partner violence and depressive symptoms. Ment Health Fam Med 9: 107–114.
62. Heim C, Newport DJ, Mletzko T, Miller AH, Nemeroff CB (2008) The link between childhood trauma and depression: insights from HPA axis studies in humans. Psychoneuroendocrinology 33: 693–710.
63. Vilhjalmsson R (1993) Life stress, social support and clinical depression: a reanalysis of the literature. Soc Sci Med 37: 331–342.

Income Inequality, Socioeconomic Deprivation and Depressive Symptoms among Older Adults

Julián Alfredo Fernández-Niño[1], Betty Soledad Manrique-Espinoza[1]*, Ietza Bojorquez-Chapela[2], Aarón Salinas-Rodríguez[1]

1 Center for Evaluation Research and Surveys, National Institute of Public Health, Cuernavaca, Morelos, Mexico, 2 Department of Population Studies, El Colegio de la Frontera Norte, Tijuana, Baja California, Mexico

Abstract

Objective: Depression is the second most common mental disorder in older adults (OA) worldwide. The ways in which depression is influenced by the social determinants of health – specifically, by socioeconomic deprivation, income inequality and social capital - have been analyzed with only partially conclusive results thus far. The objective of our study was to estimate the association of income inequality and socioeconomic deprivation at the locality, municipal and state levels with the prevalence of depressive symptoms among OA in Mexico.

Methods: Cross-sectional study based on a nationally representative sample of 8,874 OA aged 60 and over. We applied the brief seven-item version of the Center for Epidemiologic Studies Depression Scale (CES-D) to determine the presence of depressive symptoms. Additionally, to select the principal context variables, we used the Deprivation Index of the National Population Council of Mexico at the locality, municipal and state levels, and the Gini Index at the municipal and state levels. Finally, we estimated the association of income inequality and socioeconomic deprivation with the presence of depressive symptoms using a multilevel logistic regression model.

Results: Socioeconomic deprivation at the locality ($OR = 1.28$; $p<0.10$) and municipal levels ($OR = 1.16$; $p<0.01$) correlated significantly with the presence of depressive symptoms, while income inequality did not.

Conclusions: The results of our study confirm that the social determinants of health are relevant to the mental health of OA. Further research is required, however, to identify which are the specific socioeconomic deprivation components at the locality and municipal levels that correlate with depression in this population group.

Editor: Jerson Laks, Federal University of Rio de Janeiro, Brazil

Funding: These authors have no support or funding to report.

Competing Interests: The authors have declared that no competing interests exist.

* Email: bmanrique@insp.mx

Introduction

The study of depression in older adults (OA) has acquired critical importance in that it ranks as the second most common mental disorder worldwide, surpassed only by dementia [1]. According to estimates, by 2030, depression will have escalated to first place in the global burden of disease, accounting for 6% of the total disability-adjusted life years [2]. Current prevalence of clinical depression among OA fluctuates between 1% and 9% [1], exerting a high impact on quality of life, perception of health, functionality, occurrence of comorbidity and economic productivity [1].

In 2005, prevalence of clinical depression in Mexico was estimated at 5% and 9.5% among men and women, respectively [3]. Alongside major clinical depression, depressive symptoms [4] have drawn considerable attention from public health initiatives. While they share a number of probable etiological explanations with clinical depression [5–6] and have been directly associated with mortality and suicide in this age group [6–7], it is estimated that their prevalence may eventually affect four times as many individuals as clinical depression [8]. In the case of Mexico, the prevalence of subclinical depression in OA over 65 years, using the Geriatric Examination for Computer Assisted Taxonomy (GMS–AGECA), was estimated at 31.9% and 32.2% in urban and rural areas, respectively, which is more than twice that the estimated prevalence using DSM-IV or ICD-10 criteria [9].

It has been amply documented that the social determinants of health (mainly contextual poverty, income inequality and social cohesion across the social organization – from the neighborhood up to the national level-) play a prominent role in a wide array of health outcomes, including maternal and child mortality, cardiovascular disease and infectious diseases [10]. However, only recently has research recognized the impact of social determinants on mental health indicators, particularly on depression [11].

According to the ecosocial theory, the health-disease process is part of a hierarchical system where causal interactions flow organically across organization levels [12] and in consequence, social influences become literally "embodied" into individuals [13]. Kim has recently adapted this model to analyze the etiology of the depression [14] by organizing the individual and contextual factors hierarchically under an explanatory model. By interweaving the two, Kim's perspective now makes it possible to understand depression as an interaction between the social context and individual susceptibility [12,14].

Various studies have analyzed the individual and contextual aspects of depression across a variety of OA populations, with the literature identifying the following risk factors: being female, mourning as a result of a significant life event, especially the loss of a partner, functional limitations, existence of a prior depressive episode, physical pain, presence of other pathologies, an inadequate social support network, a low educational level, living alone, social isolation, a perception of being inadequately cared for, limited access to health services and, especially, a precarious economic situation [1,15–18]. On the other hand, with regard to contextual factors, it has been observed that socioeconomic disadvantage and, in general, different measures of poverty and deprivation regarding the place of residence (neighborhood, community or locality) correlate with depression in adults overall and, particularly, in OA [14].

It has been advanced that, in general, economically precarious contexts tend to generate hostile social environments (marked by insecurity and few suitable areas for recreation) [19–21], thus heightening exposure to everyday risks. In turn, these conditions are known to breed psychosocial stress, depleted social capital, limited access to resources and low-quality health services, all of which interact with individual susceptibility as catalysts of depression [14,19–21].

Acknowledging that the different levels of contextual conditions are relevant to depression not only expands the explanatory framework for this disorder by incorporating the role of social determinants, but also provides evidence for creating interventions that transcend the individual realm. The objective of this study was to estimate the association of income inequality and socioeconomic deprivation at place of residence with the occurrence of depressive symptoms in OA aged 60 and over in Mexico.

Methods

Ethics statement

The sample for our work was derived from the National Health and Nutrition Survey (ENSANUT -for its initials in Spanish). This survey was approved by the Ethics and Research Committees of the National Institute of Public Health. All subjects provided written informed consent.

Sample

ENSANUT 2012 was a probabilistic multi-phase survey conducted in Mexico in 2012 with national and state-level representativeness and a geographic breakdown by urban-rural strata. The total sample consisted of 55,008 households throughout Mexico, with only one adult aged 20 and over selected from each household to respond to an individual questionnaire. Out of the total 46,277 adults in this age bracket, 8,874 OA ages 60 and over constituted the analytical sample of our study. The survey design was developed to obtained representativeness for this age group at the national level. Therefore, this sample is representative of the overall older adult population in Mexico. A detailed description of the methodology and design of ENSANUT-2012 has been published elsewhere [22].

Data collection instruments

ENSANUT 2012 was based on two key components: nutrition and health. The latter was probed with three individual-level questionnaires involving: age groups (children aged 9 and under, adolescents from 10 to 19, and adults aged 20 and over), health service utilization, and households. We extracted the data for our study from the individual-level questionnaire for adults aged 20 and over, and the household questionnaire. The first included the following sections: sociodemographic characteristics, self-esteem and satisfaction, overweight and obesity, principal morbidities (high blood pressure, diabetes, cardiovascular disease and hypercholesterolemia), family health history, reproductive health, immunization, preventive programs, accidents, aggression and violence, and risk factors. Additionally, this questionnaire included a module for OA aged 60 and over with the following sections: cognitive status, sight and hearing impairments, functionality, depression and falls [22]. On the other hand, the household questionnaire explored sociodemographic characteristics of all household members, health service utilization, physical housing characteristics, assets and goods, expenditures, and social protection in health.

Variables

Outcome: Depressive symptoms. To measure this variable, we used the brief seven-item version of the Center for Epidemiologic Studies Depression Scale [CES-D]. The Scale covers five dimensions: dysphoric mood, motivation, concentration, loss of pleasure, and sleep disturbance [23] and it has been previously validated in Mexico [24]. The presence of clinically significant depressive symptoms was operationalized according to the total CES-D score, and a dichotomous variable was constructed where 1 (CES-D$\geq$5) indicates the presence of significant symptoms [24].

Context variables: As principal exposure variables, we considered income inequality and socioeconomic deprivation in the localities, municipalities and states where OA resided.

Income inequality. We quantified this variable using the Gini coefficient derived from the Lorenz curves [25]. As a measure of statistical dispersion for income distribution of a nation's residents, the coefficient is expressed as a number between 0 and 1, where 0 indicates perfect equality (everyone receives equal incomes), and 1, total inequality (one person receives all the incomes while the others receive none) [25]. We constructed the Gini coefficient with data from the Population and Housing Census 2010 enlarged sample, which is representative of the 2,456 municipalities in Mexico [26]. The extended questionnaire used in this sample contained the following sections: fertility, child mortality, migration, indigenous language, disability, education, health services, marital status, housing characteristics and public services, household members, and economic characteristics. With regard to the last section, respondents were asked about their total household income in the previous month, in Mexican pesos. This household-specific variable served to construct the Gini coefficient for each municipality and state in Mexico using the *ineqdeco* routine developed by Jenkins for STATA 12 [27], and in which is used the following expression:

$$1+\left(\frac{1}{n}\right)-\frac{2}{m*n^2}\left[\sum\left[n-r_i+1\right]y_i\right]$$

where n is the sample size for each group, m the arithmetic mean of incomes, r_i the rank-ordered income values for each household, and y_i the income value for each household.

Inequality indices estimated by this method have been widely used in the literature [28]. Sen [29] and Jenkins [30] provide some empirical illustrations with this same approach.

Socioeconomic deprivation. To measure this variable, we used the Mexican National Population Council (*CONAPO* for its initials in Spanish) Deprivation Index adjusted to 2010. Broadly validated and utilized in Mexico [31], this measurement groups a series of socioeconomic indicators (eight under a locality index and nine under a municipal and state index) into four major socioeconomic deprivation dimensions (plus a rurality indicator for municipalities and states). These, in turn, are estimated in three levels of geographic aggregation: by locality, municipal and state. The locality dimensions are: education (percentage of illiterate individuals aged 15 and above who lack elementary school), household (percentage of households with any level of overcrowding, earth floors, and no drainage, sanitary services, piped water or electricity), and work-related income (percentage of individuals earning less than two minimum wages, which equaled approximately 8.67 USD per month in 2010). The municipal and state index also includes a rurality indicator reflecting the percentage of individuals dwelling in localities with fewer than 5,000 inhabitants. Constructed using the principal component analysis, the municipal and state index allows identifying the intensity of deprivation and social exclusion by geographic area, specifically with regard to localities and municipalities/states [32]. The index is continuous, where the higher values denote greater socioeconomic deprivation.

Covariates: We included both -individual and household-specific variables identified by the literature as key factors associated with the occurrence of depressive symptoms in the OA population.

Individual covariates. These included: age, gender, civil status (without a partner = 1, married/cohabited = 0), paid job, schooling (years of formal education), difficulty in performing at least one of the basic activities of daily living under the Katz scale [33], difficulty in performing at least one of the instrumental activities under the Lawton scale [34], number of chronic illnesses (diabetes, high blood pressure, hypercholesterolemia, cardiovascular disease, depression, stroke and cancer), participation in household decision-making, history of any type of physical violence (broadly defined as self-reported health damage resulting from theft, aggression or battery of any type) and accidents (broadly defined as self-reported health damage resulting from an accident of any type in the last 12 months).

Household covariates. To measure the household socioeconomic level, we constructed an asset index with a total of 16 dichotomous [yes/no] variables related to a set of housing characteristics and the ownership of household assets. This index has been widely referred to in the literature and has been validated across a variety of contexts [35–37]. We built our index using a polychoric correlation matrix and the principal component analysis. The first component explained 54% of observed variance in data. The asset index was continuous, with the higher values denoting higher socioeconomic levels. We also included data on OA living arrangements using a dichotomous variable as to whether or not the OA lived alone [1 = yes].

Statistical Analysis

We used exploratory analysis techniques, including graphics (histograms and dispersion/correlation diagrams) and descriptive statistics (means and variances), to examine properties and distributions of outcome and contextual variables. Furthermore, we applied the Mann-Whitney U and chi-square tests to analyze the bivariate association between the outcome and the independent variables (continuous and categorical, respectively). Specifically, during the exploratory analysis, we tested the linearity between the outcome and continuous contextual variables.

During the statistical analysis, we also explored the pertinence of considering the data aggregated by locality, municipality and state. For this purpose, we estimated the Intraclass Correlation Coefficient (ICC) for a three-level model [38]. ICC has two main interpretations: first, the extent to which the explained percentage of variance in the outcome variable was attributable to the different aggregation levels; and second, the extent to which individual-level observations are correlated within each aggregation level. If the observations were independent (ICC = 0), nothing would be gained by incorporating different aggregation levels. Given that the outcome variable was dichotomous, we used a multilevel logistical regression model to analyze its association with the contextual variables (income inequality and socioeconomic deprivation), controlling for covariates. This allowed us to identify any relationships within the different aggregation levels which would otherwise have been biased under other statistical techniques ignoring the hierarchical nature of data. Moreover, unlike other approaches, the multilevel analysis estimates not only the relationship of each variable to the most basic aggregation level, but also the strength of the association among variables at different levels by using terms of interaction among the different levels [38].

We adjusted three consecutive models to analyze the contribution of each aggregate level: (1) one with a random intercept at the locality level; (2) other with random intercepts for localities and municipalities, and (3) the third with random intercepts for localities, municipalities and states. We also compared the performance of the different models using the log-likelihood value, the likelihood ratio test (LRT), and the Akaike Information Criterion [AIC] [39]. Finally, we explored the possibility of having models with random slopes for the continuous contextual variables, and we used the LTR to compare these last models with the first that apply just random intercepts [38]. We used the STATA 12 program (Stata Corporation, College Station, TX, USA) for all our statistical analyses.

Results

Of the 8,874 OA who participated in *ENSANUT* 2012, we excluded those who were unable to respond to the interview personally. The principal reasons for failure to respond were hearing or speech impairment (694 OA) and memory loss (320 OA). The final analytical sample thus consisted of 7,867 OA, of whom 53.4% were female, with an average age of 69.3 years (standard error (S.E). = 0.15) and 6.1 years of formal education (S.E. = 0.11). Finally, 22.3% had difficulty performing at least one of the basic activities of daily living and 18.0% at least one of the instrumental activities.

The prevalence of depressive symptoms was 35.6% (CI95%: 33.8%–37.4%). Table 1 displays the characteristics of the sample according to the presence of depressive symptoms. The following variables showed a significant association with depressive symptoms: female, absence of an intimate partner, paid job, few years of formal education, difficulty in performing basic or instrumental activities of daily living, presence of comorbidity, not being consulted about household decisions, occurrence of violent incidents or accidents in the previous 12 months, living alone, and a low household socioeconomic status ($p<0.05$). The bivariate analysis yielded no statistically significant relationship among the different income inequality levels. The estimated ICC values were: 6.3% (CI95%: 3.9%–9.6%) at the locality level; 4.0% (CI95%: 2.0%–7.7%) at the municipal level, and 1.5% (CI95%: 0.07%–3.3%) at the state level.

Table 2 presents the results of the multilevel logistic regression models. As the exploratory analysis indicated that the household asset and locality deprivation indices were not linearly associated with to the logarithm of odds on the presence of depressive symptoms, both variables were incorporated as tertiles in the regression models. Additionally, we adjusted all models using the locality and municipality population sizes as well as to the percentage of rural population at both levels.

In general, the association of the outcome variable with the individual and household variables was consistent across estimated models, in particular with regard to the following variables: female, absence of an intimate partner, not being consulted on household decisions, few years of schooling, difficulty in performing the basic or instrumental activities of daily living, presence of comorbidities and the tertiles of asset index. In comparing the three estimated models, the third (with random intercepts for the three levels) demonstrated the best fit, not only by the log-likelihood and AIC values, but also and most importantly, by the LRT results.

The third model showed a statistically significant association between the presence of depressive symptoms and the following individual variables: female (OR = 1.37; CI95%:1.23–1.54), absence of an intimate partner (OR = 1.16; CI95%; 1.03–1.32), not being consulted about household decisions (OR = 1.64; CI95%: 1.37–1.97), years of schooling (OR = 0.97; CI95%: 0.95–0.98), presence of multimorbidity (OR = 1.32; CI95%: 1.25–1.38), difficulty in performing at least one instrumental activity of daily living (OR = 1.45; CI95%: 1.26–1.68), difficulty in performing at least one basic activity of daily living (OR = 1.85; CI95%: 1.62–2.10) and self-reported accidents (OR = 1.53; CI95%: 1.26–1.85) or violent incident(s) (OR = 2.41; CI95%: 1.57–3.69) during the previous 12 months. Finally, at the household level, we observed a significant and protective association between the outcome variable and a higher socioeconomic status (OR = 0.79; CI95%: 0.66–0.94, when comparing tertiles 1 and 3).

Regarding the association of the contextual variables with the presence of depressive symptoms, on comparing tertiles 3 versus 1, the association of socioeconomic deprivation index was marginally significant at the locality level (OR = 1.28; $p<0.10$), and significant at the municipality level (OR = 1.16, $p<0.01$). While income inequality showed no association at any of the aggregation levels

Table 1. Sociodemographic characteristics according to the presence of depressive symptoms in the study sample.[‡]

	Depressive symptoms		
	No (n = 5,040)	**Yes (n = 2,827)**	**p-value†**
Individual			
Age (years)	69.27(0.19)	69.24(0.23)	n.s
Gender (Female)	0.49	0.60	***
No current intimate partner	0.35	0.42	***
Paid work	0.29	0.25	**
Years of schooling	6.42(0.15)	5.53(0.14)	***
Difficulty in performing basic activities of daily living	0.13	0.18	***
Difficulty in performing instrumental activities	0.13	0.26	***
No. of chronic illnesses	0.88(0.03)	1.14(0.03)	***
Participation in household decision-making (1 = no).	0.06	0.12	***
Accident in the last 12 months (1 = yes)	0.06	0.09	***
Violence in the last 12 months (1 = yes)	0.01	0.03	***
Household			
Asset index	−0.04 (0.02)	−0.40 (0.03)	***
Older adult lives alone	0.23	0.26	***
Locality			
Deprivation Index	−1.00(0.01)	−0.93(0.01)	***
Municipality			
Deprivation Index	−0.93(0.01)	−0.78(0.02)	***
Income inequality (Gini coefficient)	0.45(0.01)	0.45(0.01)	n.s
State			
Deprivation Index	0.01(0.01)	0.11(0.02)	***
Income inequality (Gini coefficient)	0.45(0.01)	0.45(0.01)	n.s

[‡]Share or mean (standard error].
[†]p values under the chi-square and Mann-Whitney U tests..
*$p<0.10$; **$p<0.05$; ***$p<0.01$.
n.s.: non-significant.

Table 2. Multilevel logistical regression models for the association between the presence of depressive symptoms and contextual variables: income inequality and socioeconomic deprivation‡.

Variables	Model 1			Model 2			Model 3		
	OR†	CI 95%	p	OR	CI 95%	p	OR	CI 95%	p
Individual									
Age (years)	1.00	0.99–1.00	n.s	0.99	0.99–1.00	n.s	0.99	0.99–1.00	n.s
Female gender	1.38	1.23–1.55	***	1.38	1.23–1.54	***	1.37	1.23–1.54	***
No intimate partner	1.16	1.02–1.31	**	1.16	1.02–1.32	**	1.16	1.03–1.32	**
Paid work	0.94	0.83–1.06	n.s	0.94	0.83–1.06	n.s	0.93	0.82–1.06	n.s
Not consulted in household decision-making	1.66	1.39–1.99	***	1.65	1.38–1.98	***	1.64	1.37–1.97	***
Years of Schooling	0.97	0.95–0.98	***	0.97	0.95–0.98	***	0.97	0.95–0.98	***
Number of illnesses	1.32	1.25–1.39	***	1.32	1.26–1.38	***	1.32	1.25–1.38	***
Difficulty in performing instrumental activities	1.45	1.26–1.67	***	1.46	1.26-1-68	***	1.45	1.26–1.68	***
Difficulty in performing basic activities	1.85	1.63–2.11	***	1.85	1.62–2.10	***	1.85	1.62–2.10	***
Accident in the previous 12 months	1.50	1.24–1.82	***	1.50	1.24–1.82	***	1.53	1.26–1.85	***
Violence in the previous 12 months	2.40	1.56–3.67	***	2.30	1.56–3.67	***	2.41	1.57–3.69	***
Household									
Asset index (Reference tercile 1]									
Tercile 2	0.87	0.78–0.97	**	0.87	0.77–0.97	**	0.86	0.77–0.97	**
Tercile 3	0.80	0.67–0.95	**	0.79	0.67–0.95	**	0.79	0.66–0.94	***
Older adult living alone	1.09	0.95–1.26	n.s	1.10	0.95–1.26	n.s	1.10	0.96–1.27	n.s
+ ***Locality***									
Rurality	1.10	0.89–1.36	n.s	1.08	0.88–1.33	n.s	1.06	0.86–1.31	n.s
Deprivation index (Reference tercile 1]									
Tercile 2	1.19	0.98–1.45	*	1.18	0.97–1.44	*	1.15	0.94–1.40	n.s
Tercile 3	1.33	1.02–1.73	**	1.31	1.00–1.70	**	1.28	0.98–1.67	*
Municipality									
Income inequality (Gini Coefficient)	1.68	0.40–7.03	n.s	1.72	0.40–7.52	n.s	1.68	0.37–7.30	n.s
Deprivation index	1.17	1.05–1.30	***	1.16	1.04–1.30	***	1.16	1.04–1.30	***
State level									
Income inequality (Gini coefficient)	0.41	0.03–4.88	n.s	0.49	0.04–6.54	n.s	0.45	0.01–16.14	n.s
Deprivation Index	1.01	0.93–1.09	n.s	1.01	0.93–1.09	n.s	1.00	0.91–1.11	n.s
Variance components									
	Variance	**SE**		**Variance**	**SE**		**Variance**	**SE**	
Locality	0.097	0.037		0.023	0.047		0.021	0.046	
Municipality				0.075	0.038		0.054	0.036	
State level							0.026	0.013	

Table 2. Cont.

Variables	Model 1			Model 2			Model 3		
	OR†	CI 95%	p	OR	CI 95%	p	OR	CI 95%	p
Log-likelihood value	−4745.401			−4743.051			−4738.582		
LRT				4.70 (p<0.05)¥			8.94 (p<0.01)£		
AIC	9542.802			9540.103			9533.164		

‡ Model 1: Random intercept at locality level; random intercepts for localities and municipalities; random intercepts for localities, municipalities and states.
†OR = Odds ratio; CI 95%: 95% Confidence Interval.
¥Model 2 versus Model 1.
£Model 3 versus Model 2.
*p<0.10; **p<0.05; ***p<0.01.
LRT: Likelihood Ratio Test.
AIC: Aikaike Information Criterion.
n.s.: non-significant.
+Mexico is organized politically and administratively into states, which are composed of municipalities, the smallest administrative units in the country. In turn, municipalities are composed of localities, which are defined as "any place occupied by one or more buildings utilized as housing - inhabited or not - and which are designated by a name recognized by law or custom." Rural localities are those with less than 2500 inhabitants and which are not municipal centers. Source: National Geostatistical Framework 2010. National Institute of Statistics, Geography and Data Processing.

analyzed (locality, municipality or state). Furthermore, no evidence was found to support the use of random slopes at either the municipality (LRT = 0.10; p = 0.99) or the state (LRT = 0.22; p = 0.89) levels.

Discussion

In line with other recent studies on OA, we found significant association between the presence of depressive symptoms and a number of variables at the individual level, in particular: female [17,40–43], absence of an intimate partner [17,41–43], a low educational level or illiteracy [17,41–42], lack of empowerment in household decision-making (especially with regard to financial matters) [43–44], disability or functional limitations [40–41], presence of comorbidity [40–43], and chronic exposure to psychosocial stress [42]. The latter could be an important factor in the strong connection we found between depressive symptoms and self-reported incidents of physical violence or accidents in the previous 12 months. This is consistent with a recent Brazilian study [45], which found a strong association between exposure to violent, traumatic events and the prevalence of various psychiatric disorders, including major clinical depression. Other studies have established an association between a low socioeconomic status at either the individual or household level and depression among OA [15–17,43–48].

Our principal finding was a strong link between the presence of depressive symptoms and socioeconomic deprivation at both the locality and municipality levels. Other studies have reported such a link at even more immediate aggregation levels, namely, the neighborhood [49–55]. In this regard, a recent theoretical framework for exploring the role of the social context has suggested that the highly adverse social conditions in the areas immersed in steepest socioeconomic deprivation –specifically, crime and restricted access to resources of all sorts, such as nutritional diversity, an adequate physical environment and health care– erode interpersonal relationships and social capital, interacting with individual susceptibility to heighten the risk of depression [14]. This explanatory framework could well apply to higher-level conditions, such as those characterizing the localities [43] and municipalities inhabited by our sample of OA.

The link between socioeconomic deprivation at the locality level and the presence of depressive symptoms in Mexico has already been described. OA living in deprived environments routinely confront more adverse conditions leading to feelings of impotence and hopelessness, both, recognized factors in depression [43]. Multilevel analyses in Belgium [56] and Japan [57] have reported connections between socioeconomic deprivation and depression in OA at the municipality level, while another work has correlated poverty and depression in the United States at the county level [58]. While clearly recognizing the importance of the individual-level factors identified in this study, we emphasize the need to comprehend the impact of socioeconomic disadvantages at place of residence as a critical social determinant of depression in OA.

The association found by other studies between income inequality and the presence of depressive symptoms at the state level was not encountered in our work [59]. The failure of this and other studies to find this association may stem from the fact that income inequality and socioeconomic deprivation have separate causal pathways. While socioeconomic deprivation mainly refers to the material conditions of the environment and access to various social services, income inequality is a more complex social determinant because it refers to not only the deficit but also the social distribution of available resources and the social consequences of the inequality [59].

In consequence, the effect of the first determinant would be more direct, as suggested in the Kim model [14]; while, in contrast, the effect of socioeconomic marginalization on mental health could be explained by more indirect etiologies, such as the ecological effects of social disorganization [59]. In one of the most explored theoretical models, inequality generates social corrosion, corruption and alterations in social capital, thereby creating a hostile social environment, which produces a risk to overall health, including mental health [60]. However, these pathways have not been fully elucidated and, therefore, this constitutes a promising field of research. In addition, its associations reported for this determinant vary by level and tend to be particularly salient at the aggregation levels most proximate to the event being studied.

The findings of this work can be clearly understood under the theory of the social determinants of health, particularly under the ecosocial theory [12]. The social context - measured in our study by socioeconomic deprivation at the locality and municipal levels - is a fundamental factor in the incidence of numerous chronic illnesses, such as cardiovascular disease, obesity, cancer and infant mortality [19,61]. In our work, locality and municipal level deprivation is a multidimensional construct indicative of restricted access to essential public services, such as education, housing and income, which, in turn, can be important determinants of health outcomes. Disaggregating the potential impact of the deprivation index on the presence of depressive symptoms in OA at the municipal level would probably provide more conclusive data, given that, as a summary indicator, the deprivation index simultaneously reflects the combined association of numerous interrelated social determinants –social capital, physical environment and violence - that are also known to exert an impact on depressive symptoms [40,43,49]. In fact, alternative contextual variables incorporated into our secondary analyses –homicide rates, levels of health coverage, criminality indicators, and government spending at the municipality and locality levels– revealed no significant association with the presence of depressive symptoms. On the other hand, the multidimensional character of the index may precisely constitute its strength, since it expands the conceptual horizon to encompass a host of interlocking associations, including that of depression and socioeconomic deprivation at the locality and municipal levels.

The results of our study suggest that the current public health approach to depression needs to be expanded. Policy makers might consider that transforming the social environment and generating economic development in the poorest areas could be important strategies that would have both a multidimensional impact on health promotion and protect OA from the social risks to mental health. Additionally, providing some resources in the immediate environment– such as access to health services and recreational and social support – would strengthen the individual resilience of OA to mental disorders [14].

This study has several limitations. One is related with its cross-sectional design, which does not permit drawing firm conclusion about causal associations. Our findings are thus limited to suggesting potential connections requiring more in-depth analysis in subsequent studies. Another limitation derives from the different timing of the various measurements, with the contextual and individual/household measurements conducted in 2010 and 2012, respectively. Nonetheless, it can be expected that, on the one hand, relative differences in the deprivation index would hold for two years, and most importantly, on the other, a potential effect at the municipal level would correlate more with prolonged exposure to socioeconomic deprivation than with a simultaneous event. A final weakness in our study is the fact that, due to lack of information, we were unable to explore other important factors in OA depression, such as significant life events and social networks, which have been recognized as crucial in the etiology of depression.

Conclusions

The results of this study suggest that deprivation at the municipal and locality levels is associated with depressive symptoms, thus inviting proposals for comprehensive public policy actions that view the problem of depression in older adults also as an expression or symptom of more generalized social malaise. Evidence on the role of socioeconomic deprivation will gain scientific and political importance only to the extent that epidemiologic findings translate into a transformation of the social systems [62]. Recognizing that poverty at the municipal and locality levels impacts the health of older adults should galvanize our society to undertake the profound changes required in the social structure.

Author Contributions

Conceived and designed the experiments: JAF BSM AS. Performed the experiments: JAF BSM AS. Analyzed the data: JAF BSM AS. Contributed reagents/materials/analysis tools: BSM IB AS. Wrote the paper: JAF BSM IB AS.

References

1. Rodda J, Walker Z, Carter J (2011) Depression in older adults. BMJ 343: d5219.
2. Mathers C, Fat DM, Boerma JT (2008) The global burden of disease: 2004 update. Geneva: World Health Organization.
3. Bello M, Puentes-Rosas E, Medina-Mora ME, Lozano R (2005) Prevalencia y diagnóstico de depresión en población adulta en México. Salud Pública Mex 47: S4–S11.
4. American Psychiatric Association (2000) Task Force on D-I. Diagnostic and statistical manual of mental disorders: DSM-IV-TR. Washington, DC: American Psychiatric Association.
5. Wancata J, Friedrich F (2011) Depression: a diagnosis aptly used?. Psychiatr Danub 23:406-411.
6. Chapman DP, Perry GS (2008) Depression as a major component of public health for older adults. Prev Chronic Dis 5. Avalaible: http://www.cdc.gov/pcd/issues/2008/jan/07_0150.htm. Accessed 2014 Mar 25.
7. Cho HJ, Lavretsky H, Olmstead R, Levin M, Oxman MN, et al. (2010) Prior depression history and deterioration of physical health in community-dwelling older adults: A prospective cohort study. American J Geriatr Psychiatry 18: 442–451.
8. Urbina JR, Florez JM, García MP, Torres L, Torrubias RM (2007) Depressive symptoms in the eldery. Prevalence and associtated factors. Gac Sanit 21: 37–42.
9. Guerra M, Ferri CP, Sosa AL, Salas A, Gaona C, et al. (2009) Late-life depression in Peru, Mexico and Venezuela: the 10/66 population-based study. Br J Psychiatry 195:510–515.
10. Wilkinson RG (1997) Income, inequality and social cohesion. Am J Public Health 87: 104–106.
11. Fisher M, Baum F (2010) The social determinants of mental health: implications for research and health promotion. Aust N Z J Psychiatry 44: 1057–1063.
12. Krieger N (2001) New theories for social epidemiology in the 21st century: an eco-social perspective. Int J Epidemiol 30:668–677.
13. Krieger N (2005) Embodiment: a conceptual glossary for epidemiology. J Epidemiol Community Health 59:350–355.
14. Kim D (2008) Blues from the Neighborhood? Neighborhood Characteristics and Depression. Epidemiol Rev 30:101–117.
15. Lue BH, Chen LJ, Wu SC (2010) Health, financial stresses, and life satisfaction affecting late-life depression among older adults: a nationwide, longitudinal survey in Taiwan. Arch Gerontol Geriatr 50:S34–S38.
16. Koster A, Bosma H, Kempen GI, Penninx BW, Beekman AT, et al. (2006) Socioeconomic differences in incident depression in older adults: The role of psychosocial factors, physical health status, and behavioral factors. J Psychosom Res 61:619–627.
17. Li N, Pang L, Chen G, Song X, Zhang J, et al. (2011) Risk factors for depression in older adults in Beijing. Can J Psychiatry 56:466–473.
18. Juhasz G, Eszlari N, Pap D, Gonda X (2012) Cultural differences in the development and characteristics of depression. Neuropsychopharmacol Hung 14:259–265.

19. Link BG, Phelan J (1995) Social conditions as fundamental causes of disease. J Health Soc Behav 1:80–94.
20. Wilkinson R, Marmot M (2003) Social determinants of health: the solid facts. Oxford: Oxford University Press. 31 p.
21. Rose G (2001) Sick individual and sick population. Am J Epidemiol 30:417–432.
22. Romero-Martínez M, Shamah-Levy T, Franco-Núñez A, Villalpando S, Cuevas-Nasu, et al. (2013) Encuesta Nacional de Salud y Nutrición 2012: diseño y cobertura. Salud Pública Mex 55: S332–S340.
23. Herrero J, Gracia E (2007) Una Medida Breve de la Sintomatología Depresiva (CESD-7). Salud Mental 30:40–46.
24. Salinas-Rodríguez A, Manrique-Espinoza B, Acosta-Castillo I, Franco-Núñez A, Rosas-Carrasco O, et al. (2014) Validación de un punto de corte para la versión breve de la Escala de Depresión del Centro de Estudios Epidemiológicos en adultos mayores mexicanos. Salud Pública Mex 56:279–285.
25. Farris FA (2010) The gini index and measures of inequality. Am Math Mon 117: 851–864.
26. Instituto Nacional de demografía y estadística (2010) Diseño de la muestra censal. México DF: Instituto Nacional de demografía y estadística.
27. Jenkins SP (2006) Estimation and interpretation of measures of inequality, poverty, and social welfare using Stata. Presentation at North American Stata Users' Group Meetings, Boston MA.
28. Atkinson AB (1970) On the measurement of inequality. J Econ Theory 2: 244–263.
29. Sen AK (1976) Real national income. Rev Econ Stud 43: 19–39.
30. Jenkins SP (1997) Trends in real income in Britain: a microeconomic analysis. Empirical Economics 22: 483–500.
31. Almejo R, Téllez Y, López J (2010) Índices absoluto de Marginación 2000–2010. México DF: Consejo Nacional de Población.
32. Anzaldo C, Prado M (2010) Índices de marginación 2010. México DF: Consejo Nacional de Población.
33. Katz S, Branch LG, Branson MH, Papsidero JA, Beck JC, et al. (1983) Active life expectancy. N Engl J Med 309:1218–1224.
34. Lawton MP, Brody EM (1969) Assessment of older people: self-maintaining and instrumental activities of daily living. Gerontologist 9:179–186.
35. Booysen F, van der Berg AE, Burger R, von Maltitz M, du Rand G (2008) Using an Asset Index to Assess Trends in Poverty in Seven Sub-Saharan African Countries. World Development 36:1113–1130.
36. Filmer D, Pritchett L (1998) Estimating wealth effects without expenditure data – or tears: An application to educational enrollments in states of India. In: World Bank Policy Research Working Paper No. 1994. Washington DC: World Bank.
37. Moser C (2008) Assets and livelihoods: a framework for asset-based social policy. In: Moser C, Anis D, eds. Assets, livelihoods, and social policy. Washington DC: The World Bank.
38. Snijders T, Bosker R (2012) Multilevel Analysis. An introduction to basic and advanced multilevel modeling. Oxford: SAGE Publications Ltda.
39. Akaike H (1974) A new look at the statistical model identification. IEEE Trans Automat Contr 19: 716–723.
40. Millán-Calentí JC, Sánchez A, Lorenzo T, Maseda A (2012) Depressive symptoms and other factors associated with poor self-rated health in the elderly: Gender differences. Geriatr Gerontol Int 12: 198–206.
41. Arslantas D, Unsal A, Ozbabalik D (2013) Prevalence of depression and associated risk factors among the elderly in Middle Anatolia. Turkey Geriatr Gerontol Int 14: 100-108.
42. Munhoz TM, Santos IS, Matijasevich I (2013) Major depressive episode among Brazilian adults: A cross sectional population-base study. J Affect Disord 150:401–407.
43. Bojorquez-Chapela I, Manrique-Espinoza BS, Mejia-Arango S, Téllez-Rojo MM, Salinas-Rodríguez A (2012) Effect of social capital and personal autonomy on the presence of depressive symptoms in the elderly: Evidence from a longitudinal study in Mexico. Aging Ment Health 16: 462–471.
44. Abe Y, Fujice N, Fukunaga R, Nakagawa Y, Ikeda M (2012) Comparisons of the prevalence of and risk factors for elderly depression between urban and rural populations in Japan. Int Psychogeriatr 24: 1235–1241.
45. Ribeiro WS, Mari JJ, Quintana MI, Dewey ME, Evan-Lacko S, et al. (2013) The impact of epidemic violence on the prevalence of psychiatric disorders in Sao Paulo and Rio de Janeiro, Brazil. PLoS One 8:e63545.
46. Roy K, Chaudhuri A (2008) Influence of socioeconomic status, wealth and financial empowerment on gender differences in health and healthcare utilization in later life: Evidence from India. Soc Sci Med 66: 1951–1962.
47. Bulut S (2009) Late life depression: A literature review of late-life depression and contributing factors. Anales de psicología 25: 21–26.
48. Blazer DG, Hybels CF (2005) Origins of depression in later life. Psychol Med 35: 1241–1252.
49. Ostir GV, Eschbach K, Markides KS, Goodwin JS (2003) Neighbourhood composition and depressive symptoms among older Mexican Americans. J Epidemiol Community Health 57: 987–992.
50. Kubzansky LD, Subramanian SV, Kawachi I, Fay ME, Soobader MJ, et al. (2005) Neighborhood Contextual Influences on Depressive Symptoms in the Elderly. Am J Epidemiol: 162:253-260.
51. Walters K, Breeze E, Wilkinson P, Price GM, Bulpitt CJ, et al. (2004) Local area deprivation and urban-rural differences in anxiety and depression among people older than 75 years in Britain. Am J Public Health 94:1768–1774.
52. Wight RG, Aneshensel CS, Cummings JR, Karlamangla AS (2009) Urban neighborhood context and change in depressive symptoms in late life. J Gerontol Ser B Psychol Sci Soc Sci 64:247–251.
53. Yen Y-C, Rebok GW, Yang M-J, Lung F-W (2008) A multilevel analysis of the influence of Apolipoprotein E genotypes on depressive symptoms in late-life moderated by the environment. Prog Neuropsychopharmacol Biol Psychiatry 32:479–486.
54. Hybels CF, Blazer DG, Pieper CF, Burchett BM, Hays JC, et al. (2006) Sociodemographic characteristics of the neighborhood and depressive symptoms in older adults: using multilevel modeling in geriatric psychiatry. Am J Geriatric psychiatry 14(6):498–506.
55. Menec VH, Shooshtari S, Nowicki S, Fournier S (2010) Does the relationship between neighborhood socioeconomic status and health outcomes persist into very old age? A population-based study. J Aging Health 22:27–47.
56. Patty E, Praag LV, Verhaeghe M, Levecque K, Bracke P (2011) The association between residential area characteristics and mental health outcomes among men and women in Belgium. Arch Public Health 69: 3.
57. Murata C, Kondo K, Hirai H, Ichida Y, Ojima T (2008) Association between depression and socio-economic status among community-dwelling elderly in Japan: the Aichi Gerontological Evaluation Study (AGES). Health Place 1:406–414.
58. Muramatso N (2003) County-Level Income Inequality and Depression among Older Americans. Health Serv Res 38: 1863–1884.
59. Wilkinson RG, Picket KE (2006) Income inequality and population health: A review and explanation of the evidence. Soc Sci Med 62:1768–1784.
60. Idrovo AJ, Ruiz-Rodríguez M, Manzano-Patiño AP (2010) Beyond the income inequality hypothesis and human health: a worldwide exploration. Rev Saude Publica 44:695–702.
61. Davey Smith G, Gunnell D, Ben-Shlomo Y (2001) Poverty, Inequality and Health: An International Perspective. Oxford: eds Leon D, Walt G. pp 88–124.
62. Beckfield J, Krieger N (2009) Epi + demos + cracy: Linking Political Systems and Priorities to the Magnitude of Health Inequities – Evidence, Gaps, and a Research Agenda Epidemiol Rev31: 152–77.

11

Increased Coupling of Intrinsic Networks in Remitted Depressed Youth Predicts Rumination and Cognitive Control

Rachel H. Jacobs[1], Lisanne M. Jenkins[1], Laura B. Gabriel[1], Alyssa Barba[1], Kelly A. Ryan[2], Sara L. Weisenbach[1,2,3,4], Alvaro Verges[1], Amanda M. Baker[2], Amy T. Peters[1], Natania A. Crane[1], Ian H. Gotlib[5], Jon-Kar Zubieta[2,6], K. Luan Phan[1,7,8], Scott A. Langenecker[1,2,6]*, Robert C. Welsh[5,2]

1 Department of Psychiatry, University of Illinois at Chicago, Chicago, Illinois, United States of America, **2** Department of Psychiatry, University of Michigan, Ann Arbor, Michigan, United States of America, **3** Research and Development Program, Jesse Brown VA Medical Center, Chicago, Illinois, United States of America, **4** VA Ann Arbor Healthcare System, Ann Arbor, Michigan, United States of America, **5** Department of Psychology, Stanford University, Stanford, California, United States of America, **6** Department of Radiology, Molecular and Behavioral Neuroscience Institute, Ann Arbor, Michigan, United States of America, **7** Departments of Psychology and Anatomy & Cell Biology, University of Illinois at Chicago, Chicago, Illinois, United States of America, **8** Mental Health Service Line, Jesse Brown VA Medical Center, Chicago, Illinois, United States of America

Abstract

Objective: Functional connectivity MRI (fcMRI) studies of individuals currently diagnosed with major depressive disorder (MDD) document hyperconnectivities within the default mode network (DMN) and between the DMN and salience networks (SN) with regions of the cognitive control network (CCN). Studies of individuals in the remitted state are needed to address whether effects derive from trait, and not state or chronic burden features of MDD.

Method: fcMRI data from two 3.0 Tesla GE scanners were collected from 30 unmedicated (47% medication naïve) youth (aged 18–23, modal depressive episodes = 1, mean age of onset = 16.2, SD = 2.6) with remitted MDD (rMDD; modal years well = 4) and compared with data from 23 healthy controls (HCs) using four bilateral seeds in the DMN and SN (posterior cingulate cortex (PCC), subgenual anterior cingulate (sgACC), and amygdala), followed by voxel-based comparisons of the whole brain.

Results: Compared to HCs, rMDD youth exhibited hyperconnectivities from both PCC and sgACC seeds with lateral, parietal, and frontal regions of the CCN, extending to the dorsal medial wall. A factor analysis reduced extracted data and a PCC factor was inversely correlated with rumination among rMDD youth. Two factors from the sgACC hyperconnectivity clusters were related to performance in cognitive control on a Go/NoGo task, one positively and one inversely.

Conclusions: Findings document hyperconnectivities of the DMN and SN with the CCN (BA 8/10), which were related to rumination and sustained attention. Given these cognitive markers are known predictors of response and relapse, hyperconnectivities may increase relapse risk or represent compensatory mechanisms.

Editor: Daniel Margulies, Max Planck Institute for Human Cognitive and Brain Sciences, Germany

Funding: This study was funded by NIH MH 091811 and NCATS UL1TR000050. The funders had no role in study design, data collection and analysis, decision to publish, or preparation of the manuscript.

Competing Interests: The authors have declared that no competing interests exist.

* Email: slangenecker@psych.uic.edu

Introduction

Studying individuals with a history of major depressive disorder (MDD) who are currently in the remitted state allows for a unique examination of potential trait-based mechanisms of depression and depression relapse (e.g., [1]). As such, phenotypic expressions assessed during remission may represent reliable markers of illness course, offering refined targets for future research among high-risk cohorts. Studying putative mechanisms early in the course of MDD (avoiding the chronic burden of repetitive illness scarring), during the remitted state (avoiding state effects), and towards the end of development (avoiding developmental variability in early adolescence) can provide a clearer understanding of mechanisms in relapse and recurrence given risk for depressive relapse increases as a function of previous episodes [2] and may result in greater neurobiological insults (e.g., [3]). Importantly, mechanisms identified through this approach can inform the development of early detection and primary and secondary prevention programs.

One method for understanding trait-based markers for MDD involves studying network function through measurements of network connectivity. Resting state fMRI has emerged as an approach for the identification of brain-based biomarkers, particularly in the detection of variations in network connectivity deriving from clinical features [4]. Moreover, resting state fMRI has emerged as a useful technique for studying psychiatric populations due to good signal to noise ratios, reduced participant burden, and lends itself to clinical translation [5]. Disrupted network connectivity has been documented among individuals within a major depressive episode (MDE [6,7]). In particular, disturbances in a set of regions including the posterior cingulate cortex (PCC), medial prefrontal cortex (mPFC), and inferior parietal cortex (IPC) have been reported and are hypothesized to contribute to depression [8,9]. These regions are included in a task negative default mode network (DMN), which encompasses regions demonstrating decreases in activation during performance of attention-demanding tasks and corresponding increases in activation during rest, mind-wandering, or during self-reflective thought (for a review see [10]).

In contrast, a task positive network includes regions that increase in activation during attention to demanding tasks [11]. Task positive and task negative networks act in opposition, as they have been shown to be anticorrelated during both cognitive tasks and during the resting state. Two dissociable task positive networks include the Cognitive Control Network (CCN) and salience network (SN; [12]). The SN supports emotion processing and autonomic regulation and incorporates regions such as the dorsal anterior cingulate cortex (dACC) and the orbital frontoinsula [12].

Resting state fMRI examines intrinsic network functioning by capturing temporal correlations between brain regions in the blood oxygen level-dependent (BOLD) signal, offering a reliable [13–15] method to link neural networks to traits that may make an individual vulnerable to relapse. These spontaneous low-frequency (<.1 Hz) fluctuations yield maps of neural systems that make up an individual's functional connectome [16]. The task positive network (SN, CCN) can also be studied during the resting state. Regions of the SN, including the subgenual anterior cingulate cortex (sgACC), have been observed to be hyperconnected at rest among individuals with MDD [7] and low frequency oscillations in resting state networks support biases in information processing [17]. As these networks interact and may even compete with one another to modulate attention to both the external and internal worlds [18], and given that the SN in particular may initiate switching between the CCN and DMN; understanding network functioning during rest will advance the study of MDD. For example, observed deficits in task-related activation among individuals with psychiatric disorders has led to the hypothesis that aberrant connectivity is a core feature of mental illness [19], but the lack of consistency across task-based fMRI experiments has slowed progress towards integrated models of network dysfunction in psychopathology. Aberrant network functioning is likely to underlie and support observable clinical symptoms such as rumination (DMN) and emotional reactivity (SN e.g., [8]) consistent with network models of psychopathology [19].

Increased connectivity within and between networks is hypothesized to contribute to the tendency of depressed individuals to attend to internal stimuli and to return inadvertently to internal thoughts at the expense of external tasks [6,20,21]. Moreover, depressive symptoms including maladaptive levels of internally focused thought have been associated with increased DMN connectivity [22],whereas dysfunction in the SN contributes to biases in emotion processing and autonomic regulation ([23,24], for a review see [25]). Unmedicated adults with MDD demonstrate increased connectivity of the DMN with the SN [6]. In addition, the dorsal medial and dorsal lateral portion of the PFC may represent a nexus in dysfunctional depression-associated connectivity between all three networks [22]. To date; however, the link between connectivity-related abnormalities and clinical and course features remains relatively unexplored with few positive results (but see [21]). Furthermore, only limited work has explored whether these differences exist during periods of remission [26–28]. No studies to date have been conducted with remitted late-adolescent or early adult samples – this developmental epoch may serve as a critical assessment and intervention period of near-complete neural development and network maturation prior to chronic disease progression and sequelae. Finally, investigators have explored preliminary links between network dysfunction, rumination, and cognitive control [29]; however, no studies to date directly link these mechanisms.

Thus, a critical unanswered question is whether abnormal neural connectivities represent trait markers of vulnerability to illness and recurrence that are not related to state or chronic illness scars. To address this issue, we examined functional connectivity among youth in a remitted state. This design mitigates several potential confounds including current mood state, illness severity, increased scar due to repeated episodes, and the effects of current medication. We hypothesized that hyperconnectivities would be observed within and between regions of the DMN and SN with regions of the CCN among unmedicated youth with rMDD compared to Healthy Controls (HCs), reflecting potential trait-based risk for relapse, or conversely resilience. Finally, given preliminary research correlating DMN functional connectivity with repetitive negative thoughts such as rumination (e.g., [21]) as well as evidence that the sgACC contributes to ruminative processes [30], we conducted exploratory analyses testing whether self-report rumination was correlated with aberrant connectivities among rMDD youth. Last, in order to specifically probe the clinical and behavioral correlates of hyperconnectivity with the CCN, we conducted exploratory correlations of connectivity measures with performance on the Parametric Go/No-Go Task [31,32] in light of previous work suggesting inhibitory control predicts course of illness among adults with MDD [33].

Methods

Participants

The current study was approved by the University of Michigan (UM) and the University of Illinois at Chicago (UIC) Institutional Review Boards and all participants signed consent. Participants were recruited using flyers and multiple forms of posting on the internet. All participants completed an identical assessment protocol, including the Diagnostic Interview for Genetic Studies (DIGS; [34]), the Hamilton Depression Scale (Ham-D; [35]), the Parametric Go/No-Go Test [31,32], and the Ruminative Responsiveness Scale (RRS, [36]). Participants were considered remitted from MDD if they previously met criteria for at least one MDE, but currently scored below a 7 on the Ham-D (administered during the phone screen and during the initial diagnostic interview). HCs could not meet current or past criteria (Never Mentally Ill, NMI) for MDD or any other Axis I or II psychiatric disorder and had no first degree relatives with a history of psychiatric illness. In addition, participants were required to be medication free for a period of 30 days prior to the scan and those with substance abuse or dependence within the past six months were excluded. Diagnosis of past MDD or NMI was determined with DIGS, and confirmed using a modified Family Interview for Genetic Studies completed with a parent or guardian [34]. The final sample included 30 rMDD (19 UM, 11 UIC) and 23 healthy controls (HCs; 16 UM, 7 UIC) between the ages of 18–23 years (66% Female). Participant demographics and clinical characteristics are presented in Table 1. Previous treatment history within the

Table 1. Sample Demographics and Clinical Characteristics.

	HC (n = 23)	rMDD (n = 30)
	M (SD)	M (SD)
Age	20.8 (1.6)	21.0 (1.5)
Education	14.9 (1.2)	14.5 (1.4)
HamD*	0.5 (1.1)	4.1 (7.2)
VIQ	109.0 (8.5)	109.7 (9.2)
RRS Total*	29.8 (8.5)	44.4 (15.7)
RRS Brooding*	6.8 (2.1)	9.0 (4.0)
RRS Depression Related*	16.1 (4.7)	25.1 (9.0)
RRS Reflection*	6.9 (2.7)	10.3 (3.9)
Modal Years Well	n/a	4
Modal MDE Episodes	n/a	1
% Medication Naïve	n/a	47%
Age of First Onset	n/a	16.2(2.6)
Age of Most Recent Episode	n/a	18.5(2.2)
Longest MDE Duration (weeks)	n/a	31.8(38.4)
Comorbid Anxiety Diagnosis^	2	8
Modal Number of Psychiatric Hospitalizations	n/a	0

Note. HC = Healthy Control, rMDD = remitted Major Depressive Disorder; M = Mean; SD = Standard Deviation; HamD = Hamilton Depression Rating Scale; VIQ = Verbal IQ; RRS = Ruminative Response Scale; MDE = Major Depressive Episode.
^Specific Phobia was not an exclusion for NMI.

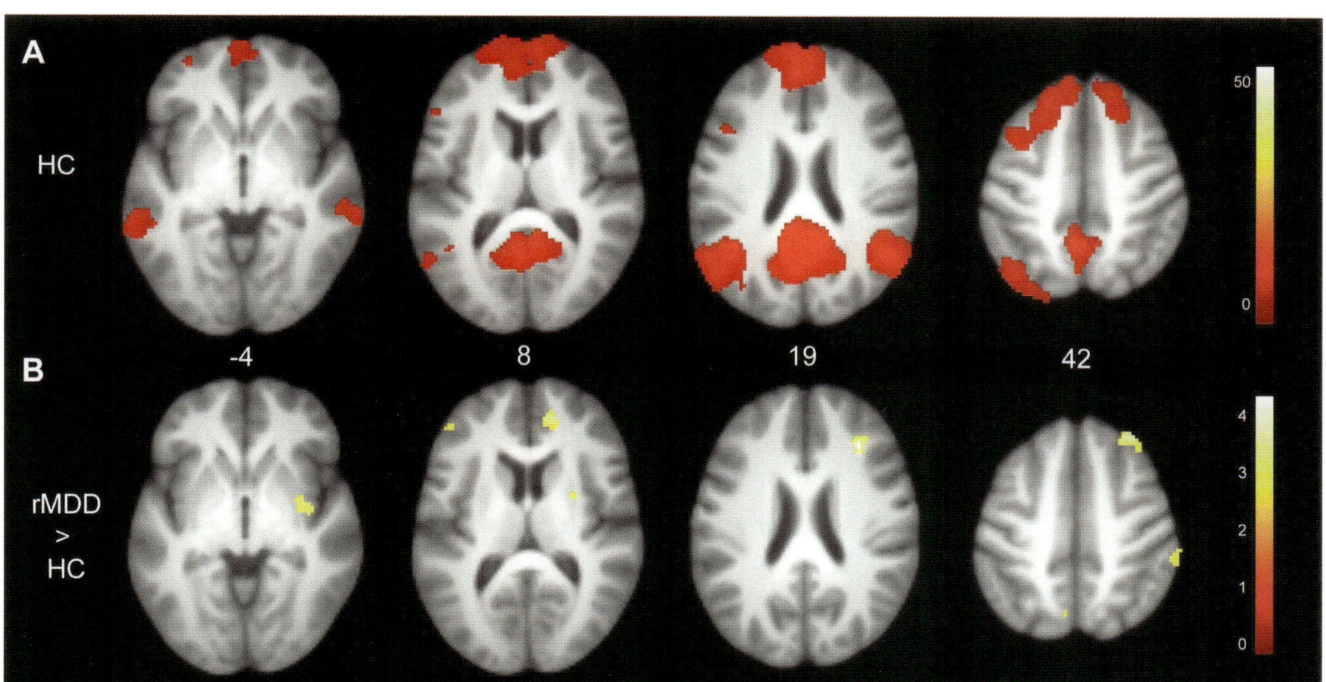

Figure 1. Connectivity of left posterior cingulate seed and between group differences. Panel A: Connectivities among HC youth illustrate the default mode network. Panel B: Youth with remitted depression demonstrated greater connectivity with the right insula, superior and middle frontal gyrus, putamen, angular gyrus, and left middle frontal gyrus.

Table 2. Differences between Healthy Controls and remitted Major Depression for left posterior cingulate seed.

Lobe/region	BA	x	y	z	Z	mm^3	Factor
Frontal							
Superior/Middle frontal	10	12	45	14	3.24	832	PCC 2*
	9	27	24	20	3.85	824	PCC1
	8	26	32	42	3.63	728	PCC 1, 2
Inferior frontal	46	−41	35	12	3.53	688	PCC 1
Parietal							
Precuneus	7	−11	−63	30	3.82	1376	PCC 1
	7	−6	−63	49	3.41	712	PCC 1
Inferior Parietal	40	43	−36	30	3.9	864	PCC 1
Subcortical							
Lentiform nucleus		17	−9	3	3.57	1384	PCC 1

Note. BA = Brodmann's Area; mm = millimeter; PCC = posterior cingulate cortex;
*PCC Factor 2 was significantly inversely correlated with Rumination Total Score, r = −.49, *p* = .03.
x, y, and z coordinates are converted and reported in Talairach space.

rMDD group (data available for n = 19) included medication (n = 13) and psychotherapy (n = 17).

Rumination

Self-report rumination was collected using the Ruminative Response Scale (RRS; [36]). Forty individuals (23 rMDD, 17 HC) completed the RRS. Individuals with scores greater than two standard deviations from the mean were given a truncated score [37]. Correlations were computed between total rumination score and extracted ROI values for regions that differed significantly between groups in seed-based connectivity.

Parametric Go/No-Go

This task (described previously, [31]) was administered to all subjects during cognitive testing prior to the scan to assess sustained attention accuracy (Go Accuracy), context-based inhibition (No-Go Accuracy), and processing speed (Reaction Time, [32]), all aspects of cognitive control. Two outliers (1 HC, 1 rMDD) were given a truncated performance score for Go Accuracy (two SDs, [37]). Exploratory correlations were computed using factors from extracted ROIs with these measures of cognitive control.

fcMRI Acquisition

At UM an eyes-open resting state scan was acquired over eight minutes on a 3.0 T GE Signa scanner (Milwaukee, WI) using T2*-weighted single shot reverse spiral sequence with the following parameters: 90 degree flip, field-of-view 20, matrix size = 64×64, slice thickness = 4 mm, 30 ms echo time, 29 slices. Eyes-open, resting scans at UIC were collected over eight minutes on a 3.0 T GE Discovery scanner (Milwaukee, WI) using parallel imaging with ASSET and T2* gradient-echo axial EPI with the following parameters: 90 degree flip, field-of-view 22, matrix size = 64×64, slice thickness = 3 mm, 22.2 ms echo time, 44 slices. At both sites, high-resolution anatomic T1 scans were obtained for spatial normalization and motion was minimized with foam pads, a visual tracking line (UIC only) and/or cross (UIC and UM) on the display, and by conveying the importance of staying still to participants, with TRs of 2000 ms and 240 TRs total. Site effects of acquisition parameters and scanner were evaluated and are reported in Supplementary Material (Figure S2).

fc-MRI Preprocessing

Several steps were taken to reduce potential sources of noise and artifact. Slice timing was completed with SPM8 (http://www.fil.ion.ucl.ac.uk/spm/doc/) and motion detection algorithms were applied using FSL (http://fsl.fmrib.ox.ac.uk/fsl/fslwiki/). Coregistration of structural images to functional images was followed by spatial normalization of the coregistered T1-spgr to the Montreal Neurological Institute (MNI) template. The resulting normalization matrix was then applied to the slice-time-corrected, physiologically corrected, time series data. These normalized T2* time-series data were spatially smoothed with a 5 mm Gaussian kernel resulting in T2* images with isotropic voxels, 2 mm on a side.

Cross-Correlation Analysis

Time series were detrended and mean centered. Physiologic correction was performed by regressing out white matter and cerebral spinal fluid signals [38]. Motion parameters were regressed out [39]. Based upon the recent literature [39,40], motion volumes were identified based on any TR to TR movement exceeding .5 mm and did not differ between groups (Figure S1) [40]. All significant differences were evaluated with

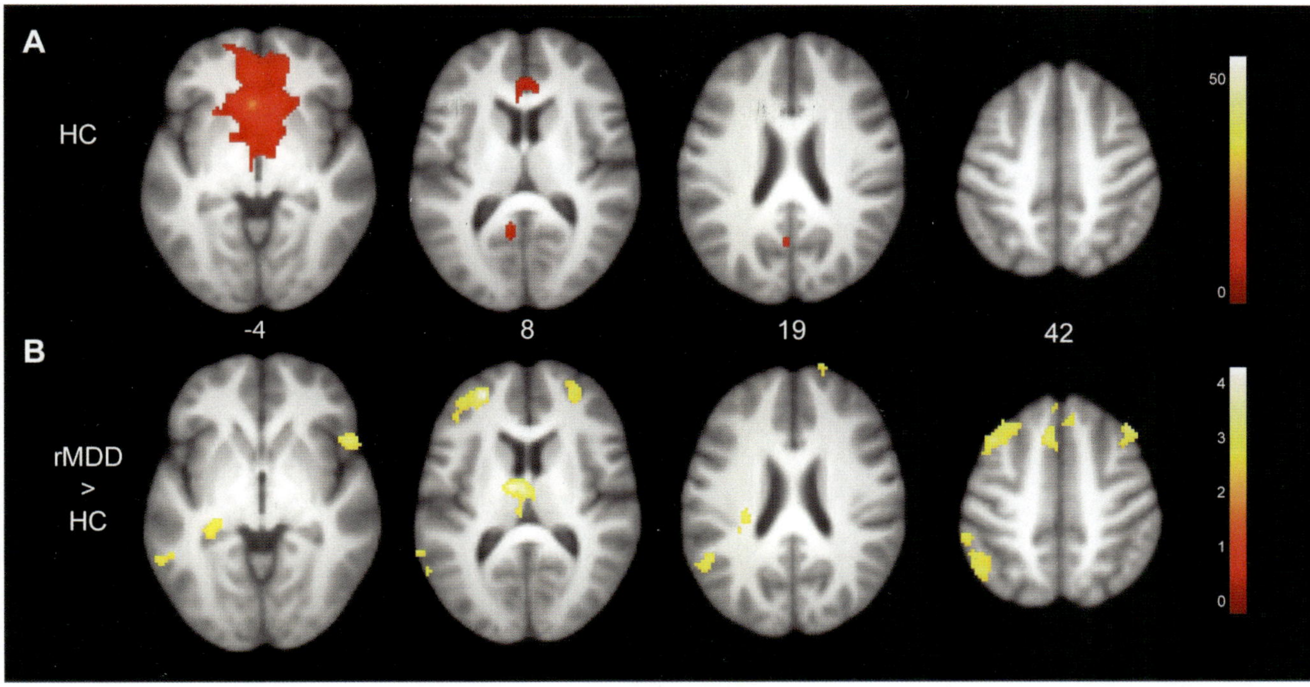

Figure 2. Connectivity of the left subgenual anterior cingulate seed and between group differences. Panel A: Connectivities among HC youth illustrate the salience network. Panel B: Youth with remitted depression demonstrated greater connectivity from the left subgenual anterior cingulate seed to the right anterior inferior frontal gyrus/insula, bilateral medial, superior and middle frontal cortex, thalamus, and left medial temporal gyrus, inferior parietal lobule, and parahippocampal gyrus.

respect to movement, and movement did not influence significant differences identified using the PCC and sgACC seeds. However, connectivities with the left amygdala seed became non-significant after covarying movement measures. Global signal was not regressed due to colinearity violations with gray matter signal, problematic mis-estimates of anticorrelations [41], and because it does not affect distance-micromovement relationships [39]. Finally time series were band-pass filtered over 0.01–0.10 Hz. Seeds were derived based on previous literature examining resting state connectivity of the amygdala [42,43], PCC [44,45], and sgACC [46,47]. The following coordinates were used: PCC (DMN, −5/5, −50, 36), amygdala (SN, −23/23, −5, −19), sgACC (SN, −4/4, 21, −8). Regions of Interest (ROIs; 2.9 mm radius, 19 voxels) were defined in MNI space and spatially averaged time course data were extracted from ROIs for each participant. Seeds were overlaid on the average warped structural anatomy of the current sample and adjusted where necessary.

Correlation coefficients were calculated between mean time course for seed regions and all other voxels of the brain, resulting in a 3-dimensional correlation coefficient image (r image). These r images were transformed to z scores using a Fisher transformation. Resulting z images were used in 2-sample Student t tests implemented in SPM8. AlphaSim was used with 1000 Monte Carlo simulations to determine whole brain correction with a joint threshold of height and extent ($p<.005$, cluster extent of 440 mm^3) for group comparisons with a corrected p value of .05. Images are displayed on an averaged brain anatomy derived from the current sample.

Importantly, movement was addressed using regression of white matter signal as recommended in the recent literature [39,40]. Further, we conducted additional analyses (see Table S3 in File S1 and Figure S1) to fully explore potential (micro) movement confounds. All PCC and sgACC clusters reported remained significant when subjects with any TR to TR movements greater than .5 mm (typically Z displacement) were excluded.

Exploratory Factor Analysis

Factor analysis is a statistical technique that can be used to discover which variables form coherent subsets that are somewhat independent. Factors are hypothesized to reflect underlying processes resulting in correlations between variables. Factor analysis differs from principal components analysis in that factor analysis examines shared variance only and attempts are made to estimate and eliminate variance that derives from error [37]. Factor analysis can be effective in data reduction and may also segregate noise from connectivity signal in fMRI [23]; therefore, exploratory factor analysis was conducted on extracted z values from each cluster of significant differences between groups separately for each seed region. The number of factors retained was determined using maximum likelihood as an extraction method and a threshold of eigenvalue >1, followed by oblique rotation. We also verified that the extracted factors surpassed 50% of total variance.

Results

PCC connectivity

Across groups, the left PCC seed was correlated with regions encompassing the DMN including the medial prefrontal cortex (PFC), posterior and superior temporal gyri, and bilateral hippocampus. Figure 1 illustrates the DMN among HC participants as well as connectivities that were greater among rMDD compared to HC participants. Table 2 details significant differences between groups. Compared to HCs, youth with rMDD demonstrated greater connectivity from the left PCC seed to the right insula and right superior and middle frontal gyrus (BA 9), as

Table 3. Differences between Healthy Controls and remitted Major Depression for left subgenual anterior cingulate seed.

Lobe/region	BA	x	y	z	Z	mm^3	Factor
Frontal							
Superior/Middle frontal	10	10	63	19	3.29	1400	sgACC 1
	8	36	24	41	3.52	2832	sgACC 1
	8	8	32	49	3.72	3664	sgACC 1,2*
	8	−36	16	45	3.58	2240	sgACC 2*
	9	−24	43	13	4.19	1944	sgACC 1,2*
	8	4	45	39	3.54	680	
Inferior frontal	47	43	14	−3	3.36	856	sgACC 2*
Limbic							
Parahippocampus	30	−22	−38	0	3.67	728	sgACC 3*
Temporal							
Inferior Temporal	37	−54	−54	−1	3.71	1536	sgACC 2*
	21	−57	−15	−19	3.51	448	sgACC 2*
Parietal							
Postcentral	3	31	−36	49	3.12	544	sgACC 3*
Angular	39	−43	−65	35	3.81	8392	sgACC 1
Subcortical							
Medial dorsal nucleus		−1	−15	6	4.01	1760	sgACC 3*
Caudate tail		−24	−30	16	3.42	592	sgACC 3*
Cerebellum							
Pyramis		−31	−83	−33	3.89	3936	sgACC 1
Inferior semi-lunar lobule		29	−71	−39	3.56	1088	sgACC 1
		15	−69	−39	3.3	1328	sgACC 1

Note. BA = Brodmann's Area; mm = millimeter; sgACC = subgenual anterior cingulate cortex;
*sgACC Factor 2 was positively correlated with Go Accuracy ($r = .40$, $p = .04$) and sgACC Factor 3 was negatively correlated with No-Go Accuracy ($r = -.44$, $p = .02$).
x, y, and z coordinates are converted and reported in Talairach space.

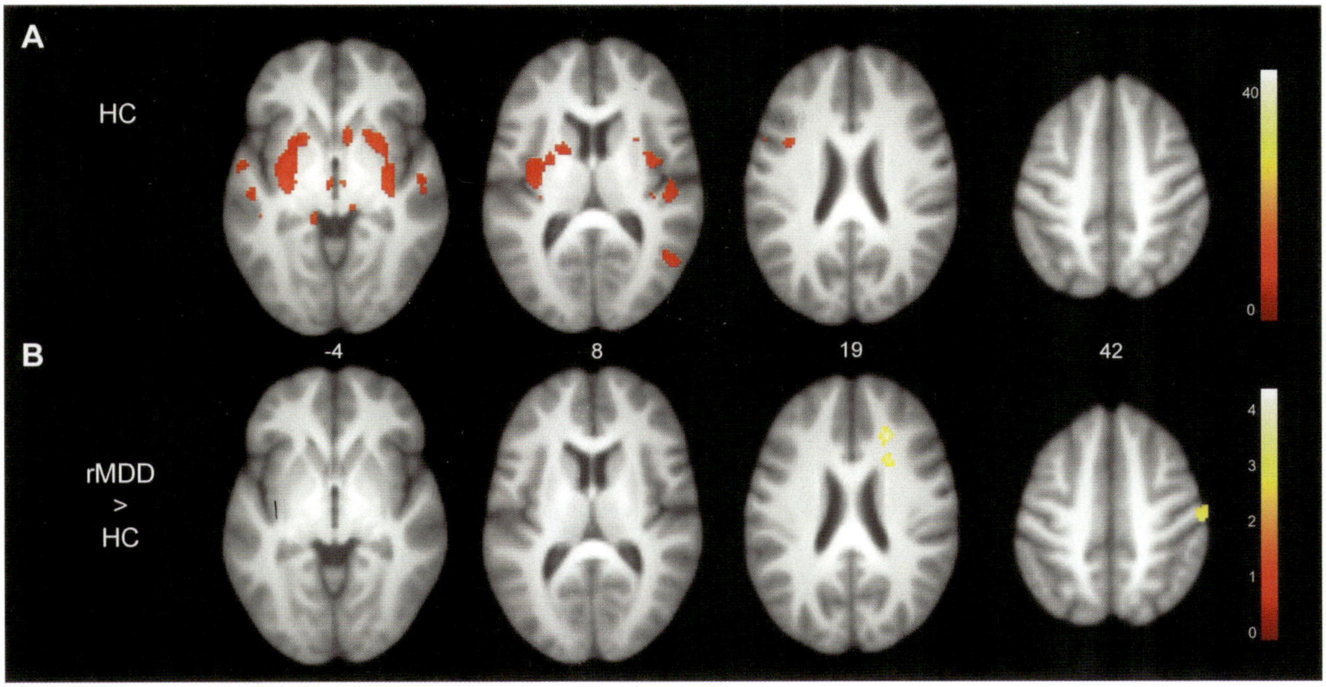

Figure 3. Connectivity of the left amygdala seed and between group differences. Figure 3 Panel A: Connectivities among HC youth with the left amygdala seed. Panel B: Youth with remitted depression demonstrated hyperconnectivities with the right medial frontal gyrus, medial parietal lobe, postcentral gyrus, and anterior cingulate cortex.

well as the left precuneus (BA 7) and left dorsolateral PFC (BA 8/10). Results for the right PCC are included as Supplementary Material for comparison (Table S1 in File S1).

sgACC connectivity

Across groups, left sgACC activation was significantly correlated with nearby areas including the orbital frontal cortex, thalamus, hippocampus, and the PCC. Figure 2 illustrates the SN among HC participants and connectivities that were greater among rMDD youth compared to HCs. Table 3 details these significant differences. rMDD youth demonstrated greater connectivity from the left sgACC seed to the bilateral superior and medial frontal cortex (BA 8/10), cerebellum, and thalamus, as well as the left medial temporal gyrus (BA 39/40), parahippocampus, and the right operculum/anterior insula when compared to HCs. Results for the right sgACC are included as Supplementary Material for comparison (Table S2 in File S1).

Amygdala hyperconnectivity

Across groups, left amygdala activation was significantly correlated with surrounding bilateral amygdaloid, hippocampal, and uncal regions. Figure 3 illustrates regions of the SN significantly connected with the left amygdala seed among HCs and those that were significantly different between rMDD and HC participants. Table 4 details these differences. The rMDD group exhibited greater connectivity between the left amygdala and the right medial frontal gyrus, medial parietal lobe, rostral ACC, and left parahippocampal gyrus (all regions not displayed in Figure 3). There were no significant between group differences for connectivity with the right amygdala.

Table 4. Differences between Healthy Controls and remitted Major Depression for left amygdala seed.

Lobe/region	BA	x	y	z	Z	mm^3
Parietal						
Postcentral	3	48	−19	39	3.04	648
Limbic						
Anterior Cingulate	32	19	24	19	4.22	784
Uncus	36	−18	−9	−27	3.81	656
Subcortical						
Caudate body		19	12	21	3.82	520

Note. BA = Brodmann's Area; mm = millimeter; amygdala clusters did not converge in factor analysis. x, y, and z coordinates are converted and reported in Talairach space.

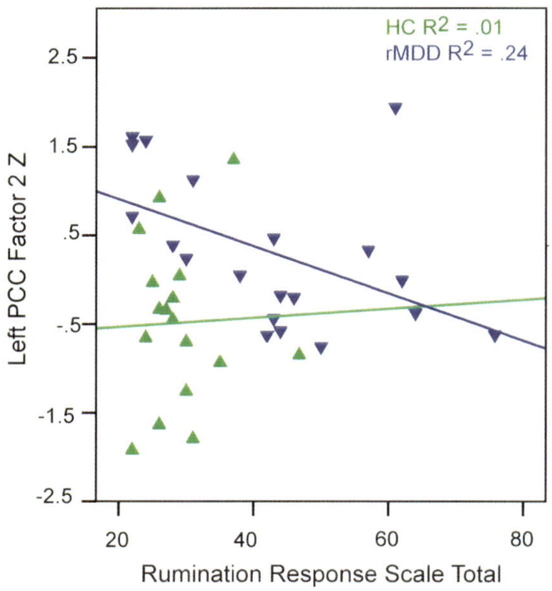

Figure 4. Correlation of Seed-based Factor with Rumination. Correlation of the left posterior cingulate Factor 2 with Rumination.

Data Reduction with Exploratory Factor Analysis

Results from exploratory factor analysis suggested a two factor solution for the PCC seed and a three factor solution for the sgACC seed. PCC Factor 1 had higher loadings on six of eight clusters, as indicated in Table 2. PCC Factor 2 had a higher loading with the right middle and medial frontal gyri and comparable loadings on a second right middle frontal gyrus cluster. sgACC Factor 1 included 11 of the 17 clusters that were hyperconnected among rMDD youth, as indicated in Table 3. Four clusters had dominant loadings on sgACC Factor 2, and four clusters had dominant loadings on sgACC Factor 3. As detailed in Tables 2 and 3, some clusters loaded highly on more than one factor. Factor analysis of the amygdala-based connectivity clusters failed to converge.

Relation of Intrinsic Networks to Rumination and Cognitive Control

As expected, rMDD youth reported higher levels of rumination than HCs ($t = -3.78$, $df = 38$, $p < .01$). For the parametric Go/No-Go, rMDD youth exhibited greater impulse control problems (No-Go Accuracy, $t = 2.30$, $df = 49$, $p = .03$), but did not differ in Go Accuracy ($t = -0.59$, $df = 49$, $p = .99$) or Go Response Time ($t = -0.70$, $df = 49$, $p = .47$). Among youth with rMDD, Go Response Time was inversely correlated with rumination ($r = -.48$, $p < .05$). Also among rMDD youth, the PCC Factor 2 (right superior and middle frontal gyrus connectivity) was inversely correlated with rumination ($r = -.49$, $p = .03$; Figure 4). Among rMDD youth only, the sgACC Factor 2 (left middle frontal, inferior temporal, right inferior frontal, and middle frontal gyri connectivity) was positively associated with Go Accuracy ($r = .40$, $p = .04$; Figure 5, Panel 1) and sgACC Factor 3 (left parahippocampal gyrus, caudate, bilateral dorsal medial thalamus, right postcentral gyri connectivity) was inversely correlated with No-Go Accuracy ($r = -.44$, $p = .02$; Figure 5, Panel B).

Potential Confounds

To rule out potential confounds, we conducted post-hoc exploratory analyses of clinical features and technological challenges and also examined the influence of participant sex (see Supplementary Material). These factors did not significantly affect between-group results for the PCC and sgACC seeds.

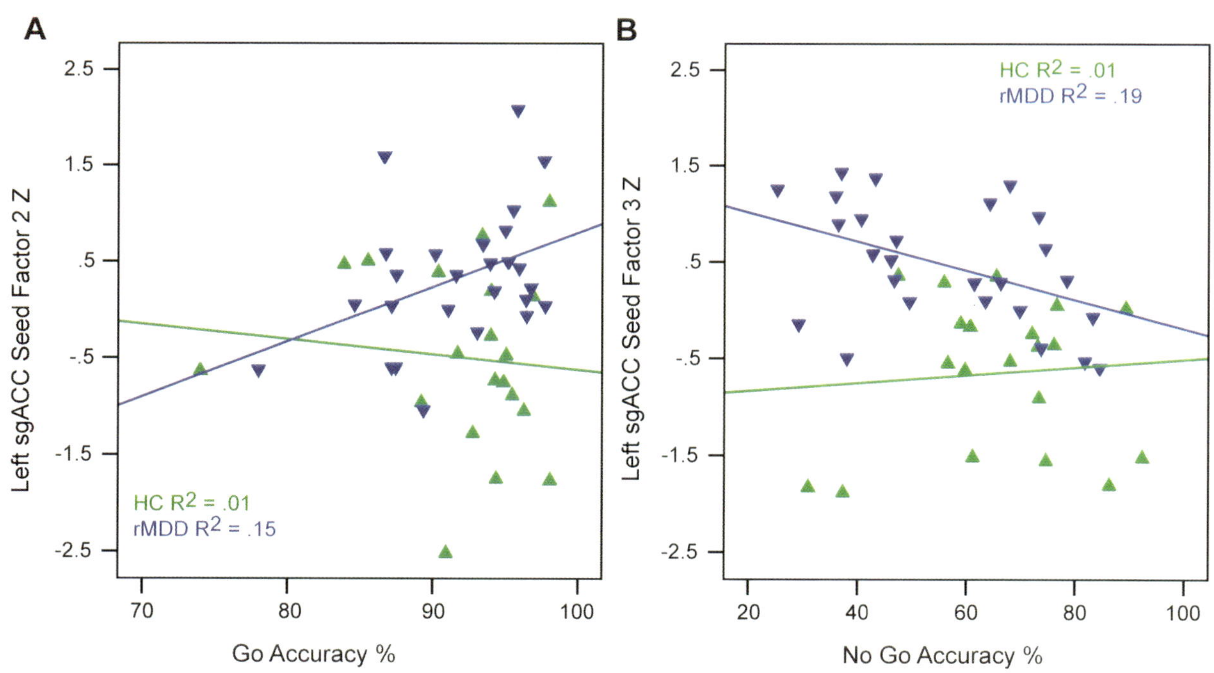

Figure 5. Correlation of Seed-based Factor with Rumination and Cognitive Control. A) Correlation of the left subgenual anterior cingulate Factor 2 with Go Accuracy and B) correlation of left subgenual anterior cingulate Factor 3 with No-Go percent accuracy.

Discussion

The current results address an understudied, yet very important set of questions regarding the dissociation of state, trait, compensatory, and scar features of MDD. To begin unravelling these questions, we obtained resting state data from a homogeneous sample of carefully characterized, unmedicated youth in a remitted state, allowing us to study MDD course in the absence of state and chronic burden features that may have confounded previous results. This is the first study of young adults with rMDD and we demonstrate hyperconnectivity of both the DMN and SN with portions of the right superior and middle frontal gyri – a central node in the CCN. Furthermore, observed hyperconnectivities were related to two known predictors of relapse: rumination (inverse correlation) and sustained attention (positive correlation).

Self-report rumination has previously been documented to correlate with sgACC-PCC connectivity during task among actively depressed adults [29]. We found an inverse correlation of rumination with hyperconnectivities suggesting that these increased temporal correlations may be protective, compensatory, or may even reduce risk for relapse. In contrast, another hypothesis is that over-enriched connections to regions outside of the CCN may be detrimental. For example, hyperconnectivity to a factor from the left sgACC to regions including the left parahippocampal gyrus, caudate, bilateral dorsal medial thalamus, and right postcentral gyri was associated with poorer inhibitory control. When interpreted in light of the strengths of the current sample, our results offer new evidence that connectivity differences may represent both protective and trait-based risk factors for relapse in MDD course.

The sgACC has long been implicated as a dysfunctional node in acute MDD and has been correlated with negative mood states, treatment response, and "treatment refractoriness" [48–50]. Our finding that this SN node is hyperconnected with both the DMN and EN among rMDD youth is noteworthy. Aberrant sgACC functioning and connectivity have been conceptualized as a *consequence* of depressive illness and sadness, as opposed to a potential risk or protective factor for future MDEs. In fact, a recent investigation of actively depressed, unmedicated adolescents found that higher levels of rumination were associated with *reduced* connectivity between the sgACC and the medial frontal gyrus [7]. Our findings suggest that *increased* connectivity between these same regions may strengthen the adolescent's ability to resist rumination and support attentional control, thereby promoting and potentially sustaining remission. Remitted youth whose CCN is overly-engaged may more effectively downregulate mind-wandering, self-referential thought supported by the DMN.

Our results extend and contextualize findings of a proposed abnormal 'dorsal nexus' in MDD [22] by suggesting that hyperconnectivity of the DMN and SN with the CCN is an early course marker observable outside of MDEs, similar to one study of DMN function among remitted preschool children [28]. The superior and middle frontal gyri may represent an extension of the CCN that modulates the DMN and SN among those with a history of MDD, which may function to ameliorate trait-based ruminative tendencies that often remain into periods of wellness [51,52].

It is also worth noting, however, that the primary factors (for both the PCC and sgACC seeds) accounting for the majority of factor variance across networks were not related to clinical features of illness or functioning in the current study – our results may reflect trait or scar biomarkers. A trait biomarker would represent a characteristic observable prior to illness and initially independent of illness, whereas a scar biomarker is a result of illness and represents a failure to achieve complete inter-episode recovery. The second and third factors, accounting for less variance, and more likely to be sample-specific, were related to cognitive markers of illness. Hyperconnectivities of the DMN and SN with portions of the CCN may result in increased neural resources directed towards emotion regulation among vulnerable individuals. Developmental hyperconnectivities may be protective to an extent, but may not always be sufficient for mounting adaptive responses to the increased adversity and stressors experienced by this population at-risk for multiple MDEs and comorbidities. We are currently following this sample longitudinally and will be able to identify predictors of both relapse and resilience.

We note several limitations of our study. First, the current data cannot discriminate between network abnormalities that render an individual vulnerable to the first-onset of MDD versus scar consequences of illness, normal maturation processes, or even protective compensatory mechanisms. In this context, prospective studies of high-risk cohorts represent an important direction for future research. Second, despite the strength of recruiting a medication-free sample, we could not examine how previous medication use or therapy exposure may have affected current results. As a related point, because our participants have had relatively fewer MDEs and have been well for relatively extended periods of time, they may represent a more mild severity or course of illness. To capture developmental trajectories that contribute to resiliency and risk in MDD, future longitudinal research can examine whether excessive coupling of intrinsic networks predicts first-onset of depression or relapse as adolescents transition into early adulthood. In addition, anatomical specificity is of concern when conducting seed-based analyses, particularly in regions such as the PCC [53,54]. We also did not specifically examine connectivity of the CCN using a CCN seed. We are currently analyzing the CCN during rest and task to more fully examine CCN function among remitted individuals. Future research involving larger samples will also specifically examine laterality. Last, examining network function both at rest and in response to task provides complementary and additive information regarding how networks function to support wellness or disease. Future directions could include inducing rumination during an fMRI task and examining how rumination impedes performance on cognitive control tasks to examine how these networks function together both at rest and in response to tasks relevant to the etiology of depression. Despite these limitations, we believe the examination of mechanisms during a relatively early phase of the disorder provides a level of protection against potential confounds including complex treatment histories and neural scarring resulting from decades of illness, making the current study innovative and important.

In sum, this study provides evidence of brain-based traits associated with MDD course that can be observed outside of a MDE, early in the course of illness. We believe the late adolescent-early adulthood transition represents a unique window for observing mechanisms of MDD, as stability of networks has been established developmentally, but opportunities remain for secondary prevention prior to the initiation of chronic illness. Thus, understanding the continuum of functional to dysfunctional connectivity patterns in the human brain is critical in elucidating the developmental psychopathology of MDD. Increased coupling between networks in our early course, remitted sample suggests that hyperconnectivities can be evaluated as developmental trait or resiliency factors, as targets for treatment, or as potential outcomes of early illness.

Supporting Information

Figure S1 Participants with movement are easily identifiable by movement deviation. Mean movement deviations among the Healthy Control and remitted Major Depressive group in the x, y, and z planes.

Figure S2 Extracted connectivity bar graphs by cluster, site, and group. rMDD = remitted Major Depressive Disorder; HC = Healthy Control; UM = University of Michigan; UIC = University of Illinois by Chicago. Tailarach coordinates corresponding to each numbered cluster: Clusters 1–7 are connectivities with the left PCC seed, Clusters 8–24 are connectivities with the left sgACC seed, Clusters 25–28 are connectivities with the left amygdala: 1 = −41, 35, 12; 2 = −6, −63, 49; 3 = 12, 45, 14; 4 = 17, −9, 3; 5 = 26, 32, 42; 6 = 27, 24, 20; 7 = 43, −36, 30; 8 = −22, −38, 0; 9 = −24, −30, 16; 9 = −24, 43, 13; 10 = −24, 43, 13; 11 = −31, −83, −33; 12 = −36, 16, 45; 13 = −43, −65, 35; 14 = −54, −54, −1; 15 = −57, −15, −19; 16 = −1, −15, 6; 17 = 8, 32, 49; 18 = 10, 63, 19; 19 = 15, −69, −39; 20 = 29, −71, −39; 21 = 31, −36, 49; 22 = 36, 24, 41; 23 = 43, 14, −3; 24 = 4, 45, 39; 25 = −18, −9, −27; 26 = 19, 12, 21; 27 = 19, 24, 19; 28 = 48, −19, 39.
(TIF)

File S1 Supplementary material containing supporting tables.

Acknowledgments

The authors would like to acknowledge the contributions of the Center for Magnetic Resonance Research 3T Program at UIC and thank Dr. F. Xavier Castellanos for his helpful feedback on the manuscript as well as Rachel Ringrose and Gloria Harrington for their data collection efforts. These data were presented in part at the 2013 annual meeting of the American College of Neuropsychopharmacology.

Author Contributions

Conceived and designed the experiments: SAL JKZ RCW. Performed the experiments: LBG AMB KAR SLW. Analyzed the data: RHJ SAL LMJ AB AV LBG NAC. Contributed reagents/materials/analysis tools: RCW. Wrote the paper: RHJ SAL LMJ KLP IHG ATP AV SLW.

References

1. Marchetti I, Koster EH, Sonuga-Barke EJ, De Raedt R (2012) The default mode network and recurrent depression: a neurobiological model of cognitive risk factors. Neuropsychology Reviews 22: 229–251.
2. Keller MB (2003) Past, present, and future directions for defining optimal treatment outcome in depression: remission and beyond. JAMA 289: 3152–3160.
3. De Raedt R, Koster EH (2010) Understanding vulnerability for depression from a cognitive neuroscience perspective: A reappraisal of attentional factors and a new conceptual framework. Cogn Affect Behav Neurosci 10: 50–70.
4. Castellanos FX, Di Martino A, Craddock RC, Mehta AD, Milham MP (2013) Clinical applications of the functional connectome. Neuroimage 80: 527–540.
5. Fox MD, Greicius M (2010) Clinical applications of resting state functional connectivity. Front Syst Neurosci 4: 19.
6. Greicius MD, Flores BH, Menon V, Glover GH, Solvason HB, et al. (2007) Resting-state functional connectivity in major depression: abnormally increased contributions from subgenual cingulate cortex and thalamus. Biol Psychiatry 62: 429–437.
7. Connolly CG, Wu J, Ho TC, Hoeft F, Wolkowitz O, et al. (2013) Resting-State Functional Connectivity of Subgenual Anterior Cingulate Cortex in Depressed Adolescents. Biol Psychiatry 12: 898–907.
8. Hamilton JP, Etkin A, Furman DJ, Lemus MG, Johnson RF, et al. (2012) Functional neuroimaging of major depressive disorder: a meta-analysis and new integration of base line activation and neural response data. American Journal of Psychiatry 169: 693–703.
9. Pizzagalli DA (2011) Frontocingulate dysfunction in depression: toward biomarkers of treatment response. Neuropsychopharmacology 36: 183–206.
10. Whitfield-Gabrieli S, Ford JM (2012) Default mode network activity and connectivity in psychopathology. Annu Rev Clin Psychol 8: 49–76.
11. Fox MD, Snyder AZ, Vincent JL, Corbetta M, Van Essen DC, et al. (2005) The human brain is intrinsically organized into dynamic, anticorrelated functional networks. Proceedings of the National Academy of Sciences of the United States of America 102: 9673–9678.
12. Seeley WW, Menon V, Schatzberg AF, Keller J, Glover GH, et al. (2007) Dissociable intrinsic connectivity networks for salience processing and executive control. J Neurosci 27: 2349–2356.
13. Shehzad Z, Kelly AMC, Reiss PT, Gee DG, Gotimer K, et al. (2009) The Resting Brain: Unconstrained yet Reliable. Cerebral Cortex 19: 2209–2229.
14. Zuo XN, Kelly C, Adelstein JS, Klein DF, Castellanos FX, et al. (2010) Reliable intrinsic connectivity networks: Test-retest evaluation using ICA and dual regression approach. Neuroimage 49: 2163–2177.
15. Zuo XN, Di Martino A, Kelly C, Shehzad ZE, Gee DG, et al. (2010) The oscillating brain: complex and reliable. Neuroimage 49: 1432–1445.
16. Biswal BB, Mennes M, Zuo XN, Gohel S, Kelly C, et al. (2010) Toward discovery science of human brain function. Proceedings of the National Academy of Sciences of the United States of America 107: 4734–4739.
17. Sadaghiani S, Scheeringa R, Lehongre K, Morillon B, Giraud AL, et al. (2010) Intrinsic connectivity networks, alpha oscillations, and tonic alertness: a simultaneous electroencephalography/functional magnetic resonance imaging study. J Neurosci 30: 10243–10250.
18. Bressler SL, Menon V (2010) Large-scale brain networks in cognition: emerging methods and principles. Trends Cogn Sci 14: 277–290.
19. Menon V (2011) Large-scale brain networks and psychopathology: a unifying triple network model. Trends Cogn Sci 15: 483–506.
20. Broyd SJ, Demanuele C, Debener S, Helps SK, James CJ, et al. (2009) Default-mode brain dysfunction in mental disorders: a systematic review. Neuroscience and Biobehavioral Reviews 33: 279–296.
21. Hamilton JP, Furman DJ, Chang C, Thomason ME, Dennis E, et al. (2011) Default-mode and task-positive network activity in major depressive disorder: implications for adaptive and maladaptive rumination. Biol Psychiatry 70: 327–333.
22. Sheline YI, Price JL, Yan Z, Mintun MA (2010) Resting-state functional MRI in depression unmasks increased connectivity between networks via the dorsal nexus. Proceedings of the National Academy of Sciences of the United States of America 107: 11020–11025.
23. Briceno EM, Weisenbach SL, Rapport LJ, Hazlett KE, Bieliauskas LA, et al. (2013) Shifted inferior frontal laterality in women with major depressive disorder is related to emotion-processing deficits. Psychol Med 43: 1433–1445.
24. Drevets WC, Price JL, Furey ML (2008) Brain structural and functional abnormalities in mood disorders: implications for neurocircuitry models of depression. Brain Structure & Function 213: 93–118.
25. Price JL, Drevets WC (2010) Neurocircuitry of Mood Disorders. Neuropsychopharmacology 35: 192–216.
26. Wang Z, Yuan Y, Bai F, You J, Li L, et al. (2012) Abnormal default-mode network in angiotensin converting enzyme D allele carriers with remitted geriatric depression. Behav Brain Res 230: 325–332.
27. Yuan Y, Zhang Z, Bai F, Yu H, Shi Y, et al. (2008) Abnormal neural activity in the patients with remitted geriatric depression: a resting-state functional magnetic resonance imaging study. J Affect Disord 111: 145–152.
28. Gaffrey MS, Luby JL, Botteron K, Repovs G, Barch DM (2012) Default mode network connectivity in children with a history of preschool onset depression. J Child Psychol Psychiatry 53: 964–972.
29. Berman MG, Peltier S, Nee DE, Kross E, Deldin PJ, et al. (2010) Depression, rumination and the default network. Soc Cogn Affect Neurosci.
30. Cooney RE, Joormann J, Eugene F, Dennis EL, Gotlib IH (2010) Neural correlates of rumination in depression. Cognitive Affective and Behavioral Neuroscience 10: 470–478.
31. Langenecker SA, Zubieta JK, Young EA, Akil H, Nielson KA (2007) A task to manipulate attentional load, set-shifting, and inhibitory control: convergent validity and test-retest reliability of the Parametric Go/No-Go Test. J Clin Exp Neuropsychol 29: 842–853.
32. Votruba KL, Langenecker SA (2013) Factor structure, construct validity, and age- and education-based normative data for the Parametric Go/No-Go Test. J Clin Exp Neuropsychol 35: 132–146.
33. Langenecker SA, Kennedy SE, Guidotti LM, Briceno EM, Own LS, et al. (2007) Frontal and limbic activation during inhibitory control predicts treatment response in major depressive disorder. Biol Psychiatry 62: 1272–1280.
34. Nurnberger JI Jr, Blehar MC, Kaufmann CA, York-Cooler C, Simpson SG, et al. (1994) Diagnostic interview for genetic studies. Rationale, unique features, and training. NIMH Genetics Initiative. Arch Gen Psychiatry 51: 849–859.
35. Hamilton M (1960) A rating scale for depression. J Neurol Neurosurg Psychiatry 23: 56–62.
36. Treynor W, Gonzalez R, Nolen-Hoeksema S (2003) Rumination reconsidered: A psychometric analysis. Cognitive Therapy and Research 27: 247–259.
37. Tabachnick BG, Fidell LS (2007) Using Multivariate Statistics. Boston, MA: Pearson Education.

38. Behzadi Y, Restom K, Liau J, Liu TT (2007) A component based noise correction method (CompCor) for BOLD and perfusion based fMRI. Neuroimage 37: 90–101.
39. Jo HJ, Gotts SJ, Reynolds RC, Bandettini PA, Martin A, et al. (2013) Effective Preprocessing Procedures Virtually Eliminate Distance-Dependent Motion Artifacts in Resting State FMRI. J Appl Math 2013: 1–9.
40. Power JD, Barnes KA, Snyder AZ, Schlaggar BL, Petersen SE (2012) Spurious but systematic correlations in functional connectivity MRI networks arise from subject motion. Neuroimage 59: 2142–2154.
41. Fox MD, Zhang D, Snyder AZ, Raichle ME (2009) The global signal and observed anticorrelated resting state brain networks. J Neurophysiol 101: 3270–3283.
42. Pannekoek JN, Veer IM, van Tol MJ, van der Werff SJ, Demenescu LR, et al. (2013) Aberrant limbic and salience network resting-state functional connectivity in panic disorder without comorbidity. J Affect Disord 145: 29–35.
43. McCabe C, Mishor Z (2011) Antidepressant medications reduce subcortical-cortical resting-state functional connectivity in healthy volunteers. Neuroimage 57: 1317–1323.
44. Bluhm RL, Clark CR, McFarlane AC, Moores KA, Shaw ME, et al. (2011) Default network connectivity during a working memory task. Hum Brain Mapp 32: 1029–1035.
45. Alexopoulos GS, Hoptman MJ, Kanellopoulos D, Murphy CF, Lim KO, et al. (2012) Functional connectivity in the cognitive control network and the default mode network in late-life depression. J Affect Disord 139: 56–65.
46. Kelly AM, Di Martino A, Uddin LQ, Shehzad Z, Gee DG, et al. (2009) Development of anterior cingulate functional connectivity from late childhood to early adulthood. Cereb Cortex 19: 640–657.
47. Margulies DS, Kelly AM, Uddin LQ, Biswal BB, Castellanos FX, et al. (2007) Mapping the functional connectivity of anterior cingulate cortex. Neuroimage 37: 579–588.
48. Konarski JZ, Kennedy SH, Segal ZV, Lau MA, Bieling PJ, et al. (2009) Predictors of nonresponse to cognitive behavioural therapy or venlafaxine using glucose metabolism in major depressive disorder. J Psychiatry Neurosci 34: 175–180.
49. Siegle GJ, Carter CS, Thase ME (2006) Use of FMRI to predict recovery from unipolar depression with cognitive behavior therapy. Am J Psychiatry 163: 735–738.
50. Keedwell P, Drapier D, Surguladze S, Giampietro V, Brammer M, et al. (2009) Neural markers of symptomatic improvement during antidepressant therapy in severe depression: subgenual cingulate and visual cortical responses to sad, but not happy, facial stimuli are correlated with changes in symptom score. J Psychopharmacol 23: 775–788.
51. Nolen-Hoeksema S, Morrow J (1991) A prospective study of depression and posttraumatic stress symptoms after a natural disaster: the 1989 Loma Prieta Earthquake. Journal of Personality and Social Psychology 61: 115–121.
52. Riso LP, Newman CF (2003) Cognitive therapy for chronic depression. J Clin Psychol 59: 817–831.
53. Margulies DS, Vincent JL, Kelly C, Lohmann G, Uddin LQ, et al. (2009) Precuneus shares intrinsic functional architecture in humans and monkeys. Proc Natl Acad Sci U S A 106: 20069–20074.
54. Lynch CJ, Uddin LQ, Supekar K, Khouzam A, Phillips J, et al. (2013) Default mode network in childhood autism: posteromedial cortex heterogeneity and relationship with social deficits. Biol Psychiatry 74: 212–219.

12

Soluble Urokinase Plasminogen Activator Receptor as a Marker for Use of Antidepressants

Eva Haastrup[1]*, Katrine Grau[2], Jesper Eugen-Olsen[3], Christian Thorball[3], Lars Vedel Kessing[4], Henrik Ullum[1]

1 Department of Clinical Immunology, the Blood bank, Rigshospitalet, University Hospital of Copenhagen, Copenhagen, Denmark, **2** Department of Epidemiology Research, Statens Serum Institut, Copenhagen, Denmark, **3** Clinical Research Centre, Hvidovre Hospital, University Hospital of Copenhagen, Copenhagen, Denmark, **4** Psychiatric Centre, Rigshospitalet, University Hospital of Copenhagen, Copenhagen, Denmark

Abstract

Objectives: Inflammation is involved in the pathogenesis of depression. A few cross-sectional population-based studies have found that depression is associated with increased levels of inflammatory markers. Soluble urokinase plasminogen activation receptor (suPAR) is known to be a stable marker for inflammation. We investigated the bidirectional association between suPAR levels and use of antidepressants.

Methods: suPAR level was measured in 9305 blood donors and analysed in relation to 5-years follow-up data on purchase of antidepressants and hospital diagnoses of depression from a nationwide Danish register.

Results: For men and women without prior use of antidepressants we found a significantly higher risk for incident use of antidepressants with higher suPAR values. For men, the risk of first use of antidepressants increased by 72% from the 1st to the 4th quartile (HR = 1.72, 95% CI: 1.11–2.69). For women, it increased by 108% from the 1st to the 4th quartile (HR = 2.08, 95% CI: 1.45–2.98). Previous use of antidepressants was also significantly associated with higher suPAR levels (p = 0.002).

Conclusions: High suPAR levels are associated with an increased risk for both previous and future use of antidepressants in healthy men and women. High suPAR are also associated with increased risk for a hospital diagnosis of depression.

Editor: Carmen Infante-Duarte, Charite Universitätsmedizin Berlin, Germany

Funding: The suPARnostic kits were kindly donated by ViroGates A/S. No additional external funding received for this study. The funder had no role in study design, data collection and analysis, decision to publish, or preparation of the manuscript.

Competing Interests: Jesper Eugen-Olsen is a founder, shareholder and board member of ViroGates, Denmark. Lars Vedel Kessing has been a consultant for Bristol-Myers Squibb, Eli Lilly, Lundbeck, AstraZenica, Pfizer, Wyeth, Servier and Janssen-Cilag.

* Email: eva.haastrup@rh.regionh.dk

Introduction

In the last decade, it has become clear that there is a biological link between inflammation and depression. In patients with depression, several studies have demonstrated increased expression of proinflammatory cytokines, chemokines, acute phase reactants, and adhesion molecules compared to non-depressed controls [1–9]. However, there is ongoing debate on whether elevated systemic inflammation is a biological mechanism leading to depression.

A few population-based studies have investigated the relationship between C-reactive protein (CRP) and de novo depression. In a study including 644 women with no prior history of depression, of whom 48 women developed depression during the 5827 person-years of follow-up, CRP was found to be an independent predictor of depressive disorder, supporting an aetiological role for inflammatory activity in the pathophysiology of depression [10]. Two larger population-based studies have investigated the direction of the depression-inflammation relationship. The SWAN study of 3292 pre- and postmenopausal women found that over a five-year observation period, higher depression scores were related to higher levels of fibrinogen and plasminogen activation inhibitor type one (PAI-1) but not CRP [11]. This was on the other hand reported by Deverts et al [12] in the CARDIA study, where depressive symptoms at baseline were positively correlated with CRP levels measured at 5-years follow-up. No association was found between CRP levels at the beginning of the observation period and subsequent depressive symptoms in any of these studies. This was however the main finding in a large study by Wium-Andersen et al [13].

The lack of consensus with regard to CRP and development of depression may in part be due to the high biological variation of CRP (hsCRP). In 38 healthy blood donors with 6 determinations over 22 days a biological variation of hsCRP of 50% was found [14]. Other studies have shown similar biological variation, ranging from 30–63% [15,16].

SuPAR is a protein that is measurable in the circulating blood of all individuals. In contrast to most pro-inflammatory and acute response biomarkers, circadian changes in plasma suPAR is minimal, and in vitro stability is also high [17–19].

Elevated levels of suPAR are associated with immune activation, inflammation and a negative outcome in patients with symptoms of infection (recently reviewed in "Usefulness of suPAR" as a biological marker in patients with systemic inflammation or infection: a systematic review [20]).

Furthermore, in an observational prospective Danish cohort (MONICA) consisting of healthy individuals, plasma suPAR levels were associated to the development of cancer, cardiovascular disease, type-2 diabetes and mortality during 12-years follow-up [21]. SuPAR and CRP seems to reflect different aspects of inflammation. A recent study suggested that CRP is associated with anthropometric measures of inflammation, whereas suPAR is linked to cellular and vascular inflammatory processes [22].

To test the hypothesis of inflammation and development of depression, we investigated whether the biomarker suPAR was associated with an increased risk of developing depression in a large cohort of Danish blood donors. As a proxy for depression, we used purchase of antidepressants, supplemented with a discharge diagnosis of depression.

Aim of the study was to test the hypothesis, that higher levels of circulating suPAR in healthy individuals are associated with an increased risk for future use of antidepressants or a hospital diagnosis of depression. From both analyses were donors with a pre-history of antidepressant use or a previous hospital diagnosis of depression excluded. We further tested the hypothesis that prior use of antidepressants was associated with higher levels of suPAR.

Methods and Materials

Ethical considerations

This study was approved by the local Medical Scientific Ethics Committee of Denmark (H-KF 01283058). All participants provided written informed consent. This study was conducted in accordance with the Declaration of Helsinki.

The cohort

Blood donors, who donated blood to the Copenhagen City Blood bank (former H:S Blood bank) during a three month period from the 14th of January to the 24th of April 2006 were invited to participate in the study. The inclusion criterion was fulfilment of the Danish criteria for blood donation (i.e. self-reported good health and lack of behavioural risks for transfusion transmissible infections). All donors were asked about medication usage. Usage of antidepressive medicine within the last two weeks prior to visiting the blood bank was an exclusion criterion for donation and thus participation. Informed written consent was obtained from 11971 donors. Blood samples were obtained from a look-back repository where samples were available for 9312 of these donors.

suPAR measurement

All blood samples were collected in 7-ml blood EDTA anticoagulated tubes with stabilising gel (Becton Dickenson, Glostrup, Denmark). Blood samples were centrifuged to separate the plasma from the cells within 1 hour and frozen within 6 hours.

Plasma suPAR was measured at Hvidovre hospital with the suPARnostic ELISA kit (ViroGates Copenhagen, Denmark) according to the manufacturer instructions. The samples were measured in singlets and the interassay variation of a control plasma sample run on all plates was $<10\%$. The kit standard curve was validated to measure suPAR levels between 0.6 and 22 ng/ml.

Danish register data

Data on purchase of antidepressive medicine and other prescription medicines from the Danish register of Medical Products [23] was linked to study participants via their central personal registration number (CPR-number). The CPR-number is a unique number ascribed to each Danish citizen. The Medical Product Register Statistics contains information on all medical prescriptions purchased in Denmark from the first of January 1995 to 31st of December 2010. In Denmark, all antidepressive or antipsychotic medications are prescribed by doctors and can only be purchased at pharmacies. The sale of prescribed medication from the pharmacies is registered with the name of the drug, Anatomical Therapeutical Chemical code (ATC code), dose, CPR-number of the patient and the identity of the doctor prescribing the medicine.

From the Danish Patient Registry we obtained data on hospitalization with depression. Diagnoses were based on the International Statistical Classification of Disease (ISCD).

Cases. Case persons were persons who filled prescriptions for antidepressive medication (any ATC code beginning with N06A registrated in the Register of Medicinal Products Statistics) or had a hospital discharge diagnose with the codes F.32 or F.33.

Exclusion. When analysing incident depression, donors who purchased antidepressants before the time of suPAR measurement were excluded.

Similarly were donors with a hospital discharge diagnosis of depression before the time of suPAR measurement, excluded from the analysis of incident hospitalization.

In the following text, references to the purchase and use of antidepressants will be used interchangeably. Other medications were all prescription medications purchased other than antidepressants.

Statistical analysis

Analysing the incident use of antidepressants. As a proxy for incident depression, we investigated the first use of antidepressants between suPAR measurement and the 31st of December 2010 in participants who never purchased antidepressants before suPAR the measurement, according to the register.

The incident use of antidepressants after suPAR measurement was illustrated according to sex-specific suPAR level quartiles by Kaplan-Meier curves and compared using a log-rank test. Cox regression analyses stratified by sex, with age as the underlying timescale, were further used to assess the effect of suPAR level on the subsequent incident use of antidepressants. The interaction between sex and suPAR in relation to time of first purchase of antidepressant medication was investigated in a model with suPAR sex and a sex-suPAR level interaction term. Analyses were conducted using the log2-transformed suPAR level as a continuous variable and with quartiles of suPAR levels. Analyses were repeated while also adjusting for the purchase of prescription medication other than antidepressants as a time-dependent variable.

The same analysis was used to examine if there was an association between the suPAR level of the donors and a hospital discharge diagnosis of depression but only with suPAR as continuous variable adjusted for sex.

Analysing prior use of antidepressants. We tested the hypothesis that a prior purchase of antidepressants was associated with increased suPAR levels. The effect of prior purchase of antidepressants on the log2-transformed suPAR level data was estimated using linear regression models adjusted for age (continuous linear variable). Separate analyses were conducted for women and men. The purchase of antidepressants was analysed as a dichotomous variable (none/any) and in categories of time from last purchase to suPAR measurement (none, less than 6 months, 6 to 12 months and 12 month or more).

Results

Descriptive statistics

A total of 9312 individuals with an available blood sample had their suPAR level measured. Seven blood samples were excluded due to outlying low values. Thus, the cohort consisted of 9305 individuals, including 4464 women and 4841 men. There were more women than men in the younger age group (18–30 years of age) while there were more men than women in all other age groups. The median age for women was 36 years (quartiles: 27–47) and the median age for men was 39.9 years (quartiles: 30–49).

The median suPAR values were 2.54 ng/ml (range 0.6–19.4) for women and 2.22 ng/ml (range 0.6–15.4) for men. suPAR levels increased with age in both men and women. In women there was an increase between the 18–30 and 31–40 age groups from 2.43 ng ml^{-1} to 2.58 ng/ml after which the level increased slowly to 2.71 ng/ml. For men the median suPAR value increased more evenly across the age groups from 2.08 ng/ml to 2.44 ng/ml (Table 1).

Data from the Danish register of Medical Products

During the observation period from the first of January 1995 to the 31st of December 2010 the 9305 donors made 387.837 purchases of prescription medications, of which 6347 were for antidepressants (ATC code 'N06A') made by 856 individuals. There were 445 donors who purchased antidepressants before suPAR measurement and 411 donors who made their first recorded purchase after suPAR measurement.

suPAR measurement and the subsequent first use of antidepressants. The 8860 donors who had previously never purchased antidepressants at the time of suPAR measurement were included in the analysis evaluating the correlation between suPAR and the subsequent first use of antidepressants. In the 5-year period from suPAR measurement to the end of follow-up in December 2010, 411 donors (247 women and 164 men) purchased antidepressant medication. The majority made less than four purchases in the period. There was a statistically significant difference in the incidence of the first use of antidepressants among the suPAR level quartiles ($p<0.0001$), Figure 1). The first use of antidepressants occurred significantly more often for individuals in the 4th suPAR level quartiles than for those in the 1st, 2nd and 3rd quartile. The association between suPAR level and first use of antidepressants persisted when stratifying by sex and adjusting for age (Table 2). Both men and women in the 4th suPAR level quartile had increased rates of first use of antidepressants compared with the rates for individuals in the lowest suPAR level quartile (Table 2). For men, the risk of first use of antidepressants increased by 72% from the 1st to the 4th quartile (HR = 1.71, 95% CI: 1.11–2.69). For women, the risk of using antidepressants for the first time increased by 108% from the 1st to the 4th quartile (HR = 2.08, 95% CI: 1.45–2.98).

The purchase of prescriptive medication other than antidepressants was not associated with an increased incidence of first antidepressant usage in men or women and the inclusion of other medication did not change the association between the suPAR level and the first use of antidepressants (Table 2). Testing for an interaction between sex and suPAR levels in relation to the first use of antidepressants revealed no statistically significant interaction ($p = 0.42$).

Analysis of data from the Danish Patient Register of hospitalization found an association between the suPAR levels and a hospital discharge diagnosis of depression (table 3). A higher suPAR levels was associated with a 28% increased risk for a hospital discharge diagnosis of depression ($p = 0.005$).

Previous use of antidepressants and suPAR. Of 9305 donors, 445 purchased antidepressant medicine in the period from January 1995 to the day of suPAR measurement in the beginning of 2006. The majority (54.4%) of those who used antidepressants had three purchases or fewer. Table 4 shows the results from the linear regression analysis with purchase of antidepressants as an explanatory variable. For men, previous use of antidepressants was associated with higher suPAR levels, when the last purchase occurred less than 12 months before suPAR measurement. The suPAR level in men who purchased their antidepressant medication more than 12 months prior to suPAR measurement was not significantly higher than that in men who never purchased antidepressant medicine. For women, suPAR levels were statistically significantly higher in those with previous use of antidepressants in all categories of time from last purchase to suPAR measurement. Women who purchased antidepressant medicine less than six month before suPAR measurement had a log2-transformed suPAR value that was 0.17 (95% CI: 0.03–0.32) higher than women who never used antidepressants. The effect was smaller for women who made their last purchase 6 to 12 months before suPAR measurement (0.06 (95% CI: 0.001–0.11)).

Thus, there was a trend towards declining effect on the suPAR level with increasing time because the last antidepressant purchase, although the associations between suPAR level and antidepressant purchase were not significantly different for the three timing categories in women.

Table 1. Soluble urokinase plasminogen activator receptor (suPAR) (ng/ml) in blood donors according to sex and age.

	Age	N	Median	Lower 25th percentile	Upper 25th percentile	Range
Men	18-30	1257	2.08	1.76	2.44	0.61–15.41
	31-40	1416	2.17	1.85	2.57	0.64–13.83
	41-50	1112	2.25	1.90	2.69	0.70–11.10
	51-65	1056	2.44	2.02	2.90	0.64–12.27
Women	18-30	1672	2.43	2.05	2.79	0.77–6.84
	31-40	1028	2.58	2.16	3.04	0.60–8.04
	41-50	978	2.62	2.18	3.12	0.88–8.64
	51-65	786	2.71	2.25	3.23	0.67–19.38

Table 2. Risk[1] of incident use of antidepressants according to the suPAR level.

	suPAR Quartiles	Analysis without other medication HR	95% CI	P-value	Analysis with other medication HR	95% CI	P-value
Men, n = 4671	q2	1.04	0.64, 1.69	0.86	1.05	0.65, 1.70	0.86
Events = 164	q3	1.34	0.89, 2.21	0.15	1.40	0.89, 2.21	0.15
	q4	1.72	1.11, 2.69	0.02	1.73	1.11, 2.70	0.02
	Other				1.24	0.90, 1.72	0.18
Women, n = 4189	q2	1.04	0.69, 1.55	0.87	1.03	0.69, 1.55	0.87
Events = 247	q3	1.37	0.94, 2.01	0.11	1.37	0.93, 2.0	0.11
	q4	2.08	1.45, 2.98	<0.0001	2.08	1.45, 2.98	0.0001
	Other				0.76	0.56, 1.03	0.08

[1]Estimates are hazard ratios from Cox regression analyses stratified by sex and with age as the underlying time scale. Purchase of antidepressants is used as proxy for depression. The analysis is performed both with and without adjustment for other medication.

Discussion

To our knowledge, this is the first larger prospective population-based study of the inflammatory marker suPAR and use of antidepressants. We investigated the association of suPAR levels and both subsequent incident use of antidepressants and prior use of antidepressants and found an association between high suPAR levels and the use of antidepressants in both directions.

When analysing the incident use of antidepressants, we found a statistically significant effect of suPAR level on the risk of subsequent use of antidepressants during a five-year observation period. To our knowledge, this is the first larger prospective population-based study of the inflammatory marker suPAR and use of antidepressants. We investigated the association of suPAR levels and both subsequent incident use of antidepressants and prior use of antidepressants and found an association between high suPAR levels and the use of antidepressants in both directions. Kaplan-Meier curves depicting suPAR quartiles indicate that a high suPAR level was associated with an increased risk of antidepressant usage throughout the observation period. This is a surprising and interesting observation, suggesting that an elevated suPAR level seems to reflect a constitutively increased risk of depression.

We also found that prior use of antidepressants was significantly associated with higher suPAR levels in both men and women. This could possibly be an example of reverse causality, as we cannot rule out that the suPAR level was already increased before the purchase of antidepressants. For men, the effect was greater when the purchase was temporally closer to the suPAR measurement. For women, the effect was independent of purchase timing. There was, however, a trend towards a decreased strength of the association when the time between suPAR measurement and the purchase of the antidepressant medicine increased. The timing categories were based on clinical guidelines for treatment in the acute and maintenance phases and are in accordance with prior studies [24,25].

Our findings are in line with studies of depression and CRP that found an association between CRP levels and prior depression [26–28]. Two of these studies, however, only detected the association in men and not in women. In this study, we found an effect for both men and women.

It is well known that there is an increased prevalence of depression among patients with diseases such as diabetes [29], myocardial infarction [30] and cancer [1,2,7,31,32]. Thus, to examine whether the relationship between suPAR levels and the subsequent use of antidepressants was caused by another underlying disease affecting both suPAR level and depression, we adjusted the analyses for prescription medications other than antidepressants. The purchase of medication, other than antidepressants, was not associated with an increased risk of antidepressant usage and did not affect the relationship between suPAR levels and the incident use of antidepressants. This does not suggests that treatment with antidepressant medicine could have been initiated in connection with an underlying other disease.

This study is for the outcome based on register data using the purchase of antidepressant medicine as a proxy for depression. The same ATC code (N06A) has previously been used in other population-based studies of depression [24,25,33,34]. Whether our use of register data on antidepressant use captures the donor with a depression is subject to discussion. However in Denmark can such medication only be prescribed by physicians and regulation and surveillance of the use of medication is quite strict. The sensitivity of antidepressant use as a proxy for major depression

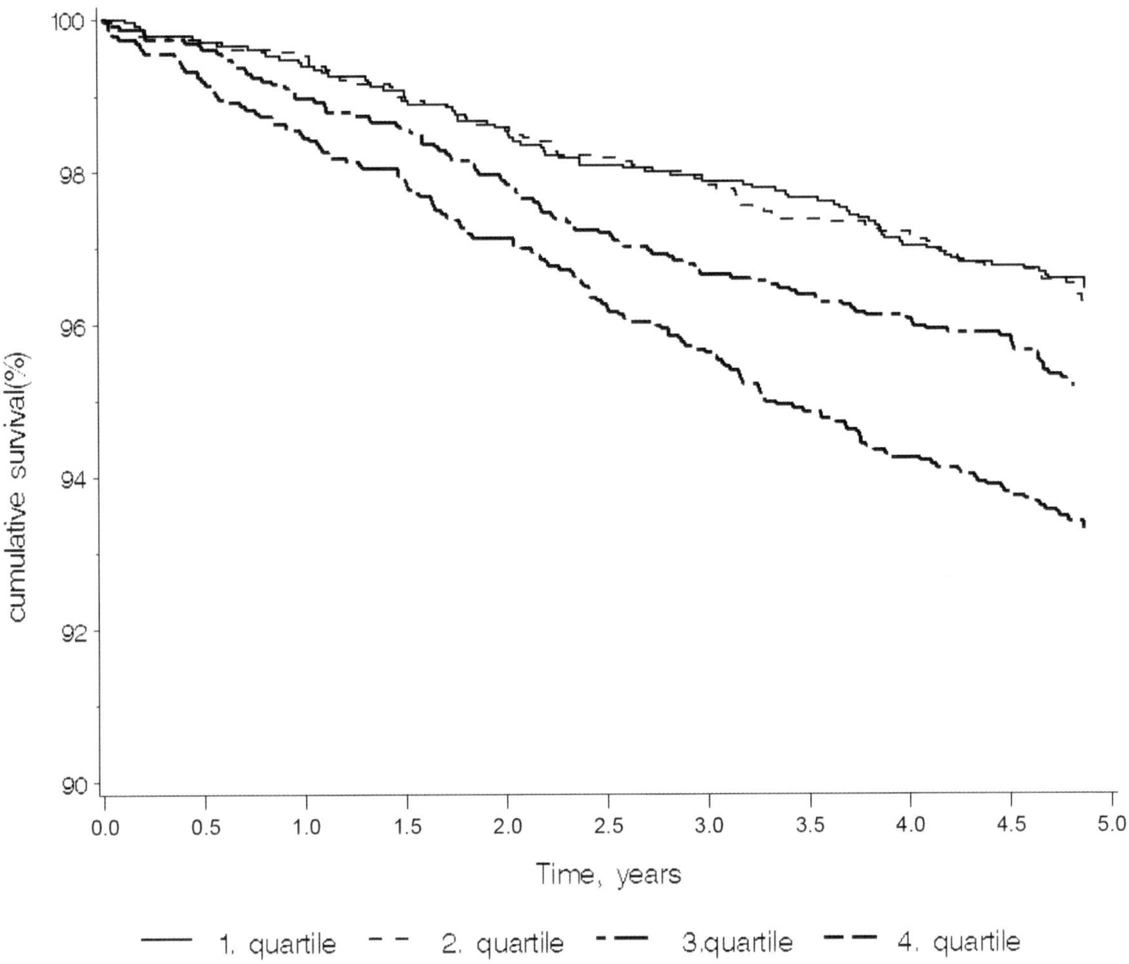

Figure 1. Kaplan-Meier plot with antidepressants as outcome and the suPAR level quartiles as explanatory variables (n = 9305). The 4th quartile is the highest values. Log-rank test: $p<0.0001$.

has been evaluated to be up to 50% [35] while, more importantly, specificity seems to be more than 90%.

Thus, it seems reasonable to use the purchase of antidepressant medicine as a proxy for depression, acknowledging that milder forms of depression may not all be recorded. The sensitivity of 50% indicates that many people with depression are not prescribed medication and there can be a long delay between the onset of depression and initiation of the antidepressant use. Further, antidepressants are used for a number of indications other than major depression. Thus, we cannot completely rule out that a proportion of participants who started using antidepressants after the suPAR measurement were already depressed or had been depressed before blood collection without receiving an antidepressant at that time. Also did we in this analysis exclude all donors who had purchased antidepressants prior to the suPAR measurement. However older donors could potentially have been treated with antidepressants before the register started in 1995.

A limitation of our study is the lack of information on relevant potential confounders such as smoking, alcohol consumption, BMI and physical activity. Smoking may lead to increased suPAR levels [36] and is common among depressed patients. Obesity has been suggested to be a potential link between depression and elevated CRP [27,37]; however, no effect of obesity on depression was found in the 12-year US national health survey [38]. The MONICA cohort study found that BMI and waist circumference were correlated with CRP but not with suPAR [21]. Thus, we cannot exclude that the suPAR level reflects lifestyle factors statistically associated with depression. On the other hand could the same factors also be acting as mediators of the association between high suPAR levels and subsequent use of antidepressants.

Table 3. Risk of an incident hospital diagnosis of depression according to the suPAR level.

		HR	95% CI	P-value
All, n = 9275	suPAR	1.28	1.08, 1.53	0.005
Events = 22	sex	0.56	0.23, 1.35	0.19

Table 4. Effect[1] of previous use of antidepressants on log2-transformed suPAR.

	Time since last purchase, (months)	Effect on suPAR	95% CI	P-value
Men, n = 4841	less than 6	0.30	0.11, 0.50	0.002
	6 to 12	0.22	0.04, 0.40	0.02
	12 or more	0.05	−0.2, 0.13	0.15
Women, n = 4463	less than 6	0.17	0.03, 0.32	0.02
	6 to 12	0.16	0.004, 0.32	0.04
	12 or more	0.06	0.001, 0.11	0.045

[1]Estimates are from linear regressions adjusting for age (continuous).

However, the cohort consists of blood donors who at each donation claim to be healthy, are able to donate blood on a voluntary basis and agree to participate in the study. In several studies blood donors are characterized as being very healthy [39,40]. Our conclusions are therefore valid in a healthy adult population only.

A second limitation of this study is the lack of a comparison between suPAR measurements and other components of the fibrinolytic system or other inflammatory markers previously shown to be associated with depression, such as CRP or IL-6 [41]. In patients with non-malignant diseases characterised by systemic immune activation, suPAR levels are correlated with TNF-α and TNFrII. Some studies have observed a positive correlation between IL-6 and suPAR level, while others have not [42,43].

suPAR has not been previously investigated in depression. In neurological diseases such as Alzheimer, multiple sclerosis, HIV dementia, cerebral malaria and Creutzfeldt-Jakob disease, the presence of uPAR in macrophages/microglia within the CNS has been described [44–48]. An animal model of cerebral inflammation with intracerebral LPS injections induced uPAR expression in microglia at both the mRNA and protein levels compared to controls [49]. Further studies are needed to investigate the role of uPAR produced in the cerebrum and its association with depression.

We conclude that high suPAR levels are associated with an increased risk of subsequent incident purchase of antidepressants and an incident hospital diagnosis of depression. Conversely, the prior purchase of antidepressants is associated with increased suPAR levels. We are not able to identify methodological drawbacks that clearly refute these findings as artefacts, though we did not have data on a number of important potential confounders. suPAR is an inflammatory marker and high levels could thus reflect a subclinical state of inflammation that increases the vulnerability to depression. Our findings support the theory that low-grade inflammation contributes to the pathogenesis of depression, adding depression to the list of diseases associated with low-grade inflammation. Further studies are needed to characterize the exact role of suPAR in depression in clinical practice.

Acknowledgments

The skilled technical assistance of Janne Amstrup, Lone Vandsø Jørgensen and Trine Baldorf Berg is highly appreciated. Mads Melbye and Henrik Hjalgrim are thanked for facilitating the epidemiological analysis at the Department of Epidemiological Research at Statens Serum Institut.

Author Contributions

Conceived and designed the experiments: EH HU LVK. Performed the experiments: EH HU. Analyzed the data: EH KG. Contributed reagents/materials/analysis tools: CT JEO. Wrote the paper: EH KG HU JEO.

References

1. Anisman H, Merali Z (1999) Anhedonic and anxiogenic effects of cytokine exposure. Adv Exp Med Biol 461: 199–233.
2. Anisman H, Merali Z (2002) Cytokines, stress, and depressive illness. Brain Behav Immun 16: 513–524.
3. Dantzer R, Bluthe RM, Laye S, Bret-Dibat JL, Parnet P, et al. (1998) Cytokines and sickness behavior. Ann N Y Acad Sci 840: 586–590.
4. Dantzer R (2004) Cytokine-induced sickness behaviour: a neuroimmune response to activation of innate immunity. Eur J Pharmacol 500: 399–411.
5. Maes M (2008) The cytokine hypothesis of depression: inflammation, oxidative & nitrosative stress (IO&NS) and leaky gut as new targets for adjunctive treatments in depression. Neuro Endocrinol Lett 29: 287–291.
6. Maes M, Meltzer HY, Bosmans E, Bergmans R, Vandoolaeghe E, et al. (1995) Increased plasma concentrations of interleukin-6, soluble interleukin-6, soluble interleukin-2 and transferrin receptor in major depression. Journal of Affective Disorders 34: 301–309.
7. Miller AH, Maletic V, Raison CL (2009) Inflammation and Its Discontents: The Role of Cytokines in the Pathophysiology of Major Depression. Biological Psychiatry 65: 732–741.
8. Raison CL, Capuron L, Miller AH (2006) Cytokines sing the blues: inflammation and the pathogenesis of depression. Trends Immunol 27: 24–31.
9. Smith RS (1991) The macrophage theory of depression. Med Hypotheses 35: 298–306.
10. Pasco JA, Nicholson GC, Williams LJ, Jacka FN, Henry MJ, et al. (2010) Association of high-sensitivity C-reactive protein with de novo major depression. Br J Psychiatry 197: 372–377.
11. Matthews KA, Schott LL, Bromberger J, Cyranowski J, Everson-Rose SA, et al. (2007) Associations between depressive symptoms and inflammatory/hemostatic markers in women during the menopausal transition. Psychosom Med 69: 124–130.
12. Deverts DJ, Cohen S, DiLillo VG, Lewis CE, Kiefe C, et al. (2010) Depressive symptoms, race, and circulating C-reactive protein: the Coronary Artery Risk Development in Young Adults (CARDIA) study. Psychosom Med 72: 734–741.
13. Wium-Andersen MK, Orsted DD, Nielsen SF, Nordestgaard BG (2013) Elevated C-reactive protein levels, psychological distress, and depression in 73, 131 individuals. JAMA Psychiatry 70: 176–184.
14. Sennels HP, Jacobsen S, Jensen T, Hansen MS, Ostergaard M, et al. (2007) Biological variation and reference intervals for circulating osteopontin, osteoprotegerin, total soluble receptor activator of nuclear factor kappa B ligand and high-sensitivity C-reactive protein. Scand J Clin Lab Invest 67: 821–835.
15. Macy EM, Hayes TE, Tracy RP (1997) Variability in the measurement of C-reactive protein in healthy subjects: implications for reference intervals and epidemiological applications. Clin Chem 43: 52–58.
16. Ockene IS, Matthews CE, Rifai N, Ridker PM, Reed G, et al. (2001) Variability and classification accuracy of serial high-sensitivity C-reactive protein measurements in healthy adults. Clin Chem 47: 444–450.
17. Andersen O, Eugen-Olsen J, Kofoed K, Iversen J, Haugaard SB (2008) Soluble urokinase plasminogen activator receptor is a marker of dysmetabolism in HIV-infected patients receiving highly active antiretroviral therapy. J Med Virol 80: 209–216.

18. Florquin S, van den Berg JG, Olszyna DP, Claessen N, Opal SM, et al. (2001) Release of urokinase plasminogen activator receptor during urosepsis and endotoxemia. Kidney Int 59: 2054–2061.
19. Sier CF, Sidenius N, Mariani A, Aletti G, Agape V, et al. (1999) Presence of urokinase-type plasminogen activator receptor in urine of cancer patients and its possible clinical relevance. Lab Invest 79: 717–722.
20. Backes Y, van der Sluijs KF, Mackie DP, Tacke F, Koch A, et al. (2012) Usefulness of suPAR as a biological marker in patients with systemic inflammation or infection: a systematic review. Intensive Care Med.
21. Eugen-Olsen J, Andersen O, Linneberg A, Ladelund S, Hansen TW, et al. (2010) Circulating soluble urokinase plasminogen activator receptor predicts cancer, cardiovascular disease, diabetes and mortality in the general population. J Intern Med 268: 296–308.
22. Lyngbaek S, Sehestedt T, Marott JL, Hansen TW, Olsen MH, et al. (2012) CRP and suPAR are differently related to anthropometry and subclinical organ damage. Int J Cardiol.
23. The Danish State Serum Institute S (2014) Medical product Statistics. Available: www.ssi.dk.
24. Kessing LV, Harhoff M, Andersen PK (2007) Treatment with antidepressants in patients with dementia–a nationwide register-based study. Int Psychogeriatr 19: 902–913.
25. Kessing LV, Harhoff M, Andersen PK (2008) Increased rate of treatment with antidepressants in patients with multiple sclerosis. Int Clin Psychopharmacol 23: 54–59.
26. Danner M, Kasl SV, Abramson JL, Vaccarino V (2003) Association between depression and elevated C-reactive protein. Psychosom Med 65: 347–356.
27. Elovainio M, Aalto AM, Kivimaki M, Pirkola S, Sundvall J, et al. (2009) Depression and C-reactive protein: population-based Health 2000 Study. Psychosom Med 71: 423–430.
28. Ford DE, Erlinger TP (2004) Depression and C-reactive protein in US adults: data from the Third National Health and Nutrition Examination Survey. Arch Intern Med 164: 1010–1014.
29. Anderson RJ, Freedland KE, Clouse RE, Lustman PJ (2001) The Prevalence of Comorbid Depression in Adults With Diabetes: A meta-analysis. Diabetes Care 24: 1069–1078.
30. Musselman DL, Miller AH, Porter MR, Manatunga A, Gao F, et al. (2001) Higher Than Normal Plasma Interleukin-6 Concentrations in Cancer Patients With Depression: Preliminary Findings. American Journal of Psychiatry 158: 1252–1257.
31. Musselman DL, Nemeroff CB (2000) Depression really does hurt your heart: stress, depression, and cardiovascular disease. Prog Brain Res 122: 43–59.
32. Raison CL, Miller AH (2003) Depression in cancer: new developments regarding diagnosis and treatment. Biol Psychiatry 54: 283–294.
33. Nielsen NO, Strom M, Boyd HA, Andersen EW, Wohlfahrt J, et al. (2013) Vitamin D status during pregnancy and the risk of subsequent postpartum depression: a case-control study. PLoS One 8: e80686. 10.1371/journal.pone.0080686 [doi];PONE-D-13-23510 [pii].
34. Manderbacka K, Sund R, Koski S, Keskimaki I, Elovainio M (2010) Diabetes and depression? Secular trends in the use of antidepressants among persons with diabetes in Finland in 1997–2007. Pharmacoepidemiol Drug Saf.
35. Thielen K, Nygaard E, Andersen I, Rugulies R, Heinesen E, et al. (2009) Misclassification and the use of register-based indicators for depression. Acta Psychiatr Scand 119: 312–319.
36. Langkilde AA, Hansen TW, Ladelund S, Linneberg A, Andersen O, et al. (2011) Increased plasma soluble uPAR level is a risk marker of respiratory cancer in initially cancer-free individuals. Cancer Epidemiol Biomarkers Prev.
37. Miller GE, Freedland KE, Carney RM, Stetler CA, Banks WA (2003) Pathways linking depression, adiposity, and inflammatory markers in healthy young adults. Brain Behav Immun 17: 276–285.
38. Gariepy G, Wang J, Lesage AD, Schmitz N (2010) The longitudinal association from obesity to depression: results from the 12-year National Population Health Survey. Obesity (Silver Spring) 18: 1033–1038.
39. Edgren G, Tran TN, Hjalgrim H, Rostgaard K, Shanwell A, et al. (2007) Improving health profile of blood donors as a consequence of transfusion safety efforts. Transfusion 47: 2017–2024.
40. Tuomainen TP, Salonen R, Nyyssonen K, Salonen JT (1997) Cohort study of relation between donating blood and risk of myocardial infarction in 2682 men in eastern Finland. BMJ 314: 793–794.
41. Langkilde A, Petersen J, Klausen HH, Henriksen JH, Eugen-Olsen J, et al. (2012) Inflammation in HIV-infected patients: impact of HIV, lifestyle, body composition, and demography - a cross sectional cohort study. PLoS One 7: e51698. 10.1371/journal.pone.0051698 [doi];PONE-D-12-21779 [pii].
42. Andersen AB, Law I, Ostrowski SR, Lebech AM, Hoyer-Hansen G, et al. (2006) Self-reported fatigue common among optimally treated HIV patients: no correlation with cerebral FDG-PET scanning abnormalities. Neuroimmunomodulation 13: 69–75.
43. Ostrowski SR, Piironen T, Hoyer-Hansen G, Gerstoft J, Pedersen BK, et al. (2005) High Plasma Levels of Intact and Cleaved Soluble Urokinase Receptor Reflect Immune Activation and Are Independent Predictors of Mortality in HIV-1-Infected Patients. J Acquir Immune Defic Syndr 39: 23–31.
44. Cinque P, Nebuloni M, Santovito ML, Price RW, Gisslen M, et al. (2004) The urokinase receptor is overexpressed in the AIDS dementia complex and other neurological manifestations. Ann Neurol 55: 687–694.
45. Deininger MH, Trautmann K, Magdolen V, Luther T, Schluesener HJ, et al. (2002) Cortical neurons of Creutzfeldt-Jakob disease patients express the urokinase-type plasminogen activator receptor. Neurosci Lett 324: 80–82.
46. Fauser S, Deininger MH, Kremsner PG, Magdolen V, Luther T, et al. (2000) Lesion associated expression of urokinase-type plasminogen activator receptor (uPAR, CD87) in human cerebral malaria. J Neuroimmunol 111: 234–240.
47. Gveric D, Hanemaaijer R, Newcombe J, van Lent NA, Sier CF, et al. (2001) Plasminogen activators in multiple sclerosis lesions: implications for the inflammatory response and axonal damage. Brain 124: 1978–1988.
48. Walker DG, Lue LF, Beach TG (2002) Increased expression of the urokinase plasminogen-activator receptor in amyloid beta peptide-treated human brain microglia and in AD brains. Brain Res 926: 69–79.
49. Cunningham O, Campion S, Perry VH, Murray C, Sidenius N, et al. (2009) Microglia and the urokinase plasminogen activator receptor/uPA system in innate brain inflammation. Glia 57: 1802–1814.

13

Physical Disability, Anxiety and Depression in People with MS: An Internet-Based Survey via the UK MS Register

Kerina H. Jones*, Philip A. Jones, Rodden M. Middleton, David V. Ford, Katie Tuite-Dalton, Hazel Lockhart-Jones, Jeffrey Peng, Ronan A. Lyons, Ann John, J. Gareth Noble

College of Medicine, Swansea University, Swansea, Wales, United Kingdom

Abstract

Introduction: People with Multiple Sclerosis are known to have a relatively high prevalence of both anxiety and depression. Studies of the relationship between physical disability and mental health in people with MS have reported mixed results, showing the need for further work.

Methods: Between May 2011 and April 2012, 4516 people completed the MSIS-29 (v.1) and HADS scales via the dedicated internet site of the UK MS Register within a 7 day time window. These responses were linked with basic demographic and descriptive data and analysed in SPSS (v.20).

Results: The proportions of people experiencing anxiety or depression increased with physical disability such that 38.0% of respondents with low, and 66.7% with high disability reported at least mild anxiety, and 17.1% of people with low, and 71.7% with high disability experienced at least mild depression. The multiple regression model explained 18.4% of the variance in anxiety with MSIS-29-PHYS score being the strongest predictor of anxiety. The model for depression explained 37.8% of the variance with MSIS-29-PHYS score being the strongest predictor. Some of the other variables included showed negative associations with anxiety and depression, indicating that the influence of physical disability on mental wellbeing could be underestimated.

Conclusions: This study indicates that there is a positive relationship between physical disability and anxiety and depression, that physical disability impacts on anxiety and depression to differing extents, and that the effects vary with gender, age, disease course and disease duration. We have shown that physical disability is a predictor of anxiety and depression, and that other factors may mask the extent of this effect. Whether the causes of anxiety and depression are reactive, organic or a combination, it is essential that mental wellbeing is given due attention in caring for people with MS so that all their health needs can be met.

Editor: Markus Reindl, Innsbruck Medical University, Austria

Funding: The UK MS Register is supported by a grant from the UK MS Society C001-13.3. The sponsor had no role in the design or conduct of the study; the interpretation or analysis of the data; or in the decision to submit for publication (http://www.mssociety.org.uk/).

Competing Interests: The authors have declared that no competing interests exist.

* Email: k.h.jones@swansea.ac.uk

Introduction

Multiple Sclerosis is a chronic, inflammatory auto-immune condition resulting in unpredictable physical and psychological difficulties over the disease course. People with MS suffer higher rates of anxiety and depression than the general population [1–4] and they have been shown to have among the lowest quality of life scores across a range of chronic conditions [5]. Studies have examined mental well-being in chronic illnesses and MS is no exception [1,2,6,7]. But, there have been mixed findings in studies of physical disability and mental health among people with MS, with some authors reporting a relationship, and some not finding one [8–13].

Advances are being made in therapeutic and biomedical MS research; however, there is an acknowledged lack of high quality evidence-based information about living with MS to inform research, policy and practice, and this led to the creation of the UK MS Register [14,15]. The development of the UK MS Register was informed by a programme of qualitative research [16–19] and it has been designed on an innovative data model that brings together datasets from: NHS neurology clinics as people attend their out-patients appointments; sources of routinely-collected data, such as GP and hospital records; and people with

MS directly via a dedicated internet portal by enrolling and providing responses to validated patient reported outcome measures (PROMs). The Register is built on the proven technologies and robust Information Governance arrangements established by the Secure Anonymised Information Linkage (SAIL) system, so that the data in the Register can be anonymously linked at the individual level and accessed for research whilst retaining privacy [20–22]. Data acquisition from clinics and routine sources is underway, subject to consent and data availability. The web portal was launched in May 2011 and, by April 2012, 8736 people with MS had enrolled, with further data collection underway as a continual process.

The portal hosts general health and disease assessment tools such as the Hospital Anxiety and Depression Scale (HADS) [23] and the EQ-5D [24], and disease-specific scales such as the MS Disease Impact Scale-29 (MSIS-29) [25]. These cover a range of topics such as: MS and mental well-being; impact of MS on daily life; lifestyle and health outcomes. Baseline information including: age, gender, date of diagnosis of MS and disease course is collected as part of the registration process and a questionnaire entitled 'You, your MS and lifestyle'. The use of internet technologies in research is increasing, and we have shown that it is feasible to collect information in this way and to use it to characterize a cohort of people with MS [26]. We have also used this method to study the mental well-being of people with MS via the HADS [27], to show that the MSIS-29 can be administered via the internet and used to predict the likely impact of disability on taking an active part in the workforce [28], and how people with MS rate their own quality of life via the EQ5D [29].

The relationship between the physical and psychological impacts of MS measured via the MSIS-29 has been documented [25,30,31] and we have confirmed this in our cohort [28]. However, the MSIS-29 is not designed to distinguish between anxiety and depression and these conditions require specific courses of treatment and care. The MSIS-29 (v.1) consists of 29 questions divided into two components: 20 in the MSIS-29-PHYS for assessing the physical impact, and 9 in the MSIS-29-PSYCH for assessing the psychological impact, of MS. The responses are scored on a Likert scale (1–5, version 1) and summed to give a maximum of 100 on MSIS-29-PHYS and 45 on MSIS-29-PSYCH. These raw scores can be transformed to create two scales each spanning 0 to 100 and expressed as percentages [25,32]. The HADS is a widely used measure of anxiety and depression, each of which are measured on a robust sub-scale of seven questions, scored from 0 to 3, giving possible maximum values of 21 [23]. The HADS has been validated for use with people who have MS [33]. Thus, by using the responses to the HADS and MSIS-29 scales, linkable within the MS Register, we are able to examine the relationships between the physical impact of MS and anxiety and depression. This is the only known study to use these scales to do this for a large cohort of people with MS. It is also novel because it is the largest known study of physical impact, anxiety and depression for MS, or any condition, conducted on data collected via the internet.

Hypothesis and research question

There are mixed results of the relationships between physical disability and mental health in people with MS, and this needs further investigation [8–13]. Previous studies involving the general population and people with MS, have shown that anxiety and depression differ with various factors [27,34]. Furthermore we showed that age and mental wellbeing can show a negative relationship, whereby there is a slight decrease in anxiety level with maturing age [27,28]. Because of this, it is postulated that when physical disability is assessed in conjunction with mental wellbeing, there may differences in how its impact relates to anxiety and depression. Therefore, we set out to use the linked responses to the HADS and MSIS-29 scales to examine the relationships between physical disability, anxiety and depression. Bearing in mind likely modifying factors, we included analysis by gender, age, disease course and disease duration, to determine if, and the extent to which, physical disability impacts upon anxiety and depression.

Methods

Research ethics and governance

The UK MS Register received peer-review via MS Society mechanisms and it ethical approval from the South West – Central Bristol Research Ethics Committee (11/SW/0160) as a research database [35]. Under the conditions of this ethical approval, the datasets collected via the portal, the neurology clinics and routine sources can be anonymously linked at the individual level via the technologies and methodologies used by SAIL, provided that agreement to the portal terms of service (via the portal) and written informed participant consent (at the clinics) have been obtained. Although identifiable information is collected, this is only used to create data linkages. The functioning UK MS Register contains only anonymous data, but facilities are in place to re-contact participants to take part in further research [36]. The Register is open to research collaborations, subject to regulatory and governance requirements. The standard model is that agreed data sub-sets are accessed and analysed within a Safe Haven environment, with scrutiny of research outputs before release [20].

Data collection and analysis

People with MS aged 18 years and over and living in the UK have been able to enrol on the web portal of the UK MS Register since its launch in May 2011. This study used the data collected up to April 2012, by which time 8736 people had joined. As we set out to compare responses to the HADS and MSIS-29, the 4516 responses to these scales completed within 7 days of each other were selected. These were collated with basic demographic and descriptive MS data and the resulting dataset was analysed in SPSS (v.20). As well as being used as continuous data, the HADS anxiety and depression components (with a maximum score of 21 for each) were classified into the accepted categories of normal ($<=7$), mild (8–11), moderate (12–15) and severe (>15), using ≥ 8 as the threshold for indicating likely caseness [37,38]. Within the MSIS-29 scale, raw scores (physical: 20 to 100, psychological: 9 to 45) and transformed scores (%) were both used for ease of reference, and the physical (MSIS-29-PHYS) and psychological (MSIS-29-PSYCH) scores were treated as separate sub-scales in all the analyses in accordance with the suggested guidance of Hobart and colleagues [25,32] and our previous findings [28]. The physical scale was also divided into tertiles with thresholds of 33.3%, 66.7% and 100% to represent low, moderate and high disability scores, respectively. Descriptive statistics were used to characterize the cohort of people with MS. Frequencies were studied using categorised data, and chi-squared tests were used to assess independence. The Kruskal-Wallis one-way analysis of variance was used because the anxiety and depression scores failed the homogeneity of variances test for an ANOVA (Levene's statistic 20.503, df 4513, $p<0.001$; 41.910, df 4513, $p<0.001$). We had previously shown that physical and mental wellbeing can vary with certain factors such as gender, age, disease course and disease duration (time since confirmation of MS by a Neurologist) [27,28], and so these variables were included in multiple regression models.

Table 1. The MSIS-29 and HADS scores of the cohort.

Categories	Mean	SD	SE	Median	IQR	Range
MSIS-29-PHYS score (raw):						
All	60.5	21.6	0.32	62.0	35	20 to 100
Men	63.5	21.0	0.58	66.0	33	20 to 100
Women	59.2	21.8	0.39	61.0	36	20 to 100
PPMS	70.0	17.9	0.70	72.0	27	22 to 100
RRMS	56.7	21.9	0.42	57.0	37	20 to 100
SPMS	73.6	16.0	0.84	74.0	22	28 to 100
DKMS	59.3	21.2	0.82	61.5	36	20 to 100
MSIS-29-PHYS score (%):						
All	50.6	27.0	0.40	52.5	44	0 to 100
Men						
Women						
PPMS	62.5	22.4	0.87	65.0	34	3 to 100
RRMS	45.9	27.3	0.52	46.3	46	0 to 100
SPMS	67.0	20.0	1.05	67.5	28	10 to 100
DKMS	49.1	26.5	1.02	51.9	45	0 to 100
MSIS-29-PSYCH score (raw):						
All	24.8	8.9	0.13	24.0	14	9 to 45
Men	24.9	8.9	0.25	24.0	14	9 to 45
Women	24.7	8.9	0.16	24	13	9 to 45
PPMS	24.7	8.6	0.33	24.0	13	9 to 45
RRMS	24.7	9.0	0.17	24.0	14	9 to 45
SPMS	26.1	8.7	0.46	25.0	13	9 to 45
DKMS	24.4	9.3	0.36	24.0	14	9 to 45
MSIS-29-PSYCH score (%):						
All	43.8	24.8	0.37	41.7	39	0 to 100
Men	44.3	24.8	0.69	41.7	39	0 to 100
Women	43.6	24.8	0.44	41.7	36	0 to 100
PPMS	43.5	23.9	0.93	41.7	36	0 to 100
RRMS	43.5	24.9	0.47	41.7	39	0 to 100
SPMS	47.5	24.1	1.27	44.4	36	0 to 100
DKMS	42.9	25.7	1.00	41.7	39	0 to 100
HADS Anxiety score:						
All	8.03	4.2	0.06	8.0	6	0 to 21
Men	7.51	4.3	0.12	7.0	7	0 to 21
Women	8.25	4.2	0.07	8.0	6	0 to 21
PPMS	7.41	4.2	0.17	7.0	6	0 to 20
RRMS	8.19	4.2	0.08	8.0	6	0 to 21
SPMS	8.08	4.3	0.23	8.0	6	0 to 21
DKMS	8.00	4.5	0.17	8.0	6	0 to 21
HADS Depression score:						
All	7.37	4.2	0.63	7.0	6	0 to 20
Men	7.90	4.3	0.12	8.0	6	0 to 20
Women	7.15	4.2	0.07	7.0	6	0 to 20
PPMS	8.00	4.2	0.16	7.0	6	0 to 20
RRMS	7.01	4.2	0.08	7.0	6	0 to 20
SPMS	8.64	4.1	0.22	8.0	7	1 to 20
DKMS	7.55	4.4	0.17	7.0	7	0 to 20

The physical (MSIS-29-PHYS) and psychological (MSIS-29-PSYCH) impact scores, assessed by the MSIS-29, and the anxiety and depression scores from the HADS of the cohort are shown. Values are included for all respondents, and by gender and disease course. N(all) =4516, N(men) =1302, N(women) =3198, N(PPMS) =654, N(RRMS)

= 2747, N(SPMS) = 360, N(DKMS) = 661). Small differences in totals for gender and disease course, compared to the overall total are due to some respondents (<2%) not providing these details.

Results

Cohort description

The 4516 respondents were comprised of 28.9% men and 71.1% women, which is a ratio of 1 man: 2.46 women. The distribution of disease courses were: 14.8% primary progressive MS (PPMS), 62.1% relapsing-remitting MS (RRMS), 8.1% secondary progressive MS (SPMS) and 14.9% did not know their type of MS (DKMS) (N = 4422). The mean age of the respondents was 50.7 years (SE 0.17, SD 11.2) with a median of 51 years (IQR 16). The mean disease duration was 10.9 years (SE 0.15, SD 8.9) with a median of 9 years (IQR 12). The basic characteristics of this cohort have been described in more detail in a previous article [29]. The mean MSIS-29-PHYS score was 60.5 (50.6%) with a median of 62 (IQR 35) and the mean MSIS-29-PSYCH score was 24.8 (43.8%) with a median of 24 (IQR 14). The mean anxiety score was 8.03 with a median of 8, and the mean depression score was 7.37 with a median of 7. Fuller details of the MSIS-29 and HADS scores, including by gender and disease course, are shown in Table 1.

Proportions and levels of anxiety and depression by physical disability

The HADS and MSIS-29-PHYS scores were divided into categories to examine frequencies and proportions (Tables S1 to S4 in the supporting information). The proportions of people reporting symptoms of anxiety increased with the MSIS-29-PHYS tertiles. Among people with low physical disability scores, the majority (62%) were not suffering from anxiety and only 1.5% were experiencing severe anxiety. However, among those with high physical disability scores only a third (33.3%) had anxiety levels in the normal category and almost a tenth (9.8%) reported severe anxiety (chi-square, $p<0.001$). A similar pattern was observed for depression. Over four fifths (82.9%) of people with low physical disability scores were not experiencing depression, and just 0.4% reported severe depression. For those with a high physical disability score, just 28.3% feel into the normal category, and 9.4% reported severe depression (chi-square, $p<0.001$). The results are illustrated in Figures 1 and 2. A similar chart displaying the relationship between the MSIS-29-PHYS and MSIS-29-PSYCH was shown in a previous article [28]. As well as differences in the frequencies of people suffering from anxiety and depression by physical disability level, differences were also found in the anxiety and depression scores. Anxiety scores were highest in respondents in the high disability category, and the pattern was repeated when depression scores were analysed. ($p<0.001$, $p<0.001$). The median and IQR values (in brackets) for anxiety by physical score in tertiles were: 6 (5) for the low, 8 (6) for the moderate and 9 (7) for the high disability groups. For depression the values were: 4 (4) for the low, 7 (5) for the moderate and 10 (6) for the high disability groups. These patterns are illustrated in Figures 3 and 4, respectively.

Initial inter-scale measures

It has been shown that there is a moderately strong positive relationship (rho = 0.6, $p<0.001$) between the physical and

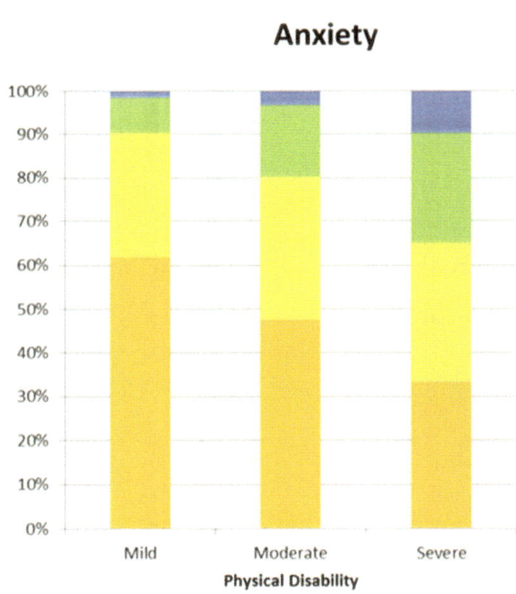

Figure 1. The proportions of people with low, moderate or high physical disability experiencing anxiety. The proportions of people reporting normal (< = 7), mild (8–11), moderate (12–15) or severe (>15) anxiety were assessed against low, moderate and high tertiles of physical disability are shown. It can be seen that greater numbers of the respondents reported symptoms of anxiety with increasing levels of disability. The numbers of people with higher levels of anxiety also increased.

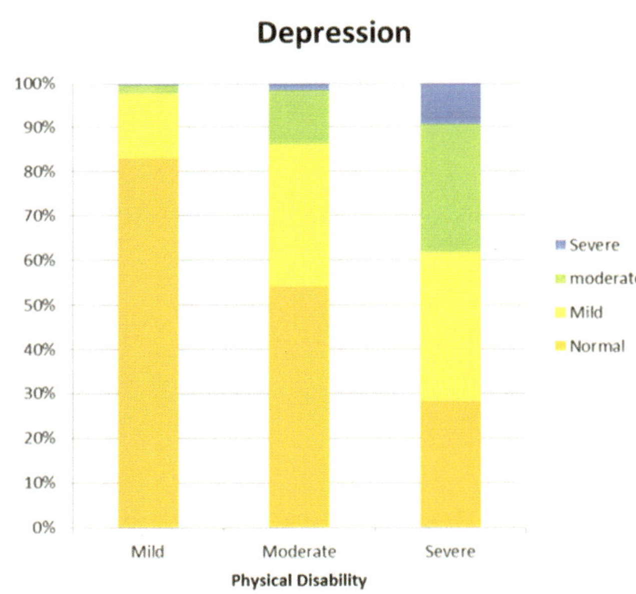

Figure 2. The proportions of people with low, moderate or high physical disability experiencing depression. This shows the proportions of people reporting normal (< = 7), mild (8–11), moderate (12–15) or severe (>15) depression were assessed against low, moderate and high tertiles of physical disability. Greater numbers of the respondents reported symptoms of depression with increasing levels of disability, and the numbers of people with higher levels of depression also increased.

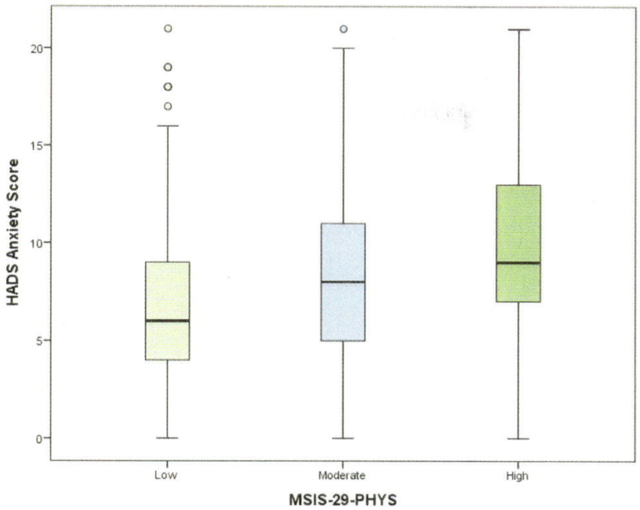

Figure 3. The variation in anxiety scores by physical disability. The variation in the median (and IQR of the) anxiety scores in relation to MSIS-29-PHYS scores divided into tertiles and categorised as low, moderate and high disability can be seen. The anxiety scores were highest for people in the high disability category and lowest in the low disability category ($p<0.001$).

psychological sub-scales of the MSIS-29 [25,28]. In beginning to explore physical disability, anxiety and depression using the MSIS-29 linked to the HADS, the relationships between the scales were assessed by comparing the scores. A weak to moderate positive relationship was found between the MSIS-29-PHYS and anxiety scores ($r = 0.301$, adjusted $r^2 = 0.090$, $p<0.001$) and a moderately strong positive relationship was found between the MSIS-29-PHYS and depression scores ($r = 0.593$, adjusted $r^2 = 0.301$, $p<0.001$). This suggested that there are differences in how physical disability impacts upon anxiety and depression, but as it was known from previous studies that mental wellbeing can vary with certain factors in a cohort such as this [27,28], further analyses were conducted including gender, age and disease course and disease duration.

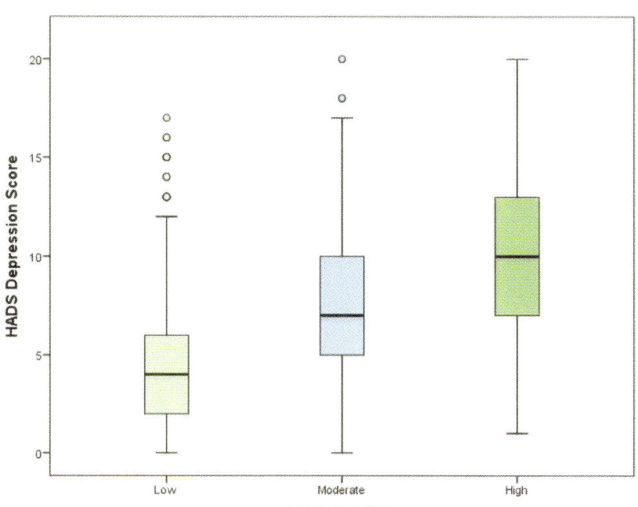

Figure 4. The variation in depression scores by physical disability. This shows the variation in the median (and IQR of the) depression scores in relation to MSIS-29-PHYS scores divided into tertiles and categorised as low, moderate and high disability. The depression scores were highest for people in the high disability category and lowest in the low disability category ($p<0.001$).

Modelling anxiety and depression

We developed multiple regression models using the HADS anxiety or depression score as the dependent variable (DV) and using the MSIS-29-PHYS score, gender, age, disease course and disease duration as the independent variables (IVs). For anxiety, the best model included the physical score, age, male gender, disease duration and a disease course of PPMS. The model excluded female gender, RRMS and SPMS due to co-linearity (all $p<0.001$). The adjusted R^2 was 0.184; Durbin-Watson 1.984; ANOVA $F = 161.508$, df = 5, $p<0.001$. The standardised coefficients β were: physical score 0.398, male gender −0.076, PPMS −0.062, disease duration −0.080, and age −0.218 (all $p<0.001$). This indicates that the MSIS-29-PHYS score is the major contributor to the increase in the anxiety score, and that the other factors actually reduce the effect, with age being the most important of these (Table 2). For depression, the best model included the physical score, age, male gender, disease duration and a disease course of SPMS. The model excluded female gender, PPMS and RRMS due to co-linearity (all $p<0.001$). The adjusted R^2 was 0.378; Durbin-Watson 1.943; ANOVA $F = 432.983$, df = 5, $p<0.001$. The standardised coefficients β were: physical score 0.636, male gender 0.040, SPMS −0.031, disease duration −0.075, and age −0.064 (all $p<0.001$, except male gender = 0.003, SPMS = 0.032). This shows that, of the variables tested, MSIS-29-PHYS score is the major contributor to the increase in the depression score. With the exception of being male, the other factors in the model actually reduce the effect to a small extent (Table 3).

Discussion

Principal Findings

This study has examined the relationships between physical disability, anxiety and depression in a large cohort of people with MS. We have found that the proportions of people experiencing anxiety and depression increase with physical disability. Among people with a low MSIS-29-PHYS score, 38% reported symptoms of anxiety, whereas among people with a high MSIS-29-PHYS score 66.7% experienced at least mild anxiety. A similar pattern was observed in the proportions suffering from depression where 17.1% with low disability and 71.7% with high disability reported at least mild symptoms. This indicates that there is a marked difference in the proportions experiencing anxiety and depression in relation to their physical disability. Furthermore, the anxiety and depression scores of the respondents were found to be higher among those reporting greater disability. The median score for anxiety was 6 in the low, and 9 in the high disability groups. An even more pronounced difference was observed in the medians for depression, with a median value of 4 for the low, and 10 for the high disability groups. So not only do larger proportions of people with greater disability experience anxiety and depression, but people who are more disabled have higher levels of these indicators of mental ill-health.

Simple linear regressions with the MSIS-29-PHYS scores as IV and depression or anxiety scores as DV showed a positive relationship; though for anxiety the model explained less than 10%

Table 2. Multiple Regression Coefficients for MSIS Physical Score for Anxiety.

Summary					
Model	R	R Square	Adjusted R Square	Std. Error of the Estimate	Durbin-Watson
Anxiety	0.420[a]	0.185	0.184	2.00474	1.984
Coefficients					
Model	B[b]	Std. Error[b]	Beta[c]	*t*	*p* value
Constant	4.772	0.203	-	23.476	<0.001
MSIS Physical Score	0.007	0.000	0.398	24.980	<0.001
Age	−0.016	0.001	−0.218	−11.684	<0.001
Length of Diagnosis	−0.128	0.029	−0.080	−4.355	<0.001
Gender	0.372	0.076	0.076	−4.917	<0.001
Disease Course	−0.389	0.102	−0.062	−3.806	<0.001

The multiple regression adjusted R2 for anxiety is 0.184 ($p<0.001$). The strongest relationship is with the MSIS Physical Score (Standardised Coefficient 0.389; $p<0.001$) and there was a negative relationship with Age (Standardised Coefficient −0.218; $p<0.001$).
[a]Predictors: (Constant), MSIS Physical Score, Age, Length of Confirmation, Gender, Disease Course.
[b]Unstandardised coefficient.
[c]Standardised coefficient.

of the change in scores. In previous studies [27,28] the relationships between physical disability, anxiety and depression were observed to vary with certain factors, and by including these, we have been able to develop better models for the impact of physical disability on anxiety and depression. Using multiple regression analyses, this study found a positive relationship between physical disability and anxiety, and between physical disability and depression. Compared to the other variables included, physical disability was found to be the strongest predictor of anxiety and of depression with standardised coefficients β of 0.398 and 0.636 respectively. Although the overall adjusted R^2 indicated that the model explained less than 20% of the variance in anxiety, the findings confirm an earlier observation that age and anxiety can be negatively related [27], and underline the importance of ensuring that moderating factors are taken into account in assessing anxiety in people with MS so that it is not masked and underestimated. However, the models still only explain part of the variance in anxiety (<20%) and depression (<40%), which leads us to conclude that there must be other significant factors involved. Even so, these results highlight the important link between physical disability, anxiety and depression in people with MS.

Limitations

This study was conducted on a self-selected sample of people with MS using self-reported measures of physical disability, anxiety and depression collected via the internet. This may introduce bias as this cohort may not be representative of the prevalent population of people with MS in the UK. For example, we have a lower than expected proportion of people reporting SPMS [26].

Table 3. Multiple Regression Coefficients for MSIS Physical Score for Depression.

Summary					
Model	R	R Square	Adjusted R Square	Std. Error of the Estimate	Durbin-Watson
Depression	0.615[a]	0.379	0.378	1.41753	1.943
Coefficients					
Model	B[b]	Std. Error[b]	Beta[c]	*t*	*p* value
Constant	2.582	0.144	-		
MSIS Physical Score	0.009	0.000	0.636	45.676	<0.001
Age	−0.004	0.001	−0.064	−3.910	<0.001
Length of Diagnosis	−0.097	0.021	−0.075	−4.676	<0.001
Gender	−0.160	0.054	−0.40	02.992	=0.003
Disease Course	−0.155	0.072	−0.031	−2.151	=0.032

The multiple regression adjusted R2 for depression is 0.378 ($p<0.001$). The strongest relationship is with the MSIS Physical Score (Standardised Coefficient 0.636; $p<0.001$) with the other factors only having a relatively small, mostly negative effect.
[a]Predictors: (Constant), MSIS Physical Score, Age, Length of Confirmation, Gender, Disease Course.
[b]Unstandardised coefficient.
[c]Standardised coefficient.

However, the mean age and gender distribution of our respondents accords with published findings, and using educational attainment as a factor that can be compared with the general UK population it was found that our cohort was of a very similar profile [26]. This needs to be recognised as a limitation but it is worth noting that the work described here is on a well characterised cohort and uses within group comparisons. In time as the MS Register builds up its data from NHS Neurology clinics, we will be able to use these data as the gold standard to validate portal data and to assess and account for bias in the self-reported responses. The MS Register has been designed on an electronic data collection model and it is possible that bias is introduced by collecting data via the internet, particularly for the technically inexperienced, elderly or socially disadvantaged [39,40]. However, the value of remote data collection methods is increasingly being recognised in epidemiologic studies, and the evidence largely supports web and mail as being comparable media for questionnaire delivery [41]. For people with MS in particular, a recent study showed that over 85% used the internet, with the majority using it as the first source of health information [42]. Another study showed that about 90% of people with MS have a personal computer and use the internet at least once a week [43]. We were only able to include some factors in our models to assess the relationship between physical disability, anxiety and depression and our models only explain part of the variance. For example, we do not currently have sufficient information on relapses or on fatigue to factor these in, and both of these have been reported to influence depression [8,44]. Another limitation of this study is that it is cross-sectional in design and so caution is needed in inferring causation. But as the MS Register continues to collect data, in the future we will be able to carry out longitudinal studies. The Register is still in early stages of its development, and although it opens up new opportunities for novel studies, some will still need more traditional data collection methods and settings [45].

Comparison with Prior Work

The relationship between chronic illness and mental wellbeing has been studied in a range of conditions [46] and people with MS have been found to experience high levels of anxiety and depression [1,2,27], often higher than among people with other chronic conditions [47]. Various studies have looked at physical disability in relation to depression among people with MS and these have produced mixed results, with some authors reporting an association and some not finding one [8–13]. This is the only study, however, that used the MSIS-29 linked to the HADS scale and at least some of the variations might be due to differing instruments, as well as to differences in size and characteristics of the samples groups. Fewer studies have been conducted on anxiety in people with MS, but it has been observed that anxiety is also of high prevalence and that it can affect the family members as well [10,11,27,48]. It has also been found that people suffering from mental ill-health are more likely to have problems in adhering to disease-modifying medications [49]. It is a matter for concern that people with MS have not in the past been adequately screened for anxiety and depression and, consequently, these conditions have been under-treated [6,50]. While this is not always the case, it is acknowledged that further studies are needed on the use and efficacy of antidepressant and anxiolytic medications among people with MS, as well as other treatments and therapies for these conditions [51]. This is an area that we will be able to address with data from the MS Register in the future as we have begun collecting medications information. Lack of social support is another factor that has been linked to depression among people with MS [52]. This, and the likely influences of co-morbidities, fatigue and relapses on anxiety and depression, are other issues we will be able to study due course. The aetiology of anxiety and depression in people with MS is the subject of much debate as to whether the main causes are organic or reactive in origin [1,12,13]. This is not something that we can examine with our data, but, whatever the causes of mental ill-health, it is imperative that people are given the treatment and care they need so that they and their families can have the best possible quality of life.

Conclusions

This novel study using >4500 responses to the MSIS-29 and HADS scales has indicated that there is a positive relationship between physical disability and anxiety and depression. It has shown that physical disability impacts on anxiety and depression to differing extents, and that the effects vary with gender, age, disease course and disease duration. By including these moderating factors in separate multiple regression models, we were able to show that physical disability is a predictor of anxiety and depression, and that other factors may actually mask the extent of this effect. Our models were able to account for some of the variance in anxiety and depression, but clearly, there must be other factors at work. These may include fatigue and relapses in relation to MS, the presence of other medical conditions, or the availability of social support [8,44,52]. Whether the causes of anxiety and depression are reactive, organic or a combination, it is essential that mental wellbeing is given due attention in caring for people with MS so that all their health needs can be met. We acknowledge the limitations of the study design in the use of self-reported data collected via the internet and in not being able to incorporate all factors that could be influential.

Supporting Information

Table S1 Proportions and frequencies: MSIS-29-PHYS. The proportions and frequencies of respondents in the low, moderate and high tertiles of the MSIS-29-PHYS, stratified by age, gender and disease course are shown.

Table S2 Proportions and frequencies: MSIS-29-PSYCH. The proportions and frequencies of respondents in the low, moderate and high tertiles of the MSIS-29-PSYCH, stratified by age, gender and disease course are shown.

Table S3 Proportions and frequencies: HADS-A. This shows the proportions and frequencies of respondents reporting normal (scores up to 7), mild (8–10), moderate (11–15) and severe anxiety (over 15), stratified by age, gender and disease course.

Table S4 Proportions and frequencies: HADS-D. This shows the proportions and frequencies of respondents reporting normal (scores up to 7), mild (8–10), moderate (11–15) and severe depression (over 15), stratified by age, gender and disease course.

Acknowledgments

The UK MS Register expresses thanks to people with MS for participating in the study by providing their data for inclusion on the Register. http://www.mssociety.org.uk/

Author Contributions

Conceived and designed the experiments: KHJ PAJ RMM DVF JGN RAL. Performed the experiments: KHJ PAJ RMM HL-J KT-D DVF. Analyzed the data: KHJ PAJ RMM JP HL-J AJ JGN. Contributed reagents/materials/analysis tools: DVF RMM HL-J JP. Contributed to the writing of the manuscript: KHJ PAJ RMM KT-D HL-J JP DVF RAL JGN.

References

1. Siegert RJ, Abernathy DA (2005) Depression in multiple sclerosis: a review. J Neurol Neurosurg Psychiatry, 76: 469–475.
2. Arnett PA, Barwick FH, Beeney JE (2008) Depression in multiple sclerosis: review and theoretical proposal. Journal of the International Psychological Society, 14: 691–724.
3. da Silva AM, Vilhena E, Lopes A, Santos E, Gonçalves MA et al. (2011) Depression and anxiety in a Portuguese MS population: associations with physical disability and severity of disease. Journal of the Neurological Sciences, 306: 66–70.
4. Michalski D, Liebig S, Thomae E, Singer S, Hinz A, et al. (2010) Anxiety, depression and impaired health-related quality of life are therapeutic challenges in patients with multiple sclerosis. Mental Illness, 2:e5.
5. Sullivan PW, Slejko JF, Sculpher MJ, Ghushchyan V (2011) Catalogue of EQ-5D Scores for the United Kingdom. Medical Decision Making 2011 31: 800.
6. Beiske AG, Svensson E, Sandanger I, Czujko B, Pedersen ED, et al. (2008) Depression and anxiety amongst multiple sclerosis patients. European Journal of Neurology, 15: 239–245.
7. Sà MJ (2008) Psychological aspects of multiple sclerosis. Clinical Neurology and Neurosurgery, 110: 868–877.
8. Minden SL1, Orav J, Reich P (1987) Depression in multiple sclerosis. General Hospital Psychiatry. Nov;9(6):426–34.
9. Chwastiak L, Ehde DM, Gibbons LE, Sullivan M, Bowen JD, et al. (2002) Depressive symptoms and severity of illness in multiple sclerosis: epidemiologic study of a large community sample. American Journal of Psychiatry, 159(11):1862–8.
10. Zorzon M, de Masi R, Nasuelli D, Ukmar M, Mucelli RP, et al. (2001) Depression and anxiety in multiple sclerosis. A clinical and MRI study in 95 subjects. Journal of Neurology, 248(5):416–421.
11. Lynch SG, Kroencke DC, Denney DR (2001) The relationship between disability and depression in multiple sclerosis: the role of uncertainty, coping, and hope. Multiple Sclerosis, 7(6):411–6.
12. Dahl OP, Stordal E, Lydersen S, Midgard R (2009) Anxiety and depression in multiple sclerosis. A comparative population-based study in Nord-Trondelag County, Norway. Multiple Sclerosis, 15(12):1495–501. doi: 10.1177/1352458509351542
13. Bakshi R, Czarnecki D, Shaikh ZA, Priore RL, Janardhan V, et al. (2000) Brain MRI lesions and atrophy are related to depression in multiple sclerosis. Neuroreport, 11(6):1153–8.
14. UK Multiple Sclerosis Society Strategy 2008 to 2012. Available: http://www.mssociety.org.uk/ms-resources/research-strategy. Accessed 2014 March 28.
15. UK Multiple Sclerosis Society Strategy 2013 to 2017. Available: http://www.mssociety.org.uk/ms-resources/ms-society-research-strategy-2013-2017. Accessed 2014 March 28.
16. Osborne LA, Middleton RM, Jones KH, Ford DV, Noble JG (2013) Desirability and expectations of the UK MS Register: Views of people with MS. International Journal of Medical Informatics 82(11): 1104–10. doi: 10.1016/j.ijmedinf.2013.07.005
17. Osborne LA, Noble JG, Lockhart-Jones H, Middleton RM, Thompson S, et al. (2013) Identifying and addressing the barriers to the use of an internet-register for Multiple Sclerosis. International Journal of Healthcare Information Systems and Informatics 8(1), 1–16, doi: 10.4018/jhisi.2013010101
18. Osborne LA, Noble JG, Lockhart-Jones H, Middleton RM, Thompson S, et al. (2012) Sources of discovery, reasons for registration, and expectations of an internet-based register for Multiple Sclerosis: Visualisations and explorations of word uses and contexts. International Journal of Healthcare Information Systems and Informatics, 7: 3.
19. Osborne LA, Noble JG, Maramba IDC, Jones KH, Middleton RM, et al. (2014) Outcome measures for Multiple Sclerosis: A review. Physical Therapy Reviews, Volume 19 Issue 1,24–38, doi: 10.1179/1743288X13Y.0000000094
20. Jones KH, Ford DV, Jones C, D'Silva R, Thompson S, et al. (2014) A case study of the Secure Anonymous Information Linkage (SAIL) Gateway: a privacy-protecting remote access system for health-related research and evaluation, Journal of Biomedical Informatics: special issue on medical data privacy. doi: 10.1016/j.jbi.2014.01.003
21. Ford DV, Jones KH, Verplancke JP, Lyons RA, John G, et al. (2009) The SAIL Databank: building a national architecture for e-health research and evaluation. BMC Health Services Research, 9(1):157.
22. Lyons RA, Jones KH, John G, Brooks CJ, Verplancke JP, et al. (2009) The SAIL databank: linking multiple health and social care datasets. BMC Medical Informatics and Decision Making, 9(1):3.
23. Zigmond AS, Snaith RP (1983) The hospital anxiety and depression scale. Acta Psychiatrica Scandinavica 67(6):361–370.
24. The EuroQol group (1990) EuroQol - a new facility for the measurement of health related quality of life. Health Policy, 16: 199–208.
25. Hobart J, Lamping D, Fitzpatrick R, Riazi A, Thompson A (2001) The Multiple Sclerosis Impact Scale (MSIS-29). Brain, 124(5):962.
26. Ford DV, Jones KH, Middleton RM, Lockhart-Jones H, Maramba IDC, et al. (2012) The feasibility of collecting information from people with Multiple Sclerosis for the UK MS Register via a web portal: characterising a cohort of people with MS. BMC Medical Informatics and Decision Making, 12(1), 73.
27. Jones KH, Ford DV, Jones PA, John A, Middleton RM, et al. (2012). A Large-scale Study of Anxiety and Depression in People with Multiple Sclerosis: a Survey via the Web Portal of the UK MS Register. PLoS One 7(7): e41910. doi:10.1371/journal.pone.0041910
28. Jones KH, Ford DV, Jones PA, John A, Middleton RM, et al. (2013) The physical and psychological impact of Multiple Sclerosis using the MSIS-29 via the web portal of the UK MS Register. PLoS One 8(1):e55422. doi: 10.1371/journal.pone.0055422
29. Jones KH, Ford DV, Jones PA, John A, Middleton RM, et al. (2013) How people with Multiple Sclerosis rate their quality of life: an EQ-5D survey via the UK MS Register. PLoS One 8(6):e65640, doi: 10.1371/journal.pone.0065640
30. Ramp M, Khan F, Misajon RA, Pallant JF (2009) Rasch analysis of the Multiple Sclerosis Impact Scale (MSIS-29). Health and Quality of Life Outcomes, 7: 58.
31. Gray OM, McDonnell GV, Hawkins SA (2009) Tried and tested: the psychometric properties of the Multiple Sclerosis Impact Scale (MSIS-29) in a population-based study. Multiple Sclerosis Journal, 15: 75–80.
32. Hobart J, Cano S (2009) Improving the evaluation of therapeutic interventions in multiple sclerosis: the role of new psychometric methods. Health Technology Assessment, vol 13, no. 12.
33. Honarmand K, Feinstein A (2009) A validation of the Hospital Anxiety and Depression Scale for use with multiple sclerosis patients. Multiple Sclerosis, 15: 1518–1524.
34. Crawford JR, Henry JD, Crombie C, Taylor EP (2001) Normative data for the HADS from a large non-clinical sample. British Journal of Clinical Psychology, 40: 429–434.
35. Health Research Authority website. Ethical review of research databases. Available: http://www.hra.nhs.uk/research-community/before-you-apply/determine-which-review-body-approvals-are-required/. Accessed 2014 March 28.
36. The UK MS Register website. Available: http://www.ukmsregister.org. Accessed 2014 March 28.
37. Snaith RP (2003) The Hospital Anxiety and Depression Scale. Health and Quality of Life Outcomes, 1(1):29.
38. Bjelland I, Dahl AA, Tangen Haug T, Neckelmann D (2002) The validity of the Hospital Anxiety and Depression Scale. An updated literature review. Journal of Psychosomatic Research 52 (2): 69–77.
39. Good A, Stokes S, Jerrams-Smith J (2007) Elderly, Novice Users and Health Information Websites: issues of accessibility and usability. Journal of Healthcare Information Management, 21:3: 72–79.
40. Boot CLR, Frans JM (2010) The public and the Internet: Multifaceted drives for seeking health information. Health Informatics Journal, 16: 145.
41. Gallacher J, Colliins R, Elliot P, Palmer S, Burton P, et al. (2013) A platform for the remote conduct of gene-environment interaction studies. PLoS One, 8(1):e54331. doi: 10.1371/journal.pone.0054331
42. Marrie RA, Salter AR, Tyry T, Fox RJ, Cutter GR (2013) Preferred Sources of Health Information in Persons With Multiple Sclerosis: Degree of Trust and Information Sought. Journal of Medical Internet Research 15(4):e67, doi:10.2196/jmir.2466
43. Haase R, Schultheiss T, Kempcke R, Thomas K, Ziemssen T (2012) Use and Acceptance of Electronic Communication by Patients With Multiple Sclerosis: A Multicenter Questionnaire Study. Journal of Medical Internet Research 14(5):e135, doi:10.2196/jmir.2133
44. Krupp LB, Alvarez LA, LaRocca NG, Scheinberg LC (1988) Fatigue in multiple sclerosis. Archives of Neurology Apr;45(4): 435–7.
45. Noble JG, Osborne LA, Jones KH, Middleton RM, Ford DV (2012) Commentary on 'Disability outcome measures in multiple sclerosis clinical trials'. Multiple Sclerosis Journal Published online before print, 11 September 2012, doi: 10.1177/1352458512457847
46. Patten SB, Williams JV, Lavorato DH, Modgill G, Jetté N, et al. (2008) Major depression as a risk factor for chronic disease incidence: longitudinal analyses in a general population cohort. General Hospital Psychiatry Oct;30(5): 407–13. doi: 10.1016/j.genhosppsych.2008.05.001
47. Egede LE (2007) Major depression in individuals with chronic medical disorders: prevalence, correlates and association with health resource utilization, lost productivity and functional disability. General Hospital Psychiatry -Oct;29(5): 409–16.
48. Janssens AC, Buljevac D, van Doorn PA, van der Meché FG, Polman CH, et al. (2006) Prediction of anxiety and distress following diagnosis of multiple sclerosis: a two-year longitudinal study. Multiple Sclerosis, 12(6): 794–801.

49. Bruce JM, Hancock LM, Arnett P, Lynch S (2010) Treatment adherence in multiple sclerosis: association with emotional status, personality, and cognition. Journal of Behavioural Medicine, (3): 219–27. doi: 10.1007/s10865-010-9247-y. Epub 2010 Feb 3.
50. Mohr DC, Hart SL, Fonareva I, Tasch ES (2006) Treatment of depression for patients with multiple sclerosis in neurology clinics. Multiple Sclerosis, 12(2): 204–8.
51. Cetin K, Johnson KL, Ehde DM, Kuehn CM, Amtmann D, et al. (2007) Antidepressant use in multiple sclerosis: epidemiologic study of a large community sample. Multiple Sclerosis, (8): 1046–53. Epub 2007 Jul 10.
52. Gilchrist AC, Creed FH (1994) Depression, cognitive impairment and social stress in multiple sclerosis. Journal of Psychosomatic Research, 38(3): 193–201.

14

Practitioner Perspectives on Strategies to Promote Longer-Term Benefits of Acupuncture or Counselling for Depression

Hugh MacPherson[1]*, Liz Newbronner[1,2], Ruth Chamberlain[2], Stewart J. Richmond[1], Harriet Lansdown[1], Sara Perren[1], Ann Hopton[1], Karen Spilsbury[1]

1 Department of Health Sciences, University of York, York, United Kingdom, **2** Firefly Research & Evaluation, North Yorkshire, United Kingdom

Abstract

Background: Non-pharmacological interventions for depression may help patients manage their condition. Evidence from a recent large-scale trial (ACUDep) suggests that acupuncture and counselling can provide longer-term benefits for many patients with depression. This paper describes the strategies practitioners reported using to promote longer-term benefits for their patients.

Methods: A qualitative sub-study of practitioners (acupuncturists and counsellors) embedded in a randomised controlled trial. Using topic guides, data was collected from telephone interviews and a focus group, altogether involving 19 counsellors and 17 acupuncturists. Data were audio recorded, transcribed verbatim and analysed using thematic content analysis.

Results: For longer-term impact, both acupuncturists and counsellors encouraged insight into root causes of depression on an individual basis and saw small incremental changes as precursors to sustained benefit. Acupuncturists stressed the importance of addressing concurrent physical symptoms, for example helping patients relax or sleep better in order to be more receptive to change, and highlighted the importance of Chinese medicine theory-based lifestyle change for lasting benefit. Counsellors more often highlighted the importance of the therapeutic relationship, emphasising the need for careful "pacing" such that the process and tools employed were tailored and timed for each individual, depending on the "readiness" to change. Our data is limited to acupuncture practitioners using the principles of traditional Chinese medicine, and counsellors using a humanistic, non-directive and person-centred approach.

Conclusions: Long-term change appears to be an important focus within the practices of both acupuncturists and counsellors. To achieve this, practitioners stressed the need for an individualised approach with a focus on root causes.

Editor: Fan Qu, Women's Hospital, School of Medicine, Zhejiang University, China

Funding: This research is supported by the National Institute for Health Research (NIHR) under Programme Grants for Applied Research (Grant No. RP-PG-0707-10186). The views expressed in this presentation are those of the author(s) and not necessarily those of the NHS, the NIHR or the Department of Health. The funders had no role in study design, data collection and analysis, decision to publish, or preparation of the manuscript.

Competing Interests: Liz Newbronner and Ruth Chamberlain worked for Firefly Research & Evaluation and were commissioned by the Department of Health Sciences, University of York, to conduct the interviews and work with the authors to analyse the data and prepare this manuscript.

* Email: hugh.macpherson@york.ac.uk

Background

Depression is a common illness in primary care. Some of the optimism regarding the potential of selective serotonin re-uptake inhibitors (SSRIs) as a treatment for depression has faded in the light of concerns about effectiveness and safety. [1] A recent meta-analysis has concluded that antidepressants have only a modest advantage over placebo, with the magnitude of benefit increasing with severity of depression. [2] There is an ongoing interest, especially among patients, in the potential of non-pharmacological treatments for depression, with the hope that they might avoid some of the concerns about antidepressants regarding safety and dependency. [3] Furthermore, for many patients, depression is a chronic and recurring illness, and non-pharmacological treatments that seek to improve longer-term outcomes are potentially of interest.

Evidence from a recent large-scale trial (ACUDep) [4] has suggested that acupuncture and counselling can provide longer-term benefits for many patients with on-going depression in primary care. The ACUDep trial recruited 755 patients with depression via 27 participating primary care practices; 302 were randomised to up to 12 acupuncture sessions; 302 to up to 12 counselling sessions; and 151 to usual care alone. The counselling was delivered within a recognised, manualised competency framework developed by Roth et al. at the University College of London's Centre for Outcomes Research and Effectiveness. [5] The acupuncture diagnosis and treatment, including selection of points, was based on the principles of traditional Chinese medicine, the details of which are reported elsewhere. [6]

Both acupuncture and counselling were found to be effective in reducing the symptoms of depression when compared to usual care, and these differences were significant at the 3 and 6 month time points, as well as when averaged over the 12 month period. [4][7] The trial focused on the effectiveness and cost effectiveness of the interventions. However, we were keen to understand the experiences of those providing treatments (acupuncture or counselling) within the trial, and in particular the aspects of these interventions that practitioners perceived to be associated with their longer-term benefit. In doing so, these insights will help understanding of the interventions and help inform both clinical practice and any future research design.

Underreported within randomised controlled trials are qualitative analyses of strategies employed by acupuncturists and counsellors within treatment for depression that are intended to promote longer-term change. In one qualitative study, interviews with patients receiving counselling in routine practice were used to identify the key characteristics of the intervention that were experienced as beneficial in the longer term. [8] In the authors' interpretation, a key component was the client's active engagement during and between counselling sessions. In turn this enabled a change to take place in the way they conducted their lives and relationships. We are unaware of any published qualitative studies of the processes of care associated with long-term change in the case of acupuncture for depression.

This qualitative study, embedded within a clinical trial, was designed to explore the perceptions and experiences of counsellors and acupuncturists who provided the treatment interventions within the trial. The aim was to understand better the key aspects of their work and their perceptions of the 'active ingredients' of counselling or acupuncture that were intended to promote longer-term benefits for the patients and may help in our understanding of the trial results. The study also provided an opportunity to identify important issues relating to professional practice and future policy, which are not reported here, including support needs and working arrangements; the acceptability and feasibility of different treatment options; the implications for the provision of acupuncture or humanistic counselling for treating depression within primary care settings; and related commissioning issues.

Methods

Recruitment of participants

To provide treatments for trial participants, 41 counsellors and 23 acupuncturists were recruited from across the regions of Yorkshire and the North East of England. Altogether these practitioners treated 497 (out of 604) patients participating in the intervention arms of the ACUDep trial. After the end of the trial's treatment phase, acupuncturists and counsellors who had consulted with at least two patients in the trial were invited to take part in the qualitative sub-study. They were sent an information sheet and consent form and asked to indicate whether they would prefer to be involved in a one-to-one telephone interview or a focus group. The aim was to recruit up to 30 counsellors and acupuncturists (approximately 15 in each group). Ethical approval was obtained from the York NHS Research Ethics Committee (REC ref: 09/H1311/75), which included approval for procedures that required written consent from all participants.

Interview and focus group data collection

The topic guides for the interviews and focus group were developed by the ACUDep research team to address the main research question of practitioner strategies intended to promote longer-term benefits for patients – a key finding of the trial results. The initial ideas were developed into topic guides for the interviews, one for each of the practitioner groups, and one for the focus group discussion which comprised both acupuncturists and counsellors. Along with questions, the topic guides also included prompts.These were then refined further at face-to-face meetings, such that the guides covered the practitioner's professional background and experience of working with depression, their approach to treating depression, their perceptions of working within the trial, and their thoughts on the implications for policy and professional practice. These issues were considered important for interpretation of the qualitative data.

All participants provided written consent. Those who agreed to take part in a telephone interview were contacted (either by telephone or email) to arrange a convenient time for the one-to-one interview. Arrangements were confirmed by email and the topic guide to be used in the interview was attached. Only small numbers of practitioners expressed a preference for a focus group discussion and so only one group discussion was held. Many issues covered in the group discussion were similar to those expressed in the individual interviews. However, the group discussion provided an opportunity for therapists to explore together any differences and similarities in their perceptions and experiences. This added to the richness of the data. The interviews and focus group were conducted by two experienced health services researchers from the research team who were not involved in the conduct of the trial itself (LN and RC). The interviews commonly lasted around 45 minutes (range 40 to 90) and the focus group 90 minutes. They were all audio-recorded (with participants' permission) and transcribed verbatim.

Data analysis

The transcripts were analysed thematically. [9] The main areas of inquiry covered in the topic guides were used for a framework approach to thematic content analysis, which involved analysing the data across the two groups of practitioners contributing to the study. [10] The framework was created in an Excel spreadsheet and coded and populated with data from the transcripts by the two researchers who had conducted the interviews (LN and RC). An inductive process was used to identify themes, drawing on shared experiences or points of difference identified from the data. As this study was intended to broaden our understanding of practice in relation to the treatment of patients with depression, the analysis also sought to draw out findings which might inform the practice of acupuncturists and counsellors.

Results

Practitioner characteristics

Forty-one therapists consented to be involved in the study but five therapists later withdrew or didn't respond when the fieldwork was being set up. The sub-study included individual telephone interviews with15 counsellors and13 acupuncturists (n = 28) and one focus group with 4 counsellors and 4 acupuncturists (n = 8) (Table 1). The sample for the qualitative sub-study included over half (56%) of the total number of therapists involved in the main trial.

The 17 participating acupuncturists were registered members of the British Acupuncture Council with at least three years' post-qualification experience and practising with the theoretical

Table 1. Breakdown of study participants.

	Number involved in main trial	Number involved in one-to-one interviews	Number involved in the focus group	Total number participating
Counsellors	41	15	4	19
Acupuncturists	23	13	4	17
Total	64	28	8	36

approach of traditional Chinese medicine. [6] The acupuncturists were predominantly male (39% were female), with an average duration of practice of 12 years. In the trial they treated on average 9 patients, who attended on average for 10 sessions. The 19 counsellors were members of the British Association for Counselling and Psychotherapy, who were accredited or were eligible for accreditation having completed 400 supervised hours post-qualification, and provided clients a humanistic style of counselling based on competences developed for Skills for Health. [11] They were predominantly female practitioners (79%), with an average duration of practice of 7 years. In the trial they treated on average 7 patients, who attended on average for 9 sessions.

Trial patient characteristics

Practitioners were treating patients in the trial who had ongoing depression for at least 3 months and a score of 20 or more on the Beck Depression Inventory (BDI-II), with 38% having depression categorised as "moderate" and 62% "severe". [4] The mean age was 44 years and 73% were female. They were (on average) 25 years old when they experienced their first episode of depression. In terms of prescribed medication, 69% were on anti-depressants and 48% were on analgesics.

Overview of the findings from thematic analysis

A cluster of eight themes emerged from the framework analysis. Almost all of the acupuncturists and counsellors stressed the importance they attached to promoting longer-term benefits. To achieve this, practitioners commonly reported on the need to focus on the root causes, to address treatment for each individual patient, and to value small incremental changes from one session to the next as precursors to sustained benefit over the longer term. Acupuncturists more commonly reported on the need to address concurrent physical symptoms, for example helping patients relax or sleep better in order to be more receptive to change. Most also highlighted the importance of Chinese medicine theory-based lifestyle change as an approach to promoting more lasting benefit. Counsellors more often highlighted the importance of the therapeutic relationship, emphasising the need for careful "pacing" such that the process and tools employed were tailored and timed for each individual, depending on the "readiness" to change. These findings are presented in more detail below.

Importance of a long-term focus

Long-term change appears to be an important focus within the practices of both acupuncturists and counsellors. Almost all of the practitioners mentioned the long-term perspective as inherent to the way they worked.

> *with something like depression, longer term for me, longer term approach is very fundamental.*(acupuncturist1)

For acupuncturists, this perspective was drawn from the theoretical approach of traditional Chinese medicine, in which long-term change needed to be facilitated by lifestyle changes related to acupuncture theory. For counsellors it was drawn from the humanistic approach, which many contrasted with what was perceived as the "quick fix" of cognitive behavioural therapy (CBT).

> *I would like to think that the whole approach is based on longer term change, in terms of the client learning ways of coping. Not just with the present crisis, whatever it might be, but hopefully that they would take something from it that they could apply in the future.*(counsellor1)

When comparing acupuncturists and counsellors, the reported long-term focus involved some differences in approach, as described above, as well as some similarities, especially with regard to encouraging insight into root causes on an individual basis and seeking small incremental changes as important precursors of overall benefit.

Identifying root causes

The commitment to identifying and addressing the root causes of depression within the treatment process was a commonly expressed factor among both acupuncturists and counsellors. Acupuncturists commonly used the theoretical concept of "root" (ben) and "branch" (biao).

> *Within Chinese Medicine we talk about treating the root and the branch. And there is merit in treating both.*(acupuncturist2)
>
> *Looking for underlying causes. Obviously there's some symptomatic stuff, but always looking at the root causes and using that as where I would start to work out my treatment principles.*(acupuncturist3)

The counsellors were more interested in "going deeper" and "further back (in time)" with their clients as a way of getting to the root causes.

> *From my experience generally, you've got to get to the root causes of depression, so it's much deeper than a CBT approach, so I think if people don't do that when clients present depression, then perhaps they are failing the clients at some level.*(counsellor2)
>
> *I suppose for me the long term change generally stems from a clear understanding of just what's been at the root of it all.*(counsellor3)

The implications of this approach, as reported by several practitioners, are that unless the underlying causes are addressed, then it is likely that there will not be the sustained long-term change that is desired.

Individualisation

When practised within the theoretical framework of traditional Chinese medicine, acupuncture treatment has been customised to the individual, such that treatment varies not only between patients but also, for the same patient, it varies over time. Likewise for the counsellors in the trial, all of whom were committed to working within the humanistic tradition, a person-centred approach was provided.

> *Everybody's different, so whenever a patient comes in, obviously, you take their full medical history. And quite often there will be other key characteristics, so not everybody gets the same points diagnosis, because of the different underlying features of their condition.*(acupuncturist4)
> *That the reason for depression for individuals and how it's processed is unique and therefore the process focuses on how the client experiences it. I also think it's useful to bear in mind the possible causes and theories to be shared with the client.*(counsellor4)

Valuing incremental change

Practitioners reported a certain amount of caution about expecting sudden or cathartic changes in their patients. More common was a sense that positive benefit required a series of small incremental changes that when combined with self-help approaches would hopefully build a more sustained improvement.

> *Well long term change can even come about from even small changes, really. If somebody can just sleep all night, it's surprising.*(acupuncturist5)
> *I think to try almost to help people take responsibility and realise that there maybe is something that they can do. I think sometimes people get trapped in feeling depressed and feeling unable to do anything. So almost helping empower them to find changes that they can start to make, to make those improvements for themselves, which over time build up and help them move forward.*(counsellor5)

Addressing concurrent physical symptoms

Acupuncturists generally stressed the importance of addressing concurrent physical symptoms, for example helping patients relax or sleep better in order to be more receptive to change.

> *What I find really interesting about working on the trial is that a lot of time people came with depression but in reality there was a host of other signs and symptoms that they were not happy in their life. Just kind of bowel, musculoskeletal, anything. So when they got a sense that I was treating them as a whole person, rather than just treating the depression........ When I'd sorted out their back, their stomach, ulcers, bad knees, you know, suddenly their depression got better. To me, that's how Traditional Chinese Medicine should be – it works with everything. Rather than, you know, like depression as a standalone thing.*(acupuncturist2)

By contrast, the counsellors were less focused on the physical symptoms, and worked more on the assumption that by treating the underlying causes of depression there should be a knock-on effect in terms of reducing physical symptoms.

> *I'm not particularly interested in just treating symptoms, but what I'm usually interested in and what people are usually asking for is that they want to understand why they're feeling the way that they are. If you can deal with that issue, then it should help them to rid themselves of the symptoms really.*(counsellor6)

Lifestyle changes

Almost all of the acupuncturists highlighted the importance of giving advice about lifestyle change that was relevant to the Chinese medicine perspective.

> *Yeah, it's overall sort of aimed at the long-term and I think people, you know, if they get further along with the acupuncture, they realise that it's all to do with lifestyle change as well and that those things are going to be the ones that bring them lasting benefit. Because often people start to feel better after a few treatments and then when they build in the lifestyle thing, when they actually start to think, oh, this acupuncture seems to be working for me, maybe I'll follow some of the advice as well.* (acupuncturist6)

Those acupuncturists who reported on the role of lifestyle change tended to stress the importance of tailoring the advice to the patient, both in terms of content related to acupuncture theory (e.g. diet, relaxation, exercise, etc) as well as likely acceptability.

The counsellors worked within a trial protocol that had a strong emphasis on working within the humanistic tradition, which included being non-directive. [11] The protocol therefore limited the extent that they could offer lifestyle advice within the trial. Some counsellors, who typically worked more eclectically elsewhere, said they might normally include lifestyle advice, especially when working with people with addictions.

Therapeutic relationship

Counsellors consistently stressed the importance of the therapeutic relationship.

> *I tend to think that lasting change requires a greater degree of insight [than CBT]. But I think the change often comes – I suppose this is what puts me very squarely in the humanistic camp, the existential camp, I think it's often the relationship itself – it's actually having a new experience of a relationship for some people can be transformative.*(counsellor3)
> *But the essence of my approach is the relationship and building good levels of rapport and trust and helping the client to feel okay with you. So it's an okay space at the start and if that forms well, that's a springboard, hopefully, for sort of therapeutic practice and change for people.*(counsellor2)

However for some acupuncturists, this was also reported as a component of the treatment process that helped engender longer-term gains.

And it's kind of like a trust relationship – if they believe in the acupuncture, they believe in what you're telling them. And that kind of gives them the impetus to carry on in the longer term.(acupuncturist6)

Careful "pacing" based on "readiness to change"

Many of the counsellors emphasised the need for careful "pacing" such that the process and tools employed were tailored and timed for each individual, depending on the "readiness" to change.

And what I'm very aware of in counselling is that people will come to therapy at different stages of readiness to change. And it's very difficult to measure how useful it's been. So for example, with one client I can think of in the trial, I think he would have – I think it was probably a first experience for him, from being listened to and from being taken seriously and I think that was huge. He was very stuck. In terms of how much that was going to affect outcomes, in terms of was he going to make the necessary changes, he might have been able to begin to identify, or briefly identify, what it was in his life that was making him depressed – in terms of outcomes he wasn't at the stage where he was going to make any massive changes. But I think just having that experience, that first experience. That kind of thing is so hard to measure, isn't it?(counsellor6)

I tend to go with the speed of the client. However, if I can – my personal approach would be to help them in as short a sessions as possible to get them to feel better. However, I'm very careful to work with their speed. So am I short or long term.(counsellor7)

A number of acupuncturists identified issues related to timing, expressing the point that as patients improve, ideally appointments should be spread out towards the end of the course of treatment and beyond, as a way of sustaining benefit over the longer term.

In summary, the themes capture both similarities and differences in approaches between acupuncture and counselling, with most practitioners of both interventions having a shared sense of the prerequisites for sustained long-term benefit. The impression formed from the interviews is that the various approaches do not operate in isolation. Although the emphasis may vary, the themes appear to be integrated into a coherent combination that uniquely informs the practice of each practitioner.

Generalisability issues

With regard to the extent that these findings are transferable to other settings, the majority of counsellors said that the severity of the depression amongst trial patients was not markedly dissimilar to the people they routinely saw. By contrast, the acupuncturists were generally less used to dealing with patients with moderate to severe depression, and many said that they less commonly saw patients who consulted primarily because of a diagnosis of depression. Several of the therapists reported that the trial patients had a different attitude towards treatment compared to their private patients, particularly a more limited knowledge of the therapeutic intervention and a lower level of motivation to help themselves. Therapists also noted that there were a greater proportion of patients in lower income brackets, with more long-standing depression, or with unmanaged drug/alcohol addictions.

Discussion

Principal findings

Both acupuncturists and counsellors generally delivered treatments with an eye to encouraging longer-term change with the intention that, ideally, any putative benefit would be sustained well beyond the 12 sessions that were provided within the trial. While both types of practitioners reported on the need to address the root causes, the approach differed. For the acupuncturists there was a focus drawn from Chinese medicine theory on treating the root cause (the *ben*) as well as the manifesting symptoms (the *biao*) with the precise details of the intervention customised to their patients at an individual level. Meanwhile the approach of the counsellors was to get below the surface of the clients' problems and to "go deeper" and "further back (in time)" as a way of getting a handle on the root cause and, as with the acupuncturists, this required an individualised approach.

There were further differences in approach to facilitating more sustained benefits. Acupuncturists were more focussed on physical symptoms, on whether these could be resolved by acupuncture in order to speed up the improvements in the symptoms of depression, and on providing lifestyle advice linked to the Chinese medicine diagnosis. Meanwhile counsellors were more explicit on the importance of a strong therapeutic relationship accompanied by a careful consideration of what might be a manageable pace of change.

Strengths and limitations

The sub-study is nested within the largest trial to date of acupuncture or counselling for depression, and provides unique access to clusters of practitioners who have reported here on the treatments that they provided. The patient group is clearly defined, all with "moderate" to "severe" depression as categorised by the Beck Depression Inventory (BDI-II). The methods used, involving interviews, verbatim transcripts, and thematic analysis, are consistent with many of the markers of quality in qualitative research. [12] We have helped establish the credibility and dependability of the results through involving an independent research team (LN and RC) to help conduct the study, by arranging meetings of stakeholders to review the research questions and the methods used, and by discussing the emerging themes and refining these through debate to agreement. A substantive report emerged from this process, from which a component is reported here. With regard to the transferability of the results, we have provided details of the practitioners as well as the patients who were the focus of our sub-study, such that readers can draw conclusions regarding relevance for other areas. In terms of limitations, our data is limited to patients receiving acupuncture as practised by those using the theories of traditional Chinese medicine and to clients receiving counselling as provided in the humanistic and non-directive and person-centred style.

Relationship to the wider literature

There is limited evidence in the literature for longer-term benefits associated with acupuncture for depression. [13] In a systematic review of RCTs, counselling for depression has been reported to be no better than GP care in the long term [14], though in a review of pre-post comparisons of client outcomes, benefits have been reported to last a year or more. [15] The trial, within which this sub-study was nested, provided some further evidence on longer-term effects beyond the period of treatment. [4] Within the wider literature there is a dearth of evidence on the acupuncture treatment factors that might be associated with longer-term change in the symptoms of depression. The findings from a small study involving interviews with six practitioners in a trial of acupuncture for back pain found that these acupuncturists had a goal of a positive long-term outcome, and developed a therapeutic partnership to support the active engagement of patients in their own recovery. [16] Consistent with many of the findings we report here, the authors reported that the key elements were: establishing rapport, using an interactive diagnostic process, matching treatment to the patient, and using explanatory models from Chinese medicine to aid a shared understanding and motivate lifestyle changes to reinforce the potential recovery.

In the counselling literature, a qualitative study reported on the long-term effects of counselling, with data drawn from 15 clients who had received counselling from between one and three years previously. [8] The authors' interpretation of the client interview data led them to describe a model of the change process and mechanisms that were perceived as essential to produce lasting benefit. They identified as key elements of the counselling process the active engagement of the client during and between sessions, and the acquisition of a "box of skills" to be built on further after the counselling was finished. Unlike in the current study, in which all clients of counsellors received humanistic counselling, the authors did not identify the counselling approach provided. Another difference between this study and ours, is that all patients in our study had been diagnosed with depression.

Implications for clinical practice and research

One implication for clinical practice is that, while both acupuncture and counselling for depression appear to be associated with longer-term benefits, the interventions seem to work in different ways. Further research is needed from the perspective of patients and clients on their experiences of treatment from these two modalities. To assist referral, a clearer understanding is needed of which type of person with depression would benefit from acupuncture and which from counselling. While taking into account patient preference, such a typology would provide referring clinicians with valuable guidance on suitability for referral.

Another question is in regard to the nature of depression, and the extent to which physical symptoms are also present. Evidence suggests that 69% of people experiencing depression in primary care initially present with physical symptoms [17] and 50% of people with depression are also in pain. [18] Our study has found that acupuncturists are interested in the physical symptoms that may accompany depression, and will routinely address these symptoms as part of the treatment.

One can speculate that this focus on physical symptoms may in part explain why the acupuncturists in this trial, who reported being less experienced in treating moderate to severe depression, nevertheless delivered just as good outcomes as the counsellors, who encountered this level of depression more commonly in routine practice. Further research is needed into the patient perspective on the treatment of depression with co-morbidities, and specifically the value they place on the comorbid symptoms being addressed concurrently.

Our research raises some important questions about the clinical practice of acupuncturists and counsellors when treating a population with depression when combined with unmanaged drug and alcohol addictions. Further research might be useful to explore appropriate strategies, which might be about ensuring the availability of options, including the involvement of other agencies, and practical support.

Conclusions

Long-term change appears to be an important focus within the practices of both acupuncturists and counsellors. Practitioners of both interventions generally stressed that, for longer-term benefit, there needs to be an individualised approach with a focus on root causes. Acupuncturists more often emphasised the importance of addressing concurrent physical symptoms and highlighted the importance of relevant lifestyle change. Counsellors commonly stressed the importance of the therapeutic relationship and emphasised the need for appropriate "pacing" such that the timing of the counselling process is geared to the "readiness" to change.

Acknowledgments

We acknowledge with appreciation the contributions of the practitioners who were interviewed or who attended the focus group, Janet Eldred for providing support for the management of both the trial and the sub-study, and Anne Burton for undertaking the transcriptions. This research is supported by the National Institute for Health Research (NIHR) under Programme Grants for Applied Research (Grant No. RP-PG-0707-10186). The views expressed in this presentation are those of the author(s) and not necessarily those of the NHS, the NIHR or the Department of Health. The funders had no role in study design, data collection and analysis, decision to publish, or preparation of the manuscript.

Author Contributions

Conceived and designed the experiments: HM LN RC SR HL SP AH KS. Performed the experiments: LN RC. Analyzed the data: HM LN RC. Contributed reagents/materials/analysis tools: HM LN RC KS. Contributed to the writing of the manuscript: HM LN RC. Revision of the manuscript: HM LN RC SR HL SP AH KS.

References

1. Parker G (2009) Antidepressants on trial: how valid is the evidence? Br J Psychiatry: 1–3.
2. Kirsch I, Deacon BJ, Huedo-Medina TB, Scoboria A, Moore TJ, et al. (2008) Initial severity and antidepressant benefits: a meta-analysis of data submitted to the Food and Drug Administration. PLoS Med 5: e45.
3. Mind (2002) My Choice: A Survey. Available: http://www.mind.org.uk/News+policy+and+campaigns/Press+archive/Mind+launches+campaign+for+more+choice+of+mental+health+services+at+GP+level.htm. Accessed 13 January 2008.
4. MacPherson H, Richmond S, Bland M, Brealey S, Gabe R, et al. (2013) Acupuncture and Counselling for Depression in Primary Care: A Randomised Controlled Trial. PLoS Medicine 10: e1001518. doi:10.1371/journal.pmed.1001518.
5. Centre for Outcomes Research & Effectiveness (CORE) (n.d.) Humanistic Psychological Therapies Competences Framework. Available: http://www.ucl.ac.uk/clinical-psychology/CORE/humanistic_framework.htm#. Accessed 30 September 2013.
6. MacPherson H, Elliot B, Hopton A, Lansdown H, Richmond S (2013) Acupuncture for Depression: Patterns of Diagnosis and Treatment within a Randomised Controlled Trial. Evid Based Complement Alternat Med 2013: 286048. doi:10.1155/2013/286048.
7. MacPherson H, Richmond S, Bland J, Lansdown H, Hopton A, et al. (2012) Acupuncture, Counselling, and Usual care for Depression (ACUDep): study protocol for a randomized controlled trial. Trials 13: 209.
8. Perren S, Godfrey M, Rowland N (2009) The long-term effects of counselling: The process and mechanisms that contribute to ongoing change from a user perspective. Counselling and Psychotherapy Research 9: 241–249. doi:10.1080/14733140903150745.
9. Braun V, Clarke V (2006) Using thematic analysis in psychology. Qualitative Research in Psychology 3: 77–101.

10. Ritchie J, Lewis J (2003) Qualitative Research Practice: A Guide for Social Science Students and Researchers. London:Sage.
11. Roth A, Hill A, Pilling S (2009) The competences required to deliver effective Humanistic Psychological Therapies. London, UK: University College London.
12. Hannes K (2011) Chapter 4: Critical appraisal of qualitative research. Supplementary Guidance for Inclusion of Qualitative Research in Cochrane Systematic Reviews of Interventions. Cochrane Collaboration Qualitative Methods Group. Available: http://cqrmg.cochrane.org/supplemental-handbook-guidance. Accessed 31 March 2014.
13. Smith CA, Hay PP, MacPherson H (2010) Acupuncture for depression. Cochrane Database Syst Rev: CD004046.
14. Bower P, Knowles S, Coventry PA, Rowland N (2011) Counselling for mental health and psychosocial problems in primary care. Cochrane Database Syst Rev: CD001025.
15. Research on humanistic-experiential psychotherapies (2013) Bergin and Garfield's handbook of psychotherapy and behavior change. Hoboken, N.J: John Wiley & Sons. pp. 495–538.
16. MacPherson H, Thorpe L, Thomas KJ (2006) Beyond needling - therapeutic processes in acupuncture care: a qualitative study nested within a low-back pain trial. J Altern Complement Med 12: 873–880.
17. Simon GE, VonKorff M, Piccinelli M, Fullerton C, Ormel J (1999) An international study of the relation between somatic symptoms and depression. N Engl J Med 341: 1329–1335. doi:10.1056/NEJM199910283411801.
18. Katona C, Peveler R, Dowrick C, Wessely S, Feinmann C, et al. (2005) Pain symptoms in depression: definition and clinical significance. ClinMed 5(4): 390–395.

15

A Prospective Cohort Study to Examine the Association between Dietary Patterns and Depressive Symptoms

Ruth Chan[1]*, Dicken Chan[2], Jean Woo[1]

1 Department of Medicine and Therapeutics, The Chinese University of Hong Kong, Shatin, Hong Kong, **2** The Jockey Club School of Public Health and Primary Care, The Chinese University of Hong Kong, Shatin, Hong Kong

Abstract

Introduction: Dietary patterns are culturally specific and there is limited data on the association of dietary patterns with late-life depression in Chinese. This study examined the associations between dietary patterns and baseline and subsequent depressive symptoms in community-dwelling Chinese older people in Hong Kong.

Methods: Participants aged ≥65 year participating in a cohort study examining the risk factors for osteoporosis completed a validated food frequency questionnaire at baseline between 2001 and 2003. Factor analysis was used to identify three dietary patterns: "vegetables-fruits" pattern, "snacks-drinks-milk products" pattern, and "meat-fish" pattern. Depressive symptoms were measured at baseline and 4-year using the validated Geriatric Depression Scale. Multiple logistic regression was used for cross-sectional analysis (n = 2,902) to assess the associations between dietary patterns and the presence of depressive symptoms, and for longitudinal analysis (n = 2,211) on their associations with 4-year depressive symptoms, with adjustment for socio-demographic and lifestyle factors.

Results: The highest quartile of "vegetables-fruits" pattern score was associated with reduced likelihood of depressive symptoms [Adjusted OR = 0.55 (95% CI: 0.36–0.83), $p_{trend} = 0.017$] compared to the lowest quartile at baseline. Similar inverse trend was observed for the highest quartile of "snacks-drinks-milk products" pattern score [Adjusted OR = 0.41 (95% CI: 0.26–0.65), $p_{trend} < 0.001$] compared to the lowest quartile. There was no association of "meat-fish" pattern with the presence of depressive symptoms at baseline. None of the dietary patterns were associated with subsequent depressive symptoms at 4-year.

Conclusion: Higher "vegetables-fruits" and "snacks-drinks-milk products" pattern scores were associated with reduced likelihood of baseline depressive symptoms in Chinese older people in Hong Kong. The longitudinal analyses failed to show any causal relationship between dietary patterns and depressive symptoms in this population.

Editor: Robert Stewart, Institute of Psychiatry, United Kingdom

Funding: This study was supported by grants from the Research Grants Council of Hong Kong, CUHK 4101/02M; the Hong Kong Jockey Club Charities Trust; the SH Ho Centre for Gerontology and Geriatric and the Centre for Nutritional Studies, The Chinese University of Hong Kong. The funders had no role in study design, data collection and analysis, decision to publish, or preparation of the manuscript.

Competing Interests: The authors have declared that no competing interests exist.

* Email: ruthchansm@cuhk.edu.hk

Introduction

Depression is a common mental health disorder. It affects over 350 million people worldwide and it is expected that depression will become the world's leading cause of disease burden by the year 2030 [1]. Depression is less prevalent among older adults than among younger counterparts [2]. However, late-life depression is considered as an important public health problem due to its devastating consequences, including increased risk of morbidity and reduced physical, cognitive, and social functioning [3,4]. As a result, to identify modifiable risk factors for depression is inevitably important [5].

Recent evidence suggests that diet modifies key biological factors associated with the development of depression, and diet rich in fruits, vegetables, whole grains and fish is in general associated with lower risk of depression [6,7]. Studies have shown that the antioxidant compounds in fruit and vegetables could reduce neuronal damage induced by oxidative-stress whereas long-chain omega-3 polyunsaturated fatty acids could possibly affect mood by an alteration of the brain serotonergic function and its immune-neuroendocrine effects [6,7]. However, the examination of diet as a risk factor for depression has traditionally focused on the effect of single foods and nutrients, and the findings thus far are inconsistent [8]. Since diet is a combination of food and nutrients, there has been an increasing interest in using dietary pattern analysis in epidemiological studies [9]. There are two main approaches to define dietary patterns [9,10]. One approach is the *a priori* approach in which dietary indices are constructed based on prevailing dietary recommendations. Another approach is the *a posteriori* approach in which dietary patterns are derived from statistical modeling, such as factor analysis, using data from dietary records or food frequency questionnaires (FFQ).

Data on the association between dietary patterns and depression are limited. Some cross-sectional studies have been carried out in Caucasians and Japanese to evaluate the association between dietary patterns and depression or depressive symptoms in adulthood [11–16]. To our knowledge, nine prospective studies have examined the role of dietary patterns and depression or depressive symptoms in adulthood [17–25] and two prospective studies have evaluated this association in adolescents [26,27]. Few studies have investigated the association between depression and diet in Chinese older people, and these studies mainly focused on the effect of single foods and nutrients [28,29]. Only one cross-sectional study has examined the association of dietary patterns with depressive symptoms in Chinese but it was done in adolescents [27].

Since dietary patterns are culturally specific and there is limited data on the association of dietary patterns with late-life depression in Chinese, we evaluated the association between dietary patterns and baseline and subsequent depressive symptoms in older Chinese people, using data from a sample of community-dwelling men and women aged 65 and over participating in a prospective study in Hong Kong. We hypothesized that dietary patterns are associated with baseline and subsequent depressive symptoms in this population.

Methods

Study population

Subjects were participants of a cohort study examining the risk factors for osteoporosis in Hong Kong [30]. 2,000 men and 2,000 women aged 65 years and over living in the community were recruited in a health survey between August 2001 and December 2003 by recruitment notices and talks in community centers and housing estates. Participants were volunteers and were able to walk or take public transport to the study site. They were recruited using a stratified sample so that approximately 33% would be in each of these age groups: 65–69, 70–74, 75+. Compared with the official population statistics, participants had higher educational level than the overall older population in Hong Kong (12–18% vs. 3–9% with tertiary education in the age groups 80+, 75–79,70–74, and 65–69 years) [31]. The 4-year follow-up was held between August 2005 and November 2007. Follow-up was done by a mailed reminder for a follow-up body check appointment. Phone reminders were given again close to the appointment dates, and defaulters were given a second appointment to enhance attendance rates. Mean (SD) follow-up year was 3.9 (0.1) years.

We excluded participants who did not have dietary data (n = 5), those with extreme daily energy intake at the first- and last-half percentiles of the sex-specific range (n = 37), those who had missing data for the variables included for the analyses (n = 6), and those who were probable dementia defined using the cognitive part of the Community Screening Instrument for Dementia (CSI-D) with the cutoff point of ≤28.4 [32] (n = 1,050). The baseline analysis was performed on 2,902 participants. For the longitudinal analysis, we further excluded 218 participants who had depressive symptoms at baseline and 473 participants who did not attend the 4-year follow-up. 2,211 participants were therefore included for the 4-year incidence analysis (Figure 1). This study was conducted in accordance with the Declaration of Helsinki. This study was approved by the Clinical Research Ethics Committee of the Chinese University of Hong Kong. Written informed consent was obtained from all participants.

Demographic and overall health characteristics

A standardized interview was performed to collect information on age, gender, education level, marital status, smoking habit, alcohol use and medical history. Information on the duration and

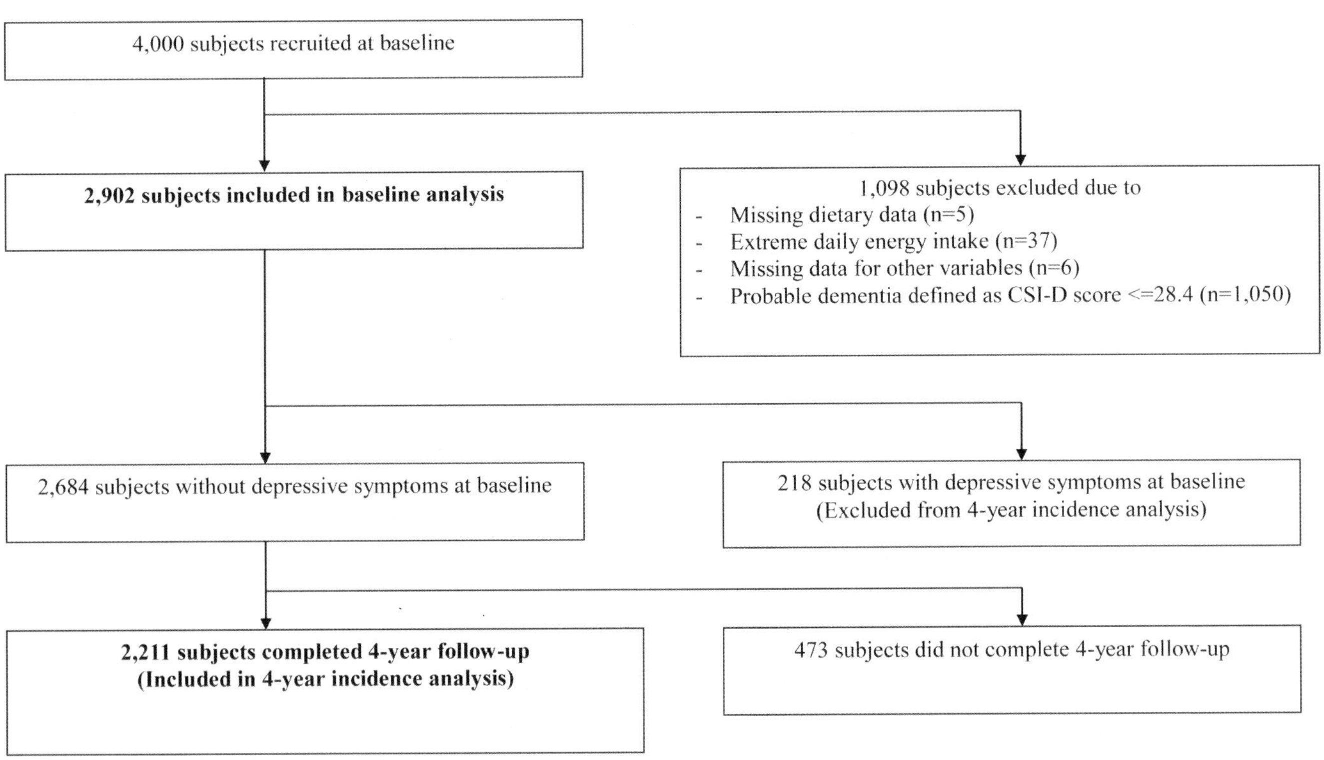

Figure 1.Number of subjects included and excluded for baseline and 4-year follow-up analyses.

level of past and current use of cigarettes, cigars and pipes was obtained. Smoking history was classified in terms of former smoking (at least 100 cigarettes smoked in a lifetime), current smoking and never smoking. Drinking status was defined as never, former (ever drank at least 5 drinks daily in a lifetime) or current drinker. Baseline disease status was obtained by self-report of their doctors' diagnoses, supplemented by the identification of drugs brought to the interviewers.

Anthropometric data

Body weight was measured to the nearest 0.1 kg with participants wearing a light gown, using the Physician Balance Beam Scale (Healthometer, Illinois, USA). Height was measured to the nearest 0.1 cm using the Holtain Harpenden stadiometer (Holtain Ltd, Crosswell, UK). Body mass index (BMI) was calculated as body weight in kg / (height in m)^2.

Physical activity assessment

Physical activity was assessed by the Physical Activity Scale for the Elderly (PASE) [33], which was adapted for use in elderly Hong Kong Chinese [34]. This is a 12-item scale measuring the average number of hours per day spent in leisure, household, and occupational physical activities over the previous 7-day period. Activity weights for each item were determined based on the amount of energy spent, and each item score was calculated by multiplying the activity weight with daily activity frequency. A composite PASE score of all the items was yielded. A higher PASE score reflects higher physical activity level.

Number of instrumental activities of daily living (IADLs) were assessed using specific questions and participants were asked to self-report of any impairment in walking two to three blocks outdoors on level ground, climbing 10 steps without resting, preparing own meals, doing heavy housework like scrubbing floors or washing windows, and shopping for groceries or clothes. A summed score from 0 to 5 was calculated from these activities as the degree of impairment in IADLs, with higher score indicating greater impairment.

Assessment of cognitive function

Since depression may be associated with cognitive impairment, in the analysis of factors associated with depression, the presence of cognitive impairment was adjusted for as a confounding factor. Cognitive function was assessed by trained research staff using the cognitive part of the Community Screening Instrument for Dementia (CSI-D) [32], validated in different cultural and educational settings [32]. The cognitive part of the CSI-D consists of 32 items in six cognitive domains: orientation to time, orientation to place, praxis, abstract thinking, language and memory. A summary score ranged from 0 to 33 was generated, with higher score meaning better cognitive function. The cutoff point for probable dementia is $\leq$28.4.

Assessment of depressive symptoms

Depressive symptoms was assessed by face-to-face interviews using a validated Chinese version of the Geriatric Depression Scale (GDS) [35,36]. The GDS short form was found to be a highly reliable (reliability coefficient of 0.90) and valid screening device (sensitivity of 96.3% and specificity of 87.5%) for assessing geriatric depression in Hong Kong Chinese [36]. The GDS short form consists of 15 questions relevant to depression, such as motivation, self-image, losses, agitation and mood. A yes/no format was designed for each question. A summary score ranged from 0 to 15 was generated, and a cut-off of 8 or more was used to define the presence of depressive symptoms.

Dietary assessment

Baseline dietary intake was assessed using a validated FFQ developed in a population survey [37]. Daily nutrient intake was calculated using food tables derived from McCance and Widdowson [38] and the Chinese Medical Sciences Institute [39]. The FFQ consisted of 280 food items. Each participant reported the frequency and the usual amount of consumption of each food item over the past year. For each food 9 different categories were given from never or seldom to more than once a day. Portion size was explained to participants using a catalogue of pictures of individual food portions. For seasonally consumed vegetables and fruits, participants were asked about the months of food consumption over the past year. The amount of cooking oil was estimated according to the usual cooking methods of preparing standardized portion of different foods and the usual portion of different foods consumed by the participants.

Dietary patterns derived by factor analysis

Details of dietary pattern scores derived by the factor analysis have been described elsewhere [40]. In brief, individual food items from the FFQ were aggregated into 32 food groups based on similarity of type of food and nutrient composition. The food groups were energy adjusted by dividing the energy intake from each food group by total energy intake and multiplying by 100, and were expressed as percentage contribution to total energy [41]. Factor analysis was conducted with varimax rotation using the 32 food groups [9]. Factors were retained based on an eigenvalues greater than 1.0, a scree plot, and the interpretability [42]. The factor scores for each pattern were calculated for each participant by summing intakes of food items weighted by their factor loadings. A higher score indicated greater conformity with the pattern being calculated.

Statistical analysis

Statistical analyses were performed using the statistical package SPSS version 21.0 (SPSS Inc., Illinois, US). Data were checked for normality using histograms and logarithmic transformation was applied whenever appropriate. Dietary pattern scores derived by factor analysis were stratified into quartiles based on the distribution of each sex. Pearson's correlation was used to examine the correlation between each dietary pattern score and intakes of various nutrients. Independent t test and chi square test were used to examine baseline differences in mean age, BMI, PASE, CSI-D score, energy intake, and also differences in the distribution of sex, education level, smoking status, alcohol use, number of IADLs, self-reported disease status, quartiles of each dietary pattern score between participants with depressive symptoms and participants without depressive symptoms at baseline. These tests were also used to examine differences in baseline characteristics between participants who included and excluded in the baseline analysis, and between participants who completed and participants who did not complete the 4-year follow-up.

Multivariate logistic regression was used to estimate the odds ratio (OR) and 95% confidence intervals (CIs) for both the baseline and the subsequent depressive symptoms according to quartiles of each dietary pattern score. Model 1 was adjusted for baseline age (years), sex, and daily energy intake (kcal). Model 2 was further adjusted for baseline BMI, PASE, number of IADLs (no difficulty/some difficulties), smoking habit (never/past/current), alcohol use (never/past/current), education level (no education/primary or below/secondary or matriculation/University or above), and marital status (married or living with a partner/widowed, separated or divorced/single). Model 3 was further adjusted for baseline self-reported history of diabetes (yes/no), hypertension (yes/no), and CVD or stroke (yes/no), and CSI-D score. Test for trend was examined by entering quartiles of each dietary pattern score in all models. An α level of 5% was used as the level of significance. Interaction between sex and quartiles of each dietary pattern score was tested by addition of cross-product terms to the multivariate models. Interactions were not significant, thus all analyses are presented in the total population.

To check the possibility of reverse causation, a sensitivity analysis excluding participants with extreme GDS at the top two percentiles (GDS≥11) was performed for the cross-sectional data. Considering that GDS is a screening scale and may be limited as a case-defining instrument compared to other diagnostic instruments [43], multivariate logistic regression models were repeated using a group whose depressive symptom levels had clearly increased over 4-year (i.e. with an increase in GDS score at 4 and over from baseline to four years) as an outcome variable. This cut-off value was chosen because 142 participants (6.4%) could be classified as the worsening cases and this number of cases may be more sufficient and powerful for statistical analysis than using an increase in GDS score at 5 and over as a cut-off value (i.e. n = 85). All models were adjusted for the same variables mentioned above.

Results

Dietary patterns of the participants

Factor analysis identified three dietary patterns (Table 1). The first factor (vegetables-fruits pattern) was dominated by frequent intake of vegetables, fruits, soy and soy products, and legumes. The second factor (snacks-drinks-milk products pattern) was composed of a mixture of healthy and unhealthy food groups. It was characterized by frequent intake of condiments, drinks, fast food, French fries, potato chips, sweets and desserts, nuts, milk products, and whole grains. The third factor (meat-fish pattern) included frequent intake of dim sum, red and processed meats, poultry, fish and seafood, and wine.

'Vegetables-fruits' dietary pattern scores were inversely associated with total fat, saturated fat, monounsaturated fat and polyunsaturated fat intakes, and positively associated with intakes of protein, fiber, isoflavones, most vitamins and minerals. 'Snacks-drinks-milk products' dietary pattern scores were inversely associated with intakes of polyunsaturated fat and vitamin K, and positively associated with intakes of carbohydrates, protein, total fat, saturated fat, monounsaturated fat, cholesterol, fiber, most minerals and vitamins. Whilst 'snacks-drinks-milk products' dietary pattern scores were also positively associated with intakes of fiber and most minerals and vitamins, the associations were less strong than those with 'vegetables-fruits' dietary pattern scores. 'Meat-fish' dietary pattern scores were weakly positively associated with intakes of polyunsaturated fat and most micronutrients, moderately positively associated with intakes of protein, total fat and monounsaturated fat, and strongly positively associated with saturated fat and cholesterol intakes. The positive associations of protein, total fat, different kinds of fat and cholesterol with 'meat-fish' dietary pattern scores were stronger than those with 'snacks-drinks-milk products' dietary pattern scores (Table 2).

Participants' characteristics by baseline depressive status

Participants who were excluded in the cross-sectional analysis were older and less physically active, had lower education level, and were more likely to be female, widowed, separated, divorced or single, and to have self-reported history of diabetes than those who were included in the cross-sectional analysis ($p<0.05$). Those who discontinued the 4-year follow-up were older, less physically active, and were more likely to be divorced or single as compared to those who completed the 4-year follow-up ($p<0.05$) (details not shown).

Among 2,902 participants included in the cross-sectional analysis, there were 218 (7.5%) participants who were classified as having depressive symptoms at baseline. For the longitudinal analysis, 81 (3.7%) cases were newly identified as having depressive symptoms out of 2,211 participants at the 4-year follow-up. The characteristics of participants with depressive symptoms and participants without depressive symptoms at baseline are shown in Table 3. Those who had depressive symptoms had lower CSI-D score, lower education level, more impairments in IADLs, and were more likely to be widowed, separated, divorced or single, and current smokers, and were more likely to have self-reported history of heart diseases or stroke. Those who had depressive symptoms also showed lower 'vegetables-fruits' dietary pattern scores and lower 'snacks-drinks-milk products' dietary pattern scores.

Dietary patterns and the presence of depressive symptoms at baseline and 4-year

In the cross-sectional analysis, participants in the highest quartile of "vegetables-fruits" pattern score had reduced likelihood of depressive symptoms [Adjusted OR = 0.55 (95% CI: 0.36–0.83), $p_{trend} = 0.017$] compared to participants in the lowest quartile. Participants in the highest quartile of "snacks-drinks-milk products" pattern score also showed reduced likelihood of depressive symptoms [Adjusted OR = 0.41 (95% CI: 0.26–0.65), $p_{trend} < 0.001$] compared to those in the lowest quartile. There was no association of "meat-fish" pattern with depressive status at baseline (Table 4). Longitudinal analysis showed that none of the dietary patterns were associated with the presence of depressive symptoms at 4-year (Table 5).

Sensitivity analysis excluding participants with extreme GDS (i.e. GDS≥11 (n = 56)) showed similar results for the cross-sectional data (details not shown). Multivariate logistic regression models that were repeated using a group with an increase in GDS score >=4 over four years as an outcome also showed no association between each dietary pattern and the presence of depressive symptoms at 4-year (details not shown).

Discussion

This study found an inverse association between "vegetables-fruits' and 'snacks-drinks-milk products' dietary pattern scores and baseline depressive symptoms. However, no significant associations between 'meat-fish' dietary pattern scores and baseline depressive symptoms were observed. Moreover, we did not observe significant associations between baseline dietary pattern scores and subsequent depressive symptoms at 4-year.

Previous cross-sectional studies have evaluated the association between dietary patterns and depression or depressive symptoms. However, the results are inconclusive [13–16,22]. Similar to our findings, two recent studies from Japan showed that a healthy Japanese dietary pattern characterized by high intakes of plant foods including vegetables, fruit, mushrooms and soy products was associated with fewer depressive symptoms [14,16]. Our results were also consistent with the findings from an Australian study which showed that a diet characterized by high intakes of fruits, vegetables, and plant based foods was associated with fewer depressive symptoms[13]. Compared to the "snacks-drinks-milk products" pattern and the "meat-fish" pattern, the "vegetables-fruits" pattern showed the highest correlations with fiber and other

Table 1. Food group factor loading[a] for three dietary patterns.

Food groups	Dietary patterns		
	Factor 1: Vegetables-fruits	Factor 2: Snacks-drinks-milk products	Factor 3: Meat-fish
Other vegetables	**0.60**	-0.08	0.03
Cruciferous vegetables	**0.48**	−0.08	−0.06
Tomatoes	**0.47**	0.05	−0.04
Soy	**0.43**	0.03	0.10
Dark green & leafy vegetables	**0.42**	−0.27	−0.04
Starchy vegetables	**0.42**	0.07	−0.03
Fruits	**0.39**	0.06	0.03
Legumes	**0.35**	−0.06	0.02
Mushroom & fungi	**0.25**	0.07	−0.06
Fats and oils	**−0.39**	−0.20	0.11
Condiments	−0.06	**0.48**	−0.06
Coffee	−0.15	**0.41**	−0.15
Nuts	0.12	**0.39**	−0.03
Fast food	−0.02	**0.35**	0.14
French fries and potato chips	−0.02	**0.34**	0.14
Milk and milk products	0.11	**0.33**	−0.10
Whole grains	0.16	**0.32**	−0.16
Sweets and desserts	0.01	**0.27**	0.19
Beverages	−0.02	**0.22**	0.10
Eggs	0.08	**0.22**	0.05
Dim sum	−0.17	−0.17	**0.51**
Red and processed meats	−0.07	−0.03	**0.47**
Poultry	0.06	0.03	**0.47**
Fish and seafood	0.20	−0.26	**0.33**
Cakes, cookies, pies and biscuits	0.07	0.12	**0.24**
Wine	−0.15	0.07	**0.22**
Refined grains	−0.24	−0.42	**−0.74**
Organ meats	−0.08	0.13	0.12
Others	0.01	0.07	0.05
Preserved vegetables	0	0.10	0.01
Soups	0	0	−0.01
Tea	−0.03	0.17	0.05
% variance explained	**6.5**	**5.2**	**5.2**

[a]Factor loadings with absolute value ≥0.2 are shown in bold (Field 2005). For food group loads more than one dietary pattern, only the highest absolute value of loading is bolded.

nutrients, such as vitamin C that are considered as beneficial for brain health [6]. It is possible that the "vegetables-fruits" pattern is associated with reduced oxidative stress, higher anti-inflammatory property, and higher antioxidant capacity, the potential biological mechanisms that are linked with better mood and brain health [44]. The potential protective effect of the 'vegetables-fruits' pattern could also come from folate that is rich in some cruciferous vegetables, leafy vegetables, and other green vegetables. There has been evidence to suggest that folate deficiency impairs the synthesis of homocysteine to methionine and S-adenosyl-methionine. The latter is a methyl donor and is involved in the synthesis and metabolism of neurotransmitters [45]. There is also substantial evidence from observational studies and randomized controlled trials to suggest that folate deficiency is associated with increased risk of depression [7,46].

Our study showed that 'snacks-drinks-milk products' dietary pattern was linked to a fewer depressive symptoms. Such an inverse association was less easy to interpret. In comparison to the 'vegetable-fruit' dietary pattern, the positive association of this pattern with intakes of fiber and most minerals and vitamins was less strong. However, this pattern was composed of healthy and unhealthy food groups. This pattern was dominated by the intake of condiments, drinks, sweets and desserts, fast food, French fries, potato chips, nuts, milk and milk products, and whole grains. Past studies have examined the role of these food groups in depression [47–49]. Greater intake of high-calorie sweet foods and fast foods appeared to be associated with more depressive symptoms [47,48].

Table 2. Pearson's correlations between each dietary pattern score and nutrient intakes at baseline (n = 2,902).

Nutrients	Vegetables-fruits		Snacks-drinks-milk products		Meat-fish	
	r	p	r	p	r	P
Energy (kcal)	−0.05	0.006	0.21	<0.001	0.22	<0.001
Carbohydrates (g)	−0.01	0.456	0.17	<0.001	−0.11	<0.001
Protein (g)	0.13	<0.001	0.21	<0.001	0.39	<0.001
Fat (g)	−0.12	<0.001	0.18	<0.001	0.48	<0.001
SFA (% energy)	−0.17	<0.001	0.14	<0.001	0.57	<0.001
MUFA (% energy)	−0.06	0.001	0.06	0.001	0.36	<0.001
PUFA (% energy)	−0.13	<0.001	−0.11	<0.001	0.15	<0.001
Cholesterol (mg) †	0.03	0.168	0.15	<0.001	0.55	<0.001
Fiber (g) †	0.60	<0.001	0.17	<0.001	0.04	0.019
Vitamin A (IU) †	0.57	<0.001	0.05	0.006	0.11	<0.001
Vitamin C (mg) †	0.52	<0.001	0.03	0.103	0.12	<0.001
Calcium (mg)	0.36	<0.001	0.31	<0.001	0.02	0.258
Phosphorus (mg)	0.19	<0.001	0.33	<0.001	0.07	<0.001
Iron (mg) †	0.28	<0.001	0.26	<0.001	0.18	<0.001
Potassium (mg) †	0.24	<0.001	0.08	<0.001	0.33	<0.001
Magnesium (mg) †	0.38	<0.001	0.07	<0.001	−0.01	0.645
Sodium (mg) †	0.12	<0.001	0.23	<0.001	0.31	<0.001
Zinc (mg)	0.20	<0.001	0.15	<0.001	0.28	<0.001
Isoflavones (mg) †	0.35	<0.001	0.09	<0.001	0.13	<0.001
Vitamin K (μg) †	0.52	<0.001	−0.13	<0.001	0.07	<0.001
Vitamin D (IU) †	0.10	<0.001	0.30	<0.001	0.06	0.001

SFA, Saturated fatty acids; MUFA, Monounsaturated fatty acids; PUFA, Polyunsaturated fatty acids.
†log transformed nutrient intake.

In contrast, there is evidence to suggest that increased intake of milk and dairy products, in particular the low-fat milk and dairy products is associated with better brain function and mood [49].

Our longitudinal analysis did not show significant associations between baseline dietary pattern scores and subsequent depressive symptoms at 4-year. Sensitivity analysis by repeating the multivariate logistic regression models with an outcome of a group with an increase in GDS score >= 4 over four years also confirmed these negative findings. Furthermore, in order to investigate the relationship between diet and depression persistence at 4-year, we tried to repeat the multivariate logistic regression models for participants with depressive symptoms at baseline. No association between dietary patterns and the presence of depressive symptoms was observed at 4-year among this group of baseline depressive participants and these findings further confirmed our negative longitudinal findings. Several prospective studies have examined the role of dietary patterns and incident depression or depressive symptoms in adulthood [17–25], and the findings generally support the role of dietary patterns in the development of depression. Most studies reported significant associations between dietary patterns and incident depression or depressive symptoms [17–19,21–25], but one recent study showed no clear associations between dietary patterns and depression incidence [20]. Using data of 3,486 men and women of the Whitehall II prospective cohort, Akbaraly and colleagues showed a higher odds of depressive symptoms with a "processed food pattern" which was heavily loaded by high intake of sweetened desserts, chocolates, fried food, processed meat, pies, refined grains, high-fat dairy products and condiments [18]. In the GAZEL cohort, Le Port et al. [19] reported that healthy pattern (characterized by vegetables consumption) were associated with fewer depressive symptoms in men and women, and traditional pattern (characterized by fish and fruit consumption) were associated with lower risk of incident depression in women. Furthermore, the highest quartile of low-fat, western, high snack and high fat-sweet diets in men and low-fat and high snack diets in women were associated with higher likelihood of depressive symptoms compared to the lowest quartile. However, recent findings among women in the Nurses' Health Study did not suggest clear associations between dietary Prudent and Western pattern scores and incident depression risk [20]. Differences in the study design, such as tools for assessing depression (i.e. self-reported scale vs. clinical diagnosis), inclusion and exclusion criteria for the subjects, and covariates that were included in the statistical models may account for the variations in the study findings [50]. Recent findings from a multicenter, randomized, primary prevention filed trial suggest that a Mediterranean diet supplemented with nuts could possibly reduce the risk of depression in patients with type 2 diabetes [51]. Therefore, the role of diet in depression warrants further investigation.

Strengths of our study are inclusion of both cross-sectional and longitudinal study design, and adjustment for several potential confounders. However, our study had several limitations. First, the use of the self-reported measure of depression (GDS) and cognitive impairment (CSI-D) may be one of the limitations. However, the sensitivity of these measures is high and has been validated in Chinese populations [32,36]. Second, the low number of participants with depressive symptoms at the 4-year follow-up

Table 3. Subject characteristics by baseline depressive status (n = 2,902).

	Subjects without depressive symptoms (GDS<8) (n = 2,684)		**Subjects with depressive symptoms (GDS> = 8) (n = 218)**		*P value*[1]
	Mean/n	**(SD/%)**	**Mean/n**	**SD/%**	
Age (years)	71.8	(4.8)	72.2	(5.0)	0.310
BMI (kg/m^2)	23.6	(3.2)	23.4	(3.3)	0.203
PASE score	94.1	(44.7)	91.5	(40.2)	0.399
CSI-D score	31.2	(0.9)	31.0	(0.8)	**0.001**
Daily energy intake (kcal)	1913.8	(571.4)	1876.3	(556.7)	0.351
Dietary pattern scores					
Vegetables-fruits	0.015	(1.002)	−0.187	(0.958)	**0.004**
Q1	651	(24.3)	76	(34.9)	**0.002**
Q2	677	(25.2)	49	(22.5)	
Q3	669	(24.9)	55	(25.2)	
Q4	687	(25.6)	38	(17.4)	
Snacks-drinks-milk products	0.022	(1.004)	−0.272	(0.915)	**<0.001**
Q1	646	(24.1)	81	(37.2)	**<0.001**
Q2	662	(24.7)	62	(28.4)	
Q3	684	(25.5)	43	(19.7)	
Q4	692	(25.8)	32	(14.7)	
Meat-fish	0.004	(0.996)	−0.045	(1.051)	0.487
Q1	669	(24.9)	56	(25.7)	0.441
Q2	665	(24.8)	61	(28.0)	
Q3	670	(25.0)	56	(25.7)	
Q4	680	(25.3)	45	(20.6)	
Female (%)	1075	(40.1)	87	(39.9)	0.967
Education level (%)					
Primary or below	1697	(63.2)	157	(72.0)	**0.014**
Secondary / Matriculation	636	(23.7)	45	(20.6)	
University or above	351	(13.1)	16	(7.3)	
Marital status (%)					
Married or living with a partner	2085	(77.7)	155	(71.1)	**0.004**
Widowed, separated or divorced	546	(20.3)	52	(23.9)	
Single	53	(2.0)	11	(5.0)	
Smoking status (%)					
Never smoke	1583	(59.0)	110	(50.5)	**0.003**
Ex-smoker	910	(33.9)	80	(36.7)	
Current smoker	191	(7.1)	28	(12.8)	
Alcohol use (%)					
Never	2203	(82.1)	181	(83.0)	0.191
Ex-drinker	55	(2.0)	8	(3.7)	
Current drinker	426	(15.9)	29	(13.3)	
Self-reported medical history (%)					
Diabetes mellitus	350	(13.0)	38	(17.4)	0.067
Hypertension	1118	(41.7)	100	(45.9)	0.225
Heart diseases or stroke	552	(20.6)	71	(32.6)	**<0.001**
IADLs					
No impairment	2141	(79.8)	138	(63.3)	**<0.001**
Some impairments	543	(20.2)	80	(36.7)	

[1]Differences between groups were assessed by independent *t* test or chi square test.

Table 4. Odds ratios (95% CI) for the cross-sectional association between dietary patterns and depressive symptoms (GDS> = 8) at baseline (n = 2,902).

Dietary pattern	Case / Control	Crude		P_{trend}[1]	Model 1[2]		P_{trend}	Model 2[3]		P_{trend}	Model 3[4]		P_{trend}
		OR	**(95% CI)**		**OR**	**(95% CI)**		**OR**	**(95% CI)**		**OR**	**(95% CI)**	
Vegetables-fruits													
Q1	76/651	1		**0.001**	1		**0.001**	1		**0.019**	1		**0.017**
Q2	49/677	0.62	0.43–0.90		0.62	0.43–0.91		0.67	0.46–0.98		0.68	0.46–0.99	
Q3	55/669	0.70	0.49–1.01		0.71	0.49–1.02		0.81	0.56–1.18		0.83	0.57–1.20	
Q4	38/687	0.47	0.32–0.71		0.48	0.32–0.72		0.56	0.37–0.84		0.55	0.36–0.83	
Snacks- drinks-milk products													
Q1	81/646	1		**<0.001**	1		**<0.001**	1		**<0.001**	1		**<0.001**
Q2	62/662	0.75	0.53–1.06		0.75	0.53–1.06		0.76	0.53–1.09		0.77	0.54–1.10	
Q3	43/684	0.50	0.34–0.74		0.51	0.34–0.74		0.51	0.34–0.76		0.52	0.35–0.78	
Q4	32/692	0.37	0.24–0.56		0.37	0.24–0.57		0.40	0.25–0.62		0.41	0.26–0.65	
Meat-fish													
Q1	56/669	1		0.221	1		0.273	1		0.269	1		0.199
Q2	61/665	1.10	0.75–1.60		1.10	0.76–1.61		1.18	0.80–1.73		1.18	0.80–1.73	
Q3	56/670	1.00	0.68–1.47		1.01	0.69–1.49		1.08	0.73–1.61		1.06	0.71–1.58	
Q4	45/680	0.79	0.53–1.19		0.81	0.54–1.22		0.80	0.53–1.22		0.77	0.51–1.18	

[1]Test for trend was examined by entering dietary pattern score quartiles as a fixed factor and testing the contrast by using the polynomial option in all models.
[2]Model 1: adjusted for age, sex and daily energy intake.
[3]Model 2: further adjusted for BMI, PASE, number of IADLs, smoking status, alcohol use, education and marital status.
[4]Model 3: further adjusted for self-reported history of diabetes mellitus, hypertension, heart disease and stroke, and CSI-D score.

Table 5. Odds ratios (95% CI) for the longitudinal association between baseline dietary patterns and 4-year incidence of depressive symptoms (GDS>=8) (n=2,211).

Dietary pattern	Case / Control	Crude		P_{trend}[1]	Model 1[2]		P_{trend}	Model 2[3]		P_{trend}	Model 3[4]		P_{trend}
		OR	(95% CI)		OR	(95% CI)		OR	(95% CI)		OR	(95% CI)	
Vegetables-fruits													
Q1	25/494	1		0.415	1		0.432	1		0.903	1		0.931
Q2	17/547	0.61	0.33–1.15		0.62	0.33–1.17		0.71	0.38–1.35		0.73	0.38–1.38	
Q3	18/534	0.67	0.36–1.24		0.66	0.36–1.24		0.77	0.41–1.45		0.80	0.42–1.50	
Q4	21/555	0.75	0.41–1.35		0.76	0.42–1.37		0.94	0.51–1.73		0.94	0.51–1.74	
Snacks- drinks-milk products													
Q1	24/494	1		0.430	1		0.569	1		0.845	1		0.824
Q2	13/514	0.52	0.26–1.03		0.54	0.27–1.07		0.61	0.31–1.21		0.62	0.31–1.24	
Q3	27/550	1.01	0.58–1.77		1.07	0.61–1.89		1.28	0.71–2.29		1.28	0.71–2.31	
Q4	17/572	0.61	0.33–1.15		0.65	0.34–1.24		0.84	0.43–1.65		0.85	0.43–1.68	
Meat-fish													
Q1	23/530	1		0.880	1		0.822	1		0.935	1		0.957
Q2	17/530	0.74	0.39–1.40		0.74	0.39–1.41		0.78	0.41–1.49		0.79	0.41–1.50	
Q3	16/533	0.69	0.36–1.32		0.71	0.37–1.36		0.74	0.38–1.44		0.75	0.39–1.45	
Q4	25/537	1.07	0.60–1.91		1.09	0.61–1.97		1.05	0.57–1.92		1.04	0.56–1.90	

[1]Test for trend was examined by entering dietary pattern score quartiles as a fixed factor and testing the contrast by using the polynomial option in all models.
[2]Model 1: adjusted for age, sex and daily energy intake at baseline.
[3]Model 2: further adjusted for BMI, PASE, number of IADLs, smoking status, alcohol use, education and marital status at baseline.
[4]Model 3: further adjusted for self-reported history of diabetes mellitus, hypertension, heart disease and stroke, and CSI-D score at baseline.

may have limited the power of the longitudinal analysis. Although we found significant associations between "vegetables-fruits" and "snacks-drinks-milk products" patterns and depressive symptoms in the cross-sectional analysis, the directionality of the associations was uncertain. The possibility of reverse causation may not be ruled out. People with major depression may change their eating behavior and food choices, either adopting an unhealthy diet (i.e. high-calorie foods) or reducing food intake [47,52], thus interpreting the relationship between diet and depression may be difficult in view of the bidirectional changes in diet as a consequence of mental health symptoms. We tried to conduct a sensitivity analysis excluding participants with extreme GDS (i.e. GDS≥11 (n = 56)) and the significant association between dietary patterns and depressive symptoms remained at baseline. These results possibly suggest that reverse causation seems an unlikely explanation for the significant findings in our cross-sectional analysis. Furthermore, we did not have dietary data at the 4-year follow-up whereas dietary patterns may have changed between baseline and follow-up. Moreover, although we controlled for various common factors and major chronic conditions in the analysis, residual potential confounding from some other factors related to the development of depression, such as family history of depression and recent life stress events might still be present. In addition, our sample as a whole was of a higher educational standard compared with the general Hong Kong population, and there were some differences in the baseline characteristics between those who included and those who excluded in the analysis, and between those who completed and those who discontinued the 4-year follow-up. Therefore, the results may not be generalized to the general population.

In conclusion, our cross-sectional analysis suggested significant associations between 'vegetables-fruits' dietary pattern and 'snacks-drinks-milk products' dietary pattern and the presence of depressive symptoms in the community-dwelling Chinese older people in Hong Kong. However, the longitudinal analyses did not support that dietary patterns are predictive of the occurrence of depressive symptoms.

Acknowledgments

We would like to give thanks for Ms Kay Yuen for coordination of this study.

Author Contributions

Conceived and designed the experiments: RC JW. Analyzed the data: RC DC JW. Contributed to the writing of the manuscript: RC DC JW

References

1. World Health Organization (2008) Global Burden of Disease: 2004 Update. Geneva: World Health Organization.
2. Hasin DS, Goodwin RD, Stinson FS, Grant BF (2005) Epidemiology of major depressive disorder: results from the National Epidemiologic Survey on Alcoholism and Related Conditions. Arch Gen Psychiatry 62: 1097–1106.
3. Blazer DG (2003) Depression in late life: review and commentary. J Gerontol A Biol Sci Med Sci 58: 249–265.
4. Fiske A, Wetherell JL, Gatz M (2009) Depression in older adults. Annu Rev Clin Psychol 5: 363–389.
5. Collins PY, Patel V, Joestl SS, March D, Insel TR, et al. (2011) Grand challenges in global mental health. Nature 475: 27–30.
6. Rogers PJ (2001) A healthy body, a healthy mind: long-term impact of diet on mood and cognitive function. Proc Nutr Soc 60: 135–143.
7. Stanger O, Fowler B, Piertzik K, Huemer M, Haschke-Becher E, et al. (2009) Homocysteine, folate and vitamin B12 in neuropsychiatric diseases: review and treatment recommendations. Expert Rev Neurother 9: 1393–1412.
8. Murakami K, Sasaki S (2010) Dietary intake and depressive symptoms: a systematic review of observational studies. Mol Nutr Food Res 54: 471–488.
9. Hu FB (2002) Dietary pattern analysis: a new direction in nutritional epidemiology. Curr Opin Lipidol 13: 3–9.
10. van Dam RM (2005) New approaches to the study of dietary patterns. Br J Nutr 93: 573–574.
11. Jacka FN, Pasco JA, Mykletun A, Williams LJ, Hodge AM, et al. (2010) Association of Western and traditional diets with depression and anxiety in women. Am J Psychiatry 167: 305–311.
12. Samieri C, Jutand MA, Feart C, Capuron L, Letenneur L, et al. (2008) Dietary patterns derived by hybrid clustering method in older people: association with cognition, mood, and self-rated health. J Am Diet Assoc 108: 1461–1471.
13. Crichton GE, Bryan J, Hodgson JM, Murphy KJ (2013) Mediterranean diet adherence and self-reported psychological functioning in an Australian sample. Appetite 70: 53–59.
14. Nanri A, Kimura Y, Matsushita Y, Ohta M, Sato M, et al. (2010) Dietary patterns and depressive symptoms among Japanese men and women. Eur J Clin Nutr 64: 832–839.
15. Sugawara N, Yasui-Furukori N, Tsuchimine S, Kaneda A, Tsuruga K, et al. (2012) No association between dietary patterns and depressive symptoms among a community-dwelling population in Japan. Ann Gen Psychiatry 11: 24 doi: 10.1186/1744-859X-11-24.
16. Suzuki T, Miyaki K, Tsutsum A, Hashimoto H, Kawakami N, et al. (2013) Japanese dietary pattern consistently relates to low depressive symptoms and it is modified by job strain and worksite supports. J Affect Disord 150: 490–498.
17. Sa' nchez-Villegas A, Delgado-Rodri'guez M, Alonso A, Schlatter J, Lahortiga F, et al. (2009) Association of the Mediterranean Dietary Pattern With the Incidence of Depression The Seguimiento Universidad de Navarra/University of Navarra Follow-up (SUN) Cohort. Arch Gen Psychiatry 66: 1090–1098.
18. Akbaraly TN, Brunner EJ, Ferrie JE, Marmot MG, Kivimaki M, et al. (2009) Dietary pattern and depressive symptoms in middle age. Br J Psychiatry 195: 408–413.
19. Le Port A, Gueguen A, Kesse-Guyot E, Melchior M, Lemogne C, et al. (2012) Association between dietary patterns and depressive symptoms over time: a 10-year follow-up study of the GAZEL cohort. PLOS ONE 7: e51593.
20. Chocano-Bedoya PO, O'Reilly EJ, Lucas M, Mirzaei F, Okereke OI, et al. (2013) Prospective study on long-term dietary patterns and incident depression in middle-aged and older women. Am J Clin Nutr 98: 813–820.
21. Lucas M, Chocano-Bedoya P, Shulze MB, Mirzaei F, O'Reilly EJ, et al. (2013) Inflammatory dietary pattern and risk of depression among women. Brain Behav Immun 36: 46–53.
22. Rienks R, Dobson AJ, Mishra GD (2013) Mediterranean dietary pattern and prevalence and incidence of depressive symptoms in mid-aged women: results from a large community-based prospective study. Eur J Clin Nutr 67: 75–82.
23. Hodge A, Almeida OP, English DR, Giles GG, Flicker L (2013) Patterns of dietary intake and psychological distress in older Australians: benefits not just from a Mediterranean diet. Int Psychogeriatr 25: 456–466.
24. Jacka FN, Cherbuin N, Anstey KJ, Butterworth P (2014) Dietary Patterns and Depressive Symptoms over Time: Examining the Relationships with Socioeconomic Position, Health Behaviours and Cardiovascular Risk. PLOS ONE 9: e87657.
25. Ruusunen A, Lehto SM, Mursu J, Tolmunen T, Tuomainen TP, et al. (2014) Dietary patterns are associated with the prevalence of elevated depressive symptoms and the risk of getting a hospital discharge diagnosis of depression in middle-aged or older Finnish men. J Affect Disord 159: 1–6.
26. Jacka FN, Kremer PJ, Berk M, de Silva-Sanigorski AM, Moodie M, et al. (2011) A prospective study of diet quality and mental health in adolescents. PLOS ONE 6: e24805.
27. Weng TT, Hao JH, Qian QW, Cao H, Fu JL, et al. (2011) Is there any relationship between dietary patterns and depression and anxiety in Chinese adolescents? Public Health Nutr 15: 673–682.
28. Tsai AC, Chang TL, Chi SH (2012) Frequent consumption of vegetables predicts lower risk of depression in older Taiwanese - results of a prospective population-based study. Public Health Nutr 15: 1087–1092.
29. Woo J, Lynn H, Lau WY, Leung J, Lau E, et al. (2006) Nutrient intake and psychological health in an elderly Chinese population. Int J Geriatr Psychiatry 21: 1036–1043.
30. Wong SY, Kwok T, Woo J, Lynn H, Griffith JF, et al. (2005) Bone mineral density and the risk of peripheral arterial disease in men and women: results from Mr. and Ms Os, Hong Kong. Osteoporos Int 16: 1933–1938.
31. Census and Statistics Department (2006) Hong Kong 2006 Population Bycensus Thematic Report: Older Persons. Hong Kong: Census and Statistics Department.
32. Prince M, Acosta D, Chiu H, Scazufca M, Varghese M, et al. (2003) Dementia diagnosis in developing countries: a cross-cultural validation study. Lancet 361: 909–917.
33. Washburn RA, Smith KW, Jette AM, Janney CA (1993) The Physical Activity Scale for the Elderly (PASE): development and evaluation. J Clin Epidemiol 46: 153–162.
34. Liu B, Woo J, Tang N, Ng K, Ip R, et al. (2001) Assessment of total expenditure in a Chinese population by a physical activity questionnaire: examination of validity. Int J Food Sci Nutr 52: 269–282.

35. Yesavage JA, Brink TL, Rose TL, Lum O, Huang V, et al. (1983) Development and validation of a geriatric depression screening scale. A preliminary report. J Psychiatr Res 17: 37–49.
36. Lee HB, Chiu HFK, Kwok WY, Leung CM, Kwong PK, et al. (1993) Chinese elderly and the GDS short form: a preliminary study. Clin Gerontol 14: 37–39.
37. Woo J, Leung SSF, Ho SC, Lam TH, Janus ED (1997) A food frequency questionnaire for use in the Chinese population in Hong Kong: Description and examination of validity. Nutr Res 17: 1633–1641.
38. Paul AA, Southgate DAT (1978) McCance & Widdowson's: The Composition of Foods. London: HMSO.
39. Yang Y, Wang G, Pan X (2002) China Food Composition 2002; Institute of Nutrition & Food Safety CC, editor. Peking: University Medical Press.
40. Chan R, Chan D, Woo J (2012) Associations between dietary patterns and demographics, lifestyle, anthropometry and blood pressure in Chinese community-dwelling older men and women. J Nutr Sci 1: e20 doi:10.1017/jns.2012.19
41. Reedy J, Wirfalt E, Flood A, Mitrou PN, Krebs-Smith SM, et al. (2010) Comparing 3 dietary pattern methods–cluster analysis, factor analysis, and index analysis–With colorectal cancer risk: The NIH-AARP Diet and Health Study. Am J Epidemiol 171: 479–487.
42. Field A (2005) Discovering Statistics Using SPSS; Wright DB, editor. London: Sage Publications.
43. Roman MW, Callen BL (2008) Screening instruments for older adult depressive disorders: updating the evidence-based toolbox. Issues Ment Health Nurs 29: 929–941.
44. Bodnar LM, Wisner KL (2005) Nutrition and depression: implications for improving mental health among childbearing-aged women. Biol Psychiatry 58: 679–685.
45. Bottiglieri T (2005) Homocysteine and folate metabolism in depression. Prog Neuro-Psychopharmacol Biol Psychiatry 29: 1103–1112.
46. Fava M, Mischoulon D (2009) Folate in depression: efficacy, safety, differences in formulations, and clinical issues. J Clin Psychiatry 70 Suppl 5: 12–17.
47. Jeffery RW, Linde JA, Simon GE, Ludman EJ, Rohde P, et al. (2009) Reported food choices in older women in relation to body mass index and depressive symptoms. Appetite 52: 238–240.
48. Crawford GB, Khedkar A, Flaws JA, Sorkin JD, Gallicchio L (2011) Depressive symptoms and self-reported fast-food intake in midlife women. Prev Med 52: 254–257.
49. Camfield DA, Owen L, Scholey AB, Pipingas A, Stough C (2011) Dairy constituents and neurocognitive health in ageing. Br J Nutr 106: 159–174.
50. Quirk SE, Williams;L.J.;, O'Neil A, Pasco JA, Jacka FN, et al. (2013) The association between diet quality, dietary patterns and depression in adults: a systematic review. BMC Psychiatry 175.
51. Sánchez-Villegas A, Martínez-González MA, Estruch R, Salas-Salvadó J, Corella D, et al. (2013) Mediterranean dietary pattern and depression: the PREDIMED randomized trial. BMC Medicine 11.
52. Lai JS, Hiles S, Bisquera A, Hure AJ, McEvoy M, et al. (2014) A systematic review and meta-analysis of dietary patterns and depression in community-dwelling adults. Am J Clin Nutr 99: 181–197.

16

Reduced Amygdala and Ventral Striatal Activity to Happy Faces in PTSD Is Associated with Emotional Numbing

Kim L. Felmingham[1,2,3]*, Erin M. Falconer[2], Leanne Williams[2,4], Andrew H. Kemp[5], Adrian Allen[2,3], Anthony Peduto[6], Richard A. Bryant[2,3]

1 School of Psychology, University of New South Wales, Sydney, Australia, **2** Brain Dynamics Centre, Westmead Millennium Institute, Westmead Hospital, Sydney, Australia, **3** School of Psychology, University of Tasmania, Hobart, Australia, **4** Western Clinical School, University of Sydney, Sydney, Australia, **5** School of Psychology, University of Sydney, Sydney, Australia, **6** MRI Unit, Department of Radiology, Westmead Hospital, Sydney, Australia

Abstract

There has been a growing recognition of the importance of reward processing in PTSD, yet little is known of the underlying neural networks. This study tested the predictions that (1) individuals with PTSD would display reduced responses to happy facial expressions in ventral striatal reward networks, and (2) that this reduction would be associated with emotional numbing symptoms. 23 treatment-seeking patients with Posttraumatic Stress Disorder were recruited from the treatment clinic at the Centre for Traumatic Stress Studies, Westmead Hospital, and 20 trauma-exposed controls were recruited from a community sample. We examined functional magnetic resonance imaging responses during the presentation of happy and neutral facial expressions in a passive viewing task. PTSD participants rated happy facial expression as less intense than trauma-exposed controls. Relative to controls, PTSD participants revealed lower activation to happy (-neutral) faces in ventral striatum and and a trend for reduced activation in left amygdala. A significant negative correlation was found between emotional numbing symptoms in PTSD and right ventral striatal regions after controlling for depression, anxiety and PTSD severity. This study provides initial evidence that individuals with PTSD have lower reactivity to happy facial expressions, and that lower activation in ventral striatal-limbic reward networks may be associated with symptoms of emotional numbing.

Editor: Michelle Hampson, Yale University, United States of America

Funding: This research was supported by a National Health and Medical Research Council (NHMRC) Program Grant (300304), and Australian Research Council Linkage Grant (LP0212048), and an NHMRC Project Grant (1050848). The funders had no role in study design, data collection and analysis, decision to publish, or preparation of the manuscript.

Competing Interests: The authors have declared that no competing interests exist.

* Email: Kim.Felmingham@utas.edu.au

Introduction

PTSD is a complex psychiatric condition with features that extend beyond conditioned fear responses to include a wider range of emotional difficulties, such as emotional numbing [1]. Emotional numbing focuses on diminished *positive* affect, including an absence of feelings of love and happiness, and a lack of response to positive environmental events [2,3]. Little is known about the neural networks associated with processing positive stimuli in PTSD. Recently, there has been a growing recognition of the importance of reward processing and in understanding its neural basis in PTSD. Emotional numbing has been shown to be the symptom that is most characteristic of chronic PTSD [4], and is strongly associated with functional and interpersonal impairment [5,6].

Two behavioral studies have reported deficient reward function in PTSD. Vietnam veterans with PTSD have been found to expend less effort in viewing beautiful female faces [7], and to have lower expectancy and satisfaction with rewards in a gambling task [8]. Two fMRI studies have examined functioning of reward networks in PTSD using monetary reward tasks [9,10]. Participants with PTSD showed lower activation in nucleus accumbens and medial prefrontal cortex (mPFC) [10] and in dorsal and ventral striatal regions (caudate and putamen) [9] compared to non-trauma exposed controls in response to gains. This pattern was interpreted to reflect deficiencies in reward function. However, it is unclear in these studies whether the lower activation in ventral striatal regions is due to PTSD specifically, or trauma-exposure, as both studies did not include a trauma-exposed control group.

Interestingly, anhedonia in patients with major depression has also been associated with lower responses in left nucleus accumbens and bilateral caudate in response to gains in a monetary incentive task [11]. Anhedonia, defined as a lack of reactivity to pleasurable stimuli, has considerable conceptual overlap to emotional numbing in PTSD. This raises the possibility that the lower ventral striatal activity seen in PTSD may at least partially be explained by the high rates of comorbid depression observed with this disorder.

Previous imaging studies in healthy controls have examined ventral striatal reactivity to gains in monetary incentive tasks [9–11], which may recruit distinctive networks from those involved in the perception of positive signals [12]. Perception of positive signals/hedonic tone appears centered on networks encompassing the nucleus accumbens [12,13], whereas networks involved in processing stimulus-reward association are associated with wider orbitofrontal-dorsal and ventral striatal networks [13]. Therefore, it is important to examine reward function in ventral striatal networks in PTSD in terms of reactivity to positive stimuli. Only one pilot study has examined neural reactivity to positive affective signals (animated film) in PTSD. Greater activation was found in right precentral and superior frontal gyrus, and lower activation in parahippocampal and superior temporal gyrus were found in the PTSD group [14]. However, this study employed small sample sizes (8 males) and did not specifically examine emotional numbing.

In the healthy brain, happy faces engage a neural network involving the ventral striatum (encompassing putamen and nucleus accumbens) [15], amygdala [16,17,18], orbitofrontal cortex [19] and anterior cingulate [16]. To date, the neural correlates of perception of innate positive signals, such as happy facial expressions, have not been examined in PTSD. Examining reactivity to facial expressions in PTSD is of particular importance, as research suggests that deficiencies in response to facial displays of affect contribute significantly to functional and social impairment [20]. Indeed, emotional numbing, which involves blunted positive affect and reactivity, has been found as the major contributor to functional impairment in PTSD [5,6].

Accordingly, the present study examined the neural networks underlying the processing of happy facial expressions in PTSD. Secondly, we examined the extent to which impairments in reactivity to positive emotional signals were associated with emotional numbing in PTSD. It was predicted there would be a lower activation in networks involved in the processing of happy faces (ventral striatum encompassing nucleus accumbens, and amygdala) in PTSD compared to trauma-exposed controls. Further, we expected lower activation in these regions to be associated with more severe symptoms of emotional numbing in PTSD.

Methods and Materials

Participants

Twenty-three individuals who developed PTSD as a result of physical assault (n = 15) or motor vehicle accidents (n = 8) were recruited for the study from the Traumatic Stress Clinic, Westmead Hospital. There were 13 female and 10 male participants with an average duration since trauma of 60.8 months (SD = 74.3). Twenty trauma-exposed controls (Trauma Controls: those who had experienced a criterion A trauma (defined by DSM-IV as being confronted with an experience that threatened physical integrity) but did not develop PTSD symptoms that reached diagnostic PTSD (or sub-clinical status) were recruited from community settings (in collaboration with the Brain Resource International Database) [21]. Ten Trauma Controls had experienced motor vehicle accidents, and 10 had experienced interpersonal assault. There was an average duration post-trauma of 110 months (SD = 139) for Trauma Controls. Participants were administered the Composite International Diagnostic Interview (CIDI) [22] to diagnose those with PTSD and identify those who were trauma-exposed controls. Trauma Controls reported symptoms that did not meet criteria for the Re-experiencing cluster (cluster B) of symptoms, or more than one PTSD symptom cluster for Avoidance or Hyperarousal. To provide an estimate of the severity and frequency of PTSD symptoms (including emotional numbing), participants with PTSD were also administered the Clinician Administered PTSD Scale (CAPS) [23]. Fifteen participants with PTSD had comorbid major depression (8 were medicated with antidepressants), 1 had comorbid panic disorder, and 1 comorbid OCD. All participants were excluded if there was any current substance abuse or dependence (within six months of testing), history of brain injury or neurological condition, psychosis or significant medical condition. To provide an estimate of current mood, all participants were administered the Depression Anxiety Stress Scales [24]. All participants provided written informed consent according to the Declaration of Helsinki. This study was approved by the Western Sydney Area Health Service Human Research Ethics Board.

Face Emotion Perception Task

The facial emotion perception task was previously established to activate networks in ventral striatum, anterior cingulate cortex and amygdala [25]. Participants viewed 240 grey-scale face stimuli selected from a standardized picture set [26]. The set consisted of four female and four male individuals depicting happy and neutral facial expressions. Face stimuli were presented in a pseudorandom sequence of 30 blocks (comprising 8 happy or 8 neutral faces each). Each stimulus was presented for 500 ms and was followed by a 767.5 ms blank screen interstimulus interval. Emotion identification accuracy and ratings of the intensity of facial emotion were assessed immediately post-scanning. Intensity ratings employed 9-point Likert scales (0 = *not at all intense*, 9 = *very intense*).

fMRI Data Acquisition

MRI scans were performed on a 1.5 T Siemens Vision Plus Scanner using an echo echoplanar protocol. A total of 90 functional T*2-weighted volumes (3 stimuli per block) were acquired for each condition, comprising 15 non-contiguous slices parallel to the intercommissural (AC-PC) line, with a 6.6 mm thickness and TR = 3.3 sec, TE = 40 ms, Flip angle = 90°; with FOV 24×24 cm^2, matrix size 128×128.

Functional MRI Data Reduction and Analysis

Pre-processing and statistical analysis of fMRI data was conducted using Statistical Parametric Mapping (SPM-2, Wellcome Department of Neurology, London, UK). Functional scans were realigned, unwarped, spatially normalized and smoothed in order to remove movement artefact and to place data into a common anatomical frame. Images were normalized into standardized MNI space and smoothed using a Gaussian kernel (FWHM: 8 mm).

An HRF-convolved boxcar model with temporal derivative was created to correspond to the experimental model, and a high pass filter was applied to remove low frequency fluctuations in the BOLD signal. Individual contrast images (fear versus neutral) were brought to the second level and examined using t-tests.

For the group voxelwise analysis, random effects independent samples t-tests comparing the PTSD and Trauma Control group to happy (-neutral) faces were conducted. To test our a priori hypotheses, analyses were undertaken using a search region of interest (ROI) approach which included regions of the amygdala and ventral striatum (caudate and putamen, including nucleus accumbens). Search regions were defined by the Automated Anatomical Labelling (AAL) Masks [27] and selected using the WFU Pickatlas (Version 1.02). We created an anatomical region of interest mask for the ventral striatum by combining caudate and putamen (including nucleus accumbens). Nucleus accumbens was identified at the inferior junction between the head of caudate and putamen, in accordance with previous studies and the Human Brain Atlas [28,29]. Coordinates of peak activations within the nucleus accumbens were confirmed with reference to the Human Brain Atlas.

Previous studies of facial emotion processing have used an uncorrected p value of $p<.05$ for determining significant activations in small structures based on a priori hypotheses [17], or p<.005 when examining ventral striatum in monetary incentive tasks [11]. Given our a priori directional hypotheses, in line with previous literature [9,17] we employed independent samples t-tests using the above ROIs, with an alpha value of p<.005, and a spatial extent threshold of 10 contiguous voxels. To examine the influence of comorbid depression, a sub-analysis (using the same analysis techniques as above) was conducted comparing PTSD_with depression (n = 15) and Trauma Controls, PTSD_no depression (n = 8) and Trauma Controls, and PTSD_with and PTSD_No depression groups using independent samples t-tests.

For the correlational analysis, intensity beta values were extracted from the most significant voxels for each individual in the ventral striatum ROI. Pearson Product moment correlations were conducted in SPM2 within the PTSD group between each individual's peak BOLD ventral striatal activity in response to happy faces and their emotional numbing score (derived from ratings on the CAPS in a procedure taken from Foa et al., (1995). To control for PTSD severity, depression and state anxiety, correlations were conducted with PTSD severity (total CAPS score), DASS depression score, and DASS anxiety score included as covariates. A probability estimate of $p<.01$ and the extent threshold >10 voxels per cluster was adopted.

Results

Demographic and Clinical Data

Demographic and clinical data are summarized in Table 1. The PTSD group were significantly older than the Trauma Controls, and there was a trend for Trauma Controls to have longer time since trauma, but there were no significant differences in gender distribution between groups. All analyses reported below were repeated taking age and time-post trauma as covariates; findings remained consistent and will not be reported. As expected, PTSD participants scored higher on the DASS depression and DASS anxiety scores.

Facial Expression Ratings Data

There were no significant differences between groups in accuracy for identification of happy (Trauma Control: 100%; PTSD: 99% correct) or neutral facial expressions (Trauma Control: 76%; PTSD: 78% correct). In terms of intensity of emotional expression, the PTSD group rated the happy faces as less intense than Trauma Controls ($F_{(1,26)} = 4.2$, $p<.05$).

fMRI Data

PTSD participants revealed lower activation in response to perception of happiness (versus neutral) left nucleus accumbens extending into putamen, and trends for lower activation in left amygdala compared to Trauma Controls (see Table 2 and Figure 1). There were no significantly greater activations in these regions of interest in the PTSD group. Examination of percentage of signal change to happy and neutral faces (see Figure 2) reveals that these group differences are most apparent in response to happy faces.

Effect of Medication. To examine the impact of medication, fMRI data was reanalyzed comparing unmedicated PTSD patients (n = 15) with Trauma Controls, and comparing medicated PTSD patients (n = 8) with Trauma Controls (see Table 3). Findings reinforced our overall group findings. Unmedicated PTSD patients displayed lower activations in left amygdala and displayed trends for lower activation in right nucleus accumbens. There were no greater activations in these regions in the PTSD group. Further, a sub-analysis of fMRI data in medicated PTSD patients (n = 8) compared to Trauma Controls revealed trends for reduced activation in right amygdala and right ventral striatum.

Effect of Depression. To examine the impact of depression, fMRI data was reanalyzed comparing PTSD with depression with Trauma Controls, and PTSD without depression to Trauma Controls. Findings are summarized in Table 4. Relative to Trauma Controls, the PTSD without depression group displayed significantly reduced activity in right amygdala and a trend for reduced activity in left ventral striatum. There were no greater activations in the PTSD group without depression over Trauma Controls. The PTSD group with depression revealed trends for reduced activation in right amygdala and significantly reduced activation in right ventral striatum. Comparing PTSD samples with and without depression revealed that PTSD patients with depression had lower activation in right caudate compared to PTSD without depression patients. PTSD patients without

Table 1. Summary of demographic and clinical characteristics of the PTSD (n = 23) and Trauma Exposed Control (n = 20) groups.

Variable	TC	PTSD	Test Statistic	p
Age	30.5(12)	38.5(11.5)	F = 5	.03*
Gender	11 M, 9 F	10 M, 13 F	$\chi^2 = .57$	.55
Time post-trauma (mths)	110 (139)	60.8 (74.3)	F = 3.8	.055
Trauma Type	10 MVA 10Assault	8 MVA 15Assault	$\chi^2 = 1.09$	.242
Comorbidity	Nil	15 MDD, 1 PD, 1 OCD	$\chi^2 = 8.6$	.004*
Medication	Nil	8 medicated 15unmedicated	$\chi^2 = 8.6$	.004*
DASS Dep	3.1 (2)	10.9 (5.2)	F = 34.5	.001*
DASS Anx	1.6(1.9)	13.1 (6.7)	F = 55	.001*

Note: Standard deviations in parentheses. TC = trauma-exposed controls, PTSD = Posttraumatic Stress Disorrder; M = male, F = female; mths = months; MVA = motor vehicle accident; MDD = major depressive disorder, PD = Panic Disorder, OCD = Obsessive Compulsive Disorder; DASS = Depression Anxiety and Stress Scale; dep = depression, anx = anxiety.
*p<.05,
**p<.001.

Table 2. Summary of between-group t-tests: Increased BOLD signal elicited by happy faces compared to neutral faces in the PTSD (n = 23) and Trauma-exposed controls (TC: n = 20; (p<.005 uncorrected).

Brain Region	Hem	MNI Coordinates			Voxels	t	p
		X	Y	Z			
TC>PTSD							
Amygdala	Left	−16	−2	−12	7	2.81	.05*
Ventral Striatum	Left	−14	0	−6	118	3.61	.000

Note: TC = trauma-exposed controls,
*trend level result.

depression displayed no significant differences in neural activation compared to PTSD with depression patients.

Correlation Analyses. Given the small samples in the depression sub-analysis, a correlation analysis was used to examine the relationships between emotional numbing symptoms and BOLD activation to happy faces in unmedicated PTSD participants, whilst taking depression and anxiety (DASS scales) and PTSD severity as covariates. Figure 3 presents a summary of findings. More severe symptoms of emotional numbing correlated negatively with activation in the right ventral striatum (putamen extending into nucleus accumbens: −32 −14 −4, 138 voxels, T = 5.7, p<.05, $r = -.709$) see Figure 3) and the culmen (−6 −52 −8, 219 voxels, T = 6.7,p<.01). A partial correlation analysis was also conducted between depression scores and activation in the right ventral striatum (putamen extending into nucleus accumbens (MNI coordinates) −32 −14 −4), whilst controlling for numbing scores. There was no significant correlation found between depression and ventral striatum activation (r = .27, p = .35).

Discussion

Our hypotheses that activation in ventral striatal reward processing networks would be lower in PTSD to happy faces, and that this would be associated with emotional numbing symptoms, were largely confirmed. The PTSD group displayed behavioural evidence of less reactivity to happy faces as they rated happy faces as less intense in expression than trauma controls. Lower activation in ventral striatal regions (putamen and nucleus accumbens) and amygdala was seen in PTSD compared to Trauma Controls in response to happy (-neutral) faces. Importantly, a correlational analysis that controlled for depression, anxiety and PTSD severity found a negative correlation between emotional numbing symptoms in PTSD and activation in ventral striatum in the PTSD group, but there was no correlation between depression symptoms and ventral striatal activation.

These findings accord with recent reports of lower activation in nucleus accumbens and ventral striatal regions in PTSD in response to gains in monetary incentive tasks [9,10], and extend this previous research by demonstrating that PTSD is associated with impaired perception of innate reward signals (happy facial expressions), with a concurrent reduction in activity within ventral striatal networks. This is significant given evidence that facial perception contributes significantly to social functioning [20], and that emotional numbing in PTSD is the most significant predictor of chronic functional and social impairment [5,6]. Importantly, this study also extends previous research by including a trauma-exposed control group – our results suggest that lower activation in ventral striatal reward networks is specifically associated with PTSD, rather than trauma exposure per se.

Despite this convergence, there was also evidence of distinctive functional networks mediating motivational incentive tasks and happy face perception. Sailer and colleagues (2009) reported lower activation in medial frontal gyrus and nucleus accumbens in PTSD, reflecting weaker mesocortical dopaminergic activity [10]. Elman and colleagues (2009) found lower activation in both ventral and dorsal striatal regions (encompassing putamen and caudate, but *not* nucleus accumbens) [9]. In contrast, we found less activation *specifically* in ventral striatum (left nucleus accumbens extending into putamen) to happy faces. Ventral striatum is thought to process salience and prediction of reward signals, whereas dorsal striatum is more involved in action planning, cognitive function and sensorimotor integration [30,31]. Nucleus accumbens is a region that is particularly associated with processing positive signals [32].

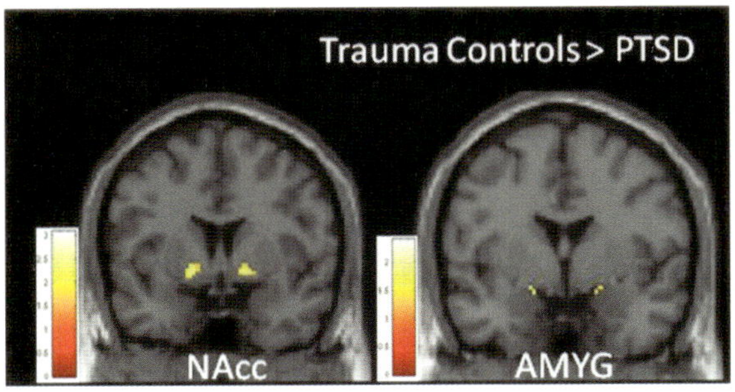

Figure 1. Reduced BOLD Activity in Ventral Striatum and Amygdala in PTSD (n = 23) compared to trauma-exposed controls (n = 20) in response to happy (- neutral) facial expressions.

The fact that lower activation in ventral striatal activity did not remain significant when removing PTSD participants with depression from the analysis, suggests that depression may contribute to the impairments in these networks. This accord with recent evidence of reduced nucleus accumbens activation to monetary rewards in major depression [11]. However, depression is not likely to be a sufficient explanation for these null findings, as although the PTSD group with depression displayed a significant reduction in activation of ventral striatum, this reduction was at trend level in the PTSD without depression group. Further, direct comparison of the PTSD with and without depression groups revealed that the PTSD with depression group displayed lower activation in more dorsal regions ofthe striatum relative to the PTSD group without depression. This lower activation may reflect impaired activation in networks governing action initiation associated with depression [30]. The failure to find lower ventral striatal activation within the PTSD group without depression compared to controls is more likely a result of limited statistical power, as the sample size for non-depressed participants was small (n = 8). This interpretation is supported by the fact that the significant negative correlation between emotional numbing and ventral striatum remained significant after controlling for depression, and there was no significant correlation between ventral striatal activity and depression whilst controlling for numbing.

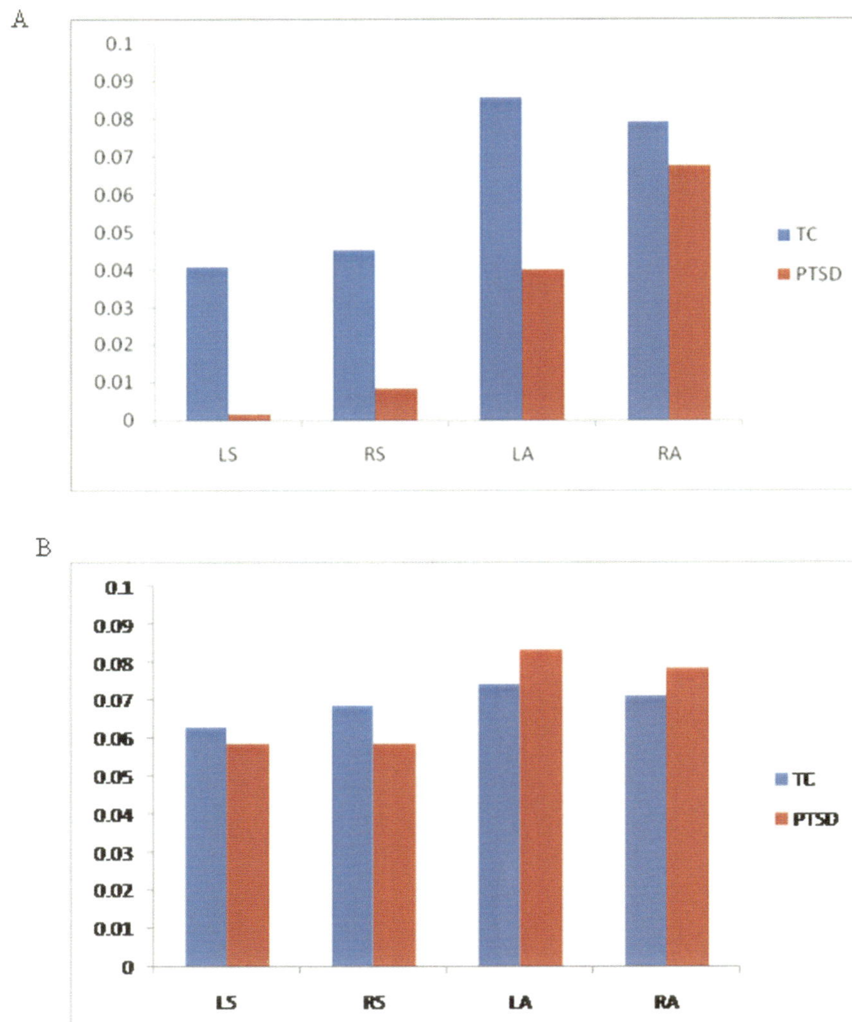

Figure 2. Percentage signal change in BOLD response to happy faces (Panel A) in Left Ventral Striatum (LS), Right ventral striatum (RS), Left Amygdala (LA), and Right Amygdala (RA), and percentage signal change in BOLD response to Neutral Faces (Panel B) in Left Ventral Striatum (LS), Right Ventral Striatum (RS), Left Amygdala (LA) and Right Amygdala (RA).

Table 3. Increased BOLD signal elicited by happy faces compared to neutral faces in the PTSD-No Medication Group (n = 15) vs Trauma-exposed controls (TC: n = 20;), and PTSD-Medication Group (n = 8) vs Trauma-exposed controls (TC: n = 20).

Brain Region	Hem	MNI Coordinates			Voxels	t	p
TC>PTSD_no medication							
Amygdala	L	−16	−2	−12	18	2.81	.004
Ventral Striatum	R	18	6	−6	110	2.60	.009
PTSD-no medication>TC							
Amygdala	-	-	-	-	-	-	-
Ventral Striatum	-	-	-	-	-	-	-
TC>Medicated PTSD							
Amygdala	R	30	−4	−28	7	2.23	.017
Ventral Striatum	R	24	20	2	49	2.32	.014
Medicated PTSD>TC							
Amygdala	-	-	-	-	-	-	-
Ventral Striatum	-	-	-	-	-	-	-

Note: TC = trauma-exposed controls,

Table 4. Increased BOLD signal elicited by happy faces compared to neutral faces in the PTSD-No Depression Group (n = 8) vs Trauma-exposed controls (TC: n = 20;), and PTSD-Depression Group (n = 15) vs Trauma-exposed controls (TC: n = 20).

Brain Region	Hem	MNI Coordinates			Voxels	t	p
TC≥PTSD-no depression							
Amygdala	R	22	−6	−12	18	2.49	.005
Ventral Striatum	L	14	4	−6	74	2.10	.009
TC≥PTSD -depression							
Amygdala	R	34	−2	−24	22	2.24	.008
Ventral Striatum	R	34	−16	0	120	2.93	.002
Non-Depressed PTSD≥Depressed PTSD							
Amygdala	R	32	−4	−20	11	2.31	.008
Ventral Striatum	R	10	14	12	843	6.19	.000
Depressed PTSD≥Non-Depressed PTSD							
Amygdala	-	-	-	-	-	-	-
Ventral Striatum	-	-	-	-	-	-	-

Note: TC = trauma-exposed controls,

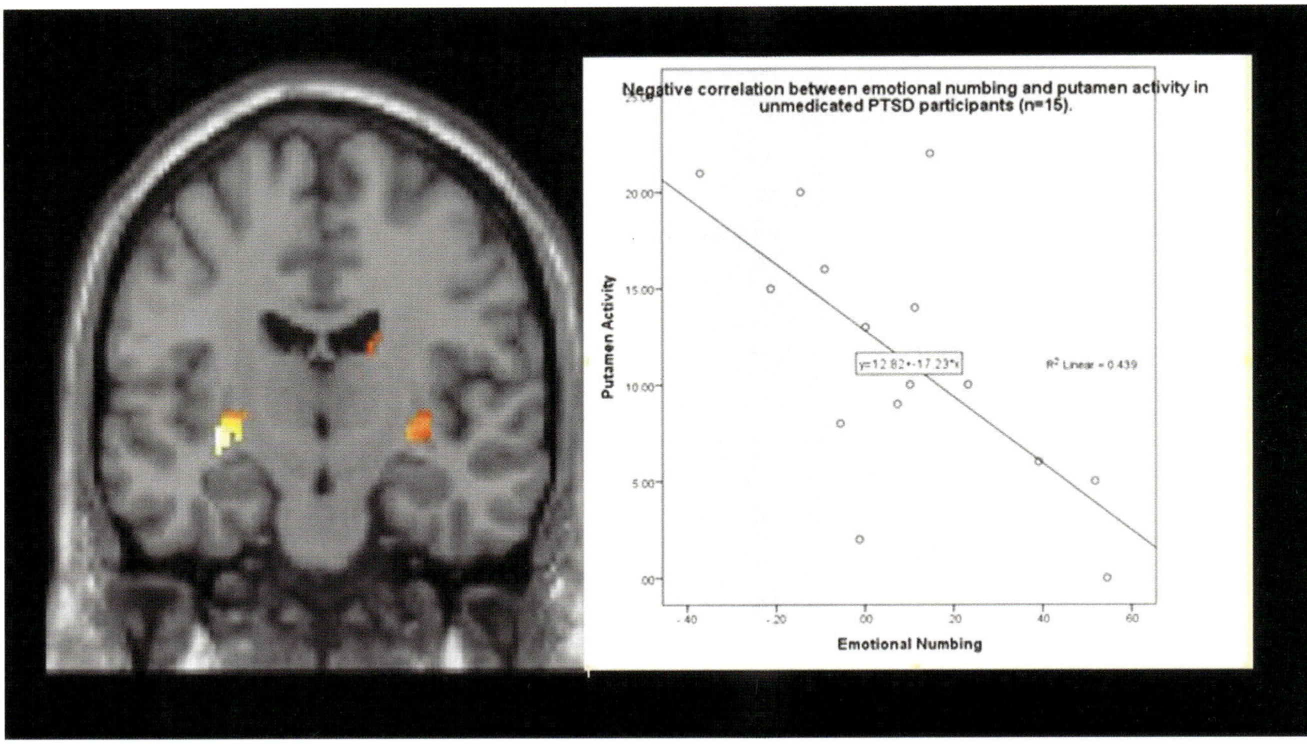

Figure 3. Correlations between BOLD activity to happy (-neutral) facial expressions in ventral striatum (putamen extending into nucleus accumbens) and CAPS emotional numbing scores in the unmedicated PTSD (n = 15) group.

Medication status does not appear to be a sufficient explanation for these findings, as comparisons between the Trauma Control group and medicated PTSD patients and unmedicated PTSD patients resulted in reduction of ventral striatal activation being reduced to trend level in both analyses. Again, however, this may relate to the smaller group sizes in these analyses. To clarify the role of depression and medication status, future research needs to examine depressed and non-depressed, medicated and non-medicated PTSD participants with larger group sizes.

There was a trend for reduced amygdala activation in the PTSD group compared to trauma controls which became significant once removing medicated PTSD participants, suggesting that medication use may have masked some amygdala effects. This reduction in amygdala activity to happy faces contrasts with reports of heightened amygdala activation to fearful faces in PTSD [33,34], suggesting that these results may not be explained by a generalized impairment in processing emotional expressions. Amygdala activation has been associated with fear perception [35], but also with a broader construct of stimulus salience [36]. There is increasing evidence that the amygdala is also responsive to happy facial expressions [16–18,37]. To the extent that amygdala activation reflects detection of salient stimuli [36], the fMRI findings suggest there is a blunted response to salient positive signals, in contrast to a heightened detection of threat (fearful face) stimuli in PTSD.

An unexpected but convergent finding was the evidence for lower activation in right orbitofrontal cortex in the non-depressed PTSD group compared to trauma controls in response to happy faces. Medial OFC has afferents to ventral striatum [38] and is thought to modulate reward related behaviours [39–43]. Anterolateral orbitofrontal cortex increases activity in response to signals of absence of reward (Ursu & Carter, 2005), and in anticipation of viewing aversive images [44,45]. Therefore, this finding suggests that PTSD without comorbid depression is associated with lower activation in reward-processing networks in the orbitofrontal cortex.

To explore predictions of the prevailing model of emotional numbing [2], future research needs to examine responses to positive and threatening stimuli concurrently. The use of a passive viewing task with a predictable series of facial expressions may have reduced our BOLD signal, as fMRI activity has been found to be greatest in response to unpredictable rewarding stimuli in nucleus accumbens and medial orbitofrontal cortex [46]. Indeed, these findings should be viewed as preliminary and require replication, as they did not survive correction for multiple comparisons. Future studies examining responses to positive signals in depressed and non-depressed PTSD samples should employ larger sample sizes and a more active emotional task to enhance BOLD signal. A more comprehensive measure of emotional numbing should be employed in future studies rather than relying on PTSD symptom scores from the CAPS. Future research should examine group differences in BOLD responses to neutral facial expressions, independently of emotional faces. Although findings may be confounded by the direct comparison of happy and neutral faces [47], examining the percentage signal change for our key ventral striatal findings suggests the main effects are driven by response to the happy face rather than the neutral face (Figure 2). Future research should employ a separate fixation baseline condition to avoid a direct comparison of happy and neutral faces. Finally, the cross-sectional design prevented us identifying if altered brain patterns preceded or followed traumatic exposure.

In conclusion, this study provides novel evidence that individuals with PTSD perceive happy facial expressions as less intense and that lower activation in ventral striatal-limbic reward networks is associated with symptoms of emotional numbing in PTSD. Importantly, these blunted responses to positive facial signals are not accounted for by trauma exposure or comorbid depression. The identification of impaired functioning of reward networks in PTSD points to the need for better understanding of these networks in PTSD and the role they play in the trajectory of PTSD. Improving the capacity to respond to positive emotional signals in PTSD is of vital therapeutic importance, given evidence that emotional numbing symptoms contribute predominantly to functional and social impairments in chronic PTSD.

Acknowledgments

We thank the Brain Resource International Database (under the auspices of the Brain Resource Company) for support in data acquisition and methodology. Kim Felmingham, Erin Falconer, Andrew Kemp, Adrian Allen, Anthony Peduto and Richard Bryant report no biomedical financial interests or potential conflicts of interest. Leanne Williams owns personal shares in the Brain Resource Company that are less than 1% of the company value. Kim Felmingham has had full access to all of the data in the study and takes responsibility for the integrity of the data and the accuracy of the data analysis.

Author Contributions

Conceived and designed the experiments: KF EF AK LW AA AP RB. Performed the experiments: AP KF. Analyzed the data: KF RB LW. Wrote the paper: KF RB EF AA LW AK.

References

1. Frewen PA, Lanius RA (2006) Toward a psychobiology of Posttraumatic self-dysregulation: Re-experiencing, hyperarousal, dissociation and emotional numbing. Ann NY Acad Sci 1071: 110–24.
2. Litz B, Gray MJ (2002) Emotional numbing in posttraumatic stress disorder: Current and future directions. Aust N Z J Psychiatry 36: 198–204.
3. Kashdan TB, Elhai JD, Frueh BC (2006) Anhedonia and emotional numbing in combat veterans with Posttraumatic Stress Disorder. Behav Res Ther 44(3): 457–67.
4. North CS, Suris AM, Davis M, Smith RP (2009) Toward validation of the diagnosis of posttraumatic stress disorder. Am J Psychiatry 166: 34–41.
5. Ruscio AM, Weathers FW, King LA, King DW (2002) Male war-zone veterans' perceived relationships with their children: the importance of emotional numbing. J Trauma Stress 15(5): 351–7.
6. Norman SB, Stein MB, Davidson JRT (2007) Profiling posttraumatic functional impairment. J Nerv Ment Dis 195: 48–53.
7. Elman I, Ariely D, Mazar N, Aharon I, Lasko NB, et al. (2005) Probing reward function in posttraumatic stress disorder with beautiful facial images. Psychiatry Res 135: 179–183.
8. Hopper JW, Pitman RK, Su Z, Heyman GM, Lasko NB, et al. (2008) Probing reward function in posttraumatic stress disorder: Expectancy and satisfaction with monetary gains and losses. J Psychiatry Res 42: 802–807.
9. Elman I, Lowen S, Frederick BB, Chi W, Becerra L, et al. (2009) Functional neuroimaging of reward circuitry responsitivity to monetary gains and losses in posttraumatic stress disorder. Biol Psychiatry 66(12): 1083–90.
10. Sailer U, Robinson S, Fischmeister FP, Konig D, Oppenauer C, et al. (2009) Altered reward processing in the nucleus accumbens and mesial prefrontal cortex of patients with posttraumatic stress disorder. Neuropsychologia 46(11): 2836–44.
11. Pizzigalli DS, Holmes AJ, Dillon DG, Goetz EL, Birk JL, et al. (2009) Reduced caudate and nucleus accumbens response to rewards in unmedicated individuals with major depressive disorder. Am J Psychiatry 166: 702–710.
12. Berridge KC, Kringelbach ML (2008) Affective neuroscience of pleasure: reward in humans and animals. Psychopharmacology 199: 457–480.
13. O'Doherty J, Dayan P, Schultz J, Deichmann R, Friston K, et al. (2004) Dissociable roles of ventral and dorsal striatum in instrumental conditioning. Science 304(5669): 452–4.
14. Jatzko A, Schmitt A, Demirakca T, Weimer E, Braus DS (2005) Disturbances in the neural circuitry underlying positive emotional processing in post-traumatic stress disorder (PTSD). Eur Arch Psychiatry Clin Neurosci 256(2): 112–114.
15. Monk CS, Klein RG, Telzer EH, Schroth FA, Mannuzza S, et al. (2008) Amygdala and nucleus accumbens activation to emotional facial expressions in adolescents at risk for major depression. Am J Psychiatry 165(2): 266.
16. Breiter H, Etcoff NL, Whalen PJ, William A, Rauch SL, et al. (1996) Response and habituation of the human amygdala during visual processing of facial expression. Neuron 17: 875–887.
17. Killgore WDS, Yurgelun-Todd DA (2004) Activation of the amygdala and anterior cingulate during nonconscious processing of sad versus happy faces. Neuroimage 21: 1215–1223.
18. Costafreda SG, Brammer MJ, David AS, Fu CH (2008) Predictors of amygdala activation during the processing of emotional stimuli: A meta-analysis of 385 PET and fMRI studies. Brain Res Rev 58(1): 57–70.
19. Rolls ET (2004) The functions of the orbitofrontal cortex. Brain Cogn 55: 11–29.
20. Addington J, Girard TA, Christensen BK, Addington D (2010) Social cognition mediates illness-related and cognitive influences on social function in patients with Schizophrenia-spectrum disorders. J Psychiatry Neurosci 35(1): 49–54.
21. Gordon E, Barnett K, Cooper NJ, Tran N, Williams LM (2008) An "Integrative Neuroscience" platform: Application to profiles of positivity and negativity bias. J Integr Neurosci 7: 345–366.
22. Robbins L, Wing J, Wittchen H, Helzer J, Babor T, et al. (1998) The Composite International Diagnostic Interview. Arch Gen Psychiatry 45: 1069–77.
23. Blake DD, Weathers FW, Nagy LM, Kaloupek DG, Klauminzer G, et al. (1990) A clinician rating scale for assessing current and lifetime PTSD: The CAPS-1. Behav Ther 13: 187–188.
24. Lovibond SF, Lovibond PF (1995) Manual for the Depression Anxiety Stress Scales (2nd Ed.). Sydney: Psychology Foundation.
25. Williams LM, Das P, Liddell BJ, Kemp AH, Rennie CJ, et al. (2006) Mode of functional connectivity in amygdala pathways dissociates level of awareness for signals of fear. J Neurosci 26(36): 9264–71.
26. Gur RC, Sara R, Hagendoorn M, Maron O, Hughgett P, et al. (2002) A method for obtaining 3-dimensional facial expressions and its standardization for use in neurocognitive studies. J Neurosci Methods 115: 137–143.
27. Tzourio-Mazoyer N, Landeaum B, Papathanassioum D, Crivello F, Etard O, et al. (2002) Automated anatomical labeling of activations in SPM using a macroscopic anatomical parcellation of the MNI MRI single-subject brain. Neuroimage 15: 273–289.
28. Mai JK, Assheuer J, Paxinos G (2004) Atlas of the Human Brain (Second Edition). London: Elsevier Academic Press.
29. Ernst M, Nelson EE, Jazbec S, McClure EB, Monk CS, et al. (2005) Amygdala and nucleus accumbens in responses to receipt and omission of gains in adults and adolescents. Neuroimage 25: 1279–91.
30. Balleine BW, Delgado MR, Hiksaka O (2007) The role of the dorsal striatum in reward and decision making. J Neurosci 27: 8161–65.
31. Romero MC, Bermudez MA, Vicente AF, Perez R, Gonzalez F (2008) Activity of neurons in the caudate and putamen during a visuomotor task. Neuroreport 19: 1141–45.
32. Elliot R, Friston KJ, Dolan RJ (2000) Dissociable neural responses in human reward systems. J Neurosci 20: 6159–65.
33. Shin LM, Wright CI, Cannistraro PA, Wedig MM, McMullin K, et al. (2005). A functional magnetic resonance imaging study of amygdala and medial prefrontal cortex responses to overtly presented fearful faces in Posttraumatic Stress Disorder. Arch Gen Psychiatry 62: 273–281.
34. Williams LM, Kemp AH, Felmingham KL, Barton M, Olivieri G, et al. (2006). Trauma modulates amygdala and medial prefrontal responses to consciously attended fear. Neuroimage 29(2): 347–357.
35. Phan KL, Wager T, Taylor SF, Liberzon I (2002) Functional neuroanatomy of emotion: A meta-analysis of emotional activation studies in PET and fMRI. Neuroimage 16(2): 331–348.
36. Davis M, Whalen PJ (2003) The amygdala: vigilance and emotion. Mol Psychiatry 6: 13–34.
37. Fusar-Poli P, Placentino A, Carletti F, Landi P, Allen P, et al. (2009). Functional analyses of emotional faces processing: A voxel-based meta-analysis of 105 functional magnetic resonance imaging studies. J Psychiatry Neurosci 34(6): 418–52.
38. Ferry AT, Lu XC, Price JL (2000) Effects of excitotoxic lesions in the ventral striatopallidal-thalamocortical pathway on odor reversal learning: Inability to extinguish extinguish an incorrect response. Exp Brain Res 131: 320–335.
39. O'Doherty J, Winston J, Critchley H, Perrett D, Burt DM (2003) Beauty in a smile: The role of medial orbitofrontal cortex in facial attractiveness. Neuropsychologia 41: 147–155.
40. Ursu S, Carter CS (2005) Outcome representations, counterfactual comparisons and the human orbitofrontal cortex: implications for neuroimaging studies of decision-making. Brain Res Cogn Brain Res 23: 51–60
41. Galvan A, Hare TA, Davidson M, Spicer J, Glover G, et al. (2005) The role of ventral frontostriatal circuitry in reward-based learning in humans. J Neurosci 25: 8650–8656.
42. Winston JS, O'Doherty J, Kilner JM, Perrett DI, Dolan RJ (2007) Brain systems for assessing facial attractiveness. Neuropsychologia 45: 195–206.

43. Milad MR, Rauch SL (2007) The role of the orbitofrontal cortex in anxiety disorders. Ann NY Acad Sci 1121: 546–61.
44. Kringelbach ML, Rolls ET (2004) The functional neuroanatomy of the human orbitofrontal cortex: Evidence from neuroimaging and neuropsychology. Prog Neurobiol 72: 341–72.
45. Nitschke JB, Sarinopoulos KL, Mackiewicz KL (2006) Functional neuroanatomy of aversion and its anticipation. Neuroimage 29: 106–116.
46. Berns GS, McClure SM, Pagnoni G, Montague PR (2001) Predictability modulates human brain response to reward. J Neurosci 21(8): 2793–8.
47. Somerville LH, Kim H, Johnstone T, Alexander AL, Whalen PJ (2004). Human amygdala responses during presentation of happy and neutral faces: correlations with state anxiety. Biological Psychiatry 55(9): 897–903.

Effects of Deletion of Mutant Huntingtin in Steroidogenic Factor 1 Neurons on the Psychiatric and Metabolic Phenotype in the BACHD Mouse Model of Huntington Disease

Barbara Baldo*⁹, Rachel Y. Cheong⁹, Åsa Petersén

Translational Neuroendocrine Research Unit, Department of Experimental Medical Science, Lund University, Lund, Sweden

Abstract

Psychiatric and metabolic features appear several years before motor disturbances in the neurodegenerative Huntington's disease (HD), caused by an expanded CAG repeat in the *huntingtin* (*HTT*) gene. Although the mechanisms leading to these aspects are unknown, dysfunction in the hypothalamus, a brain region controlling emotion and metabolism, has been suggested. A direct link between the expression of the disease causing protein, huntingtin (HTT), in the hypothalamus and the development of metabolic and psychiatric-like features have been shown in the BACHD mouse model of HD. However, precisely which circuitry in the hypothalamus is critical for these features is not known. We hypothesized that expression of mutant HTT in the ventromedial hypothalamus, an area involved in the regulation of metabolism and emotion would be important for the development of these non-motor aspects. Therefore, we inactivated mutant HTT in a specific neuronal population of the ventromedial hypothalamus expressing the transcription factor steroidogenic factor 1 (SF1) in the BACHD mouse using cross-breeding based on a Cre-loxP system. Effects on anxiety-like behavior were assessed using the elevated plus maze and novelty-induced suppressed feeding test. Depressive-like behavior was assessed using the Porsolt forced swim test. Effects on the metabolic phenotype were analyzed using measurements of body weight and body fat, as well as serum insulin and leptin levels. Interestingly, the inactivation of mutant HTT in SF1-expressing neurons exerted a partial positive effect on the depressive-like behavior in female BACHD mice at 4 months of age. In this cohort of mice, no anxiety-like behavior was detected. The deletion of mutant HTT in SF1 neurons did not have any effect on the development of metabolic features in BACHD mice. Taken together, our results indicate that mutant HTT regulates metabolic networks by affecting hypothalamic circuitries that do not involve the SF1 neurons of the ventromedial hypothalamus.

Editor: Hoon Ryu, Boston University School of Medicine, United States of America

Funding: This work was supported by grants from the Swedish Medical Research Council (K2011-62X-20404-05-6), the Ragnar Söderberg foundation, the province of Skåne ALF grant, the Kungliga Fysiografiska foundation and the Blanceflor Boncompagni Ludovisi foundation. The funders had no role in study design, data collection and analysis, decision to publish or preparation of the manuscript.

Competing Interests: The authors have declared that no competing interests exist.

* Email: barbara.baldo@med.lu.se

⁹ These authors contributed equally to this work.

Introduction

Huntington's disease (HD) is a devastating neurodegenerative disorder caused by an expanded CAG repeat in the *huntingtin* (*HTT*) gene [1]. It is clinically diagnosed when an individual presents with typical involuntary movements in combination with a positive gene test. The disease then progresses over 15–25 years, inevitably leading to death. It is now well recognized that individuals with the mutant HTT gene often manifest psychiatric and cognitive disturbances many years before the motor onset of the disease [2,3]. Other non-motor features are also common including metabolic dysfunction, changes in the circadian rhythm as well as sleep disturbances [4]. The motor symptoms and the cognitive changes have been associated with the pathology in the basal ganglia as well in the cerebral cortex [5,6], but less is known about the neural substrate of other non-motor aspects of the disease.

The hypothalamus is a region in the brain involved in the regulation of important functions such as emotion, metabolism and circadian rhythm [7]. Neuropathological analyses have revealed effects on different neuropeptide populations regulating emotion and metabolism in human postmortem tissue from HD patients [8–11]. Hypothalamic changes have indeed been shown in clinical HD prior to motor dysfunction using magnetic resonance imaging (MRI) and positron emission tomography (PET) [12,13], suggesting that this region may be affected early in the HD process. Interestingly, recent studies in experimental models of HD have established a direct link between the expression of mutant HTT in the hypothalamus and the development of non-motor signs [14,15]. Expression of mutant

HTT by the use of stereotactic injections of recombinant adeno-associated viral (rAAV) vectors in the hypothalamus of wild-type (WT) mice led to increased body weight as well as insulin and leptin resistance. Another experiment used the BACHD mouse model of HD expresses, which human full-length mutant HTT with a floxed exon1 with 97 CAG, allowing selective deletion of mutant HTT in the presence of Cre-recombinase (Cre; [16]). The mouse model displays both depressive and anxiety-like behaviors as well as a robust metabolic phenotype with leptin and insulin resistance at an early age [14,17]. Interestingly, inactivation of mutant HTT in the hypothalamus of the BACHD mouse using rAAV-Cre prevented the development of both the metabolic phenotype as well as the depressive-like behavior [14,15]. These studies were conducted by either expressing or inactivating mutant HTT in around 30% of the neurons in the hypothalamus [14,15]. Additional experiments carried out by inactivating mutant HTT only in leptin receptor-expressing neurons in the hypothalamus of BACHD mice did not have any effect on the phenotype [18]. Hence, the critical neuronal circuitry in the hypothalamus responsible for the development of the non-motor features remains to be determined.

The ventromedial hypothalamus (VMH) plays a crucial role in the control of metabolism, energy expenditure and anxiety-like behavior [19,20]. The neurons expressing steroidogenic factor 1 (SF1) represent a large part of the neurons in the VMH [21]. SF1 is a transcription factor belonging to the subfamily of transcription factors known as nuclear receptor subfamily 5 and has a fundamental role for VMH development [22–26]. Most importantly, SF1-expressing neurons contribute in the regulation of energy homeostasis and body weight mainly through the leptin circuitry [27–30]. Along with their key role in the regulation of metabolism, SF1-expressing neurons have been proposed to control the development of psychiatric-like behavior since SF1 controls the transcription of cannabinoid receptor 1 and SF1 knock-out mice present anxiety-like features [21,23,29]. Therefore, we hypothesized that expression of mutant HTT in the SF1-expressing neuronal population of the VMH would be critical for the development of the metabolic and emotional dysfunction in BACHD mice. In order to answer this question, we crossed BACHD mice with animals expressing Cre under the SF1 promoter and performed a battery of behavioral and metabolic analysis at 4 months of age. Our results suggest that deletion of mutant HTT in the VMH and specifically in the SF1-expressing neurons is not sufficient for preventing the onset of metabolic and psychiatric-like signs in BACHD mice.

Materials and Methods

Ethics statement

All the experimental procedures were approved by the Regional Ethical Committee in Lund, Sweden (Permit number: M360-12).

Animals

BACHD mice, expressing human full-length HTT with 97 polyQ (FVB/N strain) and Tg(Nr5a1-Cre)7Lowl/J mice expressing Cre under the SF1 promoter (SF1; mixed FVB/N and C57BL6/J background) were obtained from Jacksons Laboratories (Bar Harbor, Maine, USA) [27]. Heterozygous SF1 males were crossed with FVB/N females obtained from Charles Rivers Laboratories (Sulzfeld, Germany). SF1 mice have no overt phenotype. SF1 females from the F1 generation were further crossed with BACHD males in order to obtain the generation used for all the experiments in this study (See Figure S1). The genotype of the offspring was determined from tail samples using PCR primers for Cre (5′–3′): forward GCGGTCTGGCAGTAAAAACTATC and reverse GTGAAACAGCATTGCTGTCACTT or for the BACHD transgene (5′–3′): forward CCGCTCAGGTTCTGCTTTTA and reverse AGGTCGGTGCAGAGGCTCCTC. The mice obtained from the F1 generation of the crossing BACHD-SF1 was tested for multiple behavioral and metabolic readouts (see paragraphs below) at 4 months of age. It is known that BACHD mice manifest psychiatric-like behaviors as well as metabolic changes as early as at 2 months of age and this phenotype is maintained until at least 12 months of age [14,15,31,32]. The number of animals for each genotype and sex was between 11 and 28 in all experimental groups. The animals were culled at 4 months of age by decapitation for the collection of fresh frozen tissue or an overdose of anesthesia with sodium-pentobarbital (Apoteksbolaget) for perfusion with paraformaldehyde (PFA). All mice were housed in groups at a 12 h light/dark cycle with ad libitum access to normal chow diet.

To verify the selective expression and activity of Cre in the VMH, SF1 animals were crossed with B6.129X1-Gt(ROSA)26-Sortm1(EYFP)Cos/J (ROSA-EYFP) and yellow fluorescent protein (EYFP) expression was evaluated by immunofluorescence (see paragraph below). ROSA-EYFP animals present a loxP-flanked STOP codon inserted before the EYFP gene, in the Gt(ROSA)26Sor locus, therefore expressing EYFP only in presence of active Cre-recombinase (C57BL/6 strain; Jackson laboratories).

PCR for Cre-recombinase excision validation

In order to verify the successful deletion of mutant HTT exon 1 in BACHD-SF1 animals, we performed PCR analysis from genomic DNA extracted from selected brain regions. 300 µm thick slices of fresh frozen tissue from brains of animals belonging to each of the four genotypes were cut using a cryostat. Selected brain regions were rapidly collected using a puncher of 2 mm diameter (Miltex). Genomic DNA was extracted from the tissue with the DNeasy Blood and Tissue kit (Qiagen) according to manufacturer's instructions. 1 µl of DNA was the used for the PCR reaction, which was performed using a PX2 Thermal Cycler (Thermo Electron Corporation). The PCR products were run on a 1% agarose gel for 40 min, with SYBR Safe DNA gel stain (Invitrogen). The primers were designed to detect the loxP flanked HTT exon 1 of the BACHD mice. Forward primer 5′-ATTCATTGCCCCGGTGCTGA-3′ and reverse primer 5′-AGCCCTCTTCCCTCTCAGACTAGAAGAGG-3′.

Metabolic Analyses

Body weight of the animals and content of body fat were measured at 4 months of age. The body fat content was assessed under isoflurane anesthesia using a whole body dual energy x-ray absorptiometry (DEXA) scanner (Lunar PIXImus2, Lunar Corporation, Madison, WI, USA). Percentage of body fat was then calculated with the PIXImus2 2.10 software (Lunar Corporation, Madison, WI, USA).

Whole blood was collected from the right ventricle during deep anesthesia using an 18G syringe needle and kept at room temperature for 30 min allowing the blood to clot. The blood was then spun for 15 min at 2000×g and the serum collected and stored at −80°C until further analysis. Serum levels of leptin and insulin were measured using ELISA kits (CrystalChem Inc.) according to manufacturer's instructions. Samples were diluted according to need and measured in duplicates.

Behavioral Analyses

Animals belonging to the four genotypes were assessed for general activity as well as anxiety- and depressive- like behavior at

4 months of age. All behavioral tests were performed during the light phase of the circadian rhythm according to procedures described previously. All arenas were wiped with ethanol after each trial.

Total activity was assessed with the Open field test (OF) using the PAS-Open field system (San Diego Instruments) as previously described [15]. The animals were placed in the center of the activity box (40.6×40.6×38.1 cm) and their movements across the arena were recorded for 1 hour and scored as infrared beam crossings (16×16 beams).

Elevated Plus Maze (EPM) and Novelty-induced suppressed feeding test (NSFT) were used to assess anxiety-like behaviors [15,33,34]. EPM was performed in using the Ethovision 3.1 Software system (Noldus Information Technology). The EPM consisted of four 30 cm long and 6 cm wide arms (two open and two closed) and it was elevated 50 cm above its base. The closed arms were surrounded by 30 cm high walls. Each mouse was placed in the center of the maze and its movements recorded for 5 minutes. The Ethovision software calculated the percentage of time spent on the open or closed arms over this time interval.

NSFT was performed using an arena constituted by a plastic box (90×90 cm), with about 40 cm high walls and containing a light (approx. 800 lux) directed to the center of the arena, where the food pellet was located. Prior to the trial, the animals were food-deprived for 12 hours but they had ad libitum access to water. The body weight was measured pre- and post-food deprivation. Individual animals were placed in one corner of the arena and the latency to approach and eat the food was measured within a 5 min time frame. When the animal would start feeding it would be removed from the arena and placed back into the home cage. There they would be allowed to feed for 5 minutes from a single food pellet with known weight. The latency to eat in the home cage was measured and the food pellet weighed, to determine the food consumption in 5 min.

The Porsolt Forced Swim Test (FST) was used to assess depressive-like behavior. Each mouse was placed in a 17 cm wide and 18 cm high glass cylinder filled with 10–12 cm of water at 25°C. The mice were filmed for 6 min with a digital video camera and then dried with a towel. The total time spent immobile during the last 4 min of the trial was calculated manually. Immobility was defined by an absence of swimming movements (movements of two or more paws). Slow movements of a single paw aimed to keep the head above the water surface were included in the time of immobility, as described by Porsolt [35]. The mice were scored blinded by the same rater.

Immunofluorescence and confocal imaging

In order to verify the presence of functional Cre activity, we crossed ROSA-EYFP mice with SF1 and visualized EYFP expression in the VMH. The cull of the mice was performed by transcardial perfusion with 4% PFA after deep anesthesia with sodium-pentobarbital (Apoteksbolaget). After 24 h post-fixation in 4% PFA, the brains were transferred to a 25% sucrose solution for cryopreservation and cut in 30 μm thick slices on a freezing microtome. Free floating slices were then processed with immunofluorescence for EYFP expression. After 1 h blocking with 5% normal donkey serum (NDS) in 0.25% Triton-X in KPBS (KPBS-T), the sections were incubated overnight in primary antibody chicken anti-GFP (*Abcam,* 1:100000) in 5% NDS in KPBS-T at room temperature. The sections were washed 3 times in KPBS-T and then incubated with DyLight 488-conjugated AffiniPure donkey anti-chicken (*Jackson ImmunoResearch Laboratories, Inc.*, 1:200) for 2 h at room temperature. After a final washing in KPBS the sections were mounted on gelatin-coated glass slides (Thermo Scientific) and cover-slipped with PVA-DABCO. The glasses were kept at 4°C in the dark till the acquisition of the images. GFP expression was visualized using a Nikon inverted confocal microscope with a 488 nm laser (*Coherent Sapphire).* Z-stacks images were acquired using a 4X (NA 0.13) objective and NIS Elements (Nikon) software.

Statistical Analyses

The data are presented as mean+SEM. Statistical analyses were performed using Prism 6. Statistical difference was considered at $p<0.05$. Normal distribution of the data was first verified using the Kolmogorov–Smirnov test. When normally distributed, the data were analyzed using one-way analysis of variance (ANOVA) followed by Tukey post hoc test. When not normally distributed, the data were analyzed using Kruskal–Wallis one-way analysis of variance followed by Dunn's post hoc test. Power analysis was performed using the program PS: Power and Sample Size Calculation version 3.0, 2009 (http://biostat.mc.vanderbilt.edu/wiki/Main/PowerSampleSize). Further details on statistical analyses are available in Statistical Results S1.

Results

No effect of inactivation of mutant HTT in SF1-expressing neurons on the metabolic phenotype of BACHD mice

To examine the role of SF1-expressing neurons in the development of metabolic and psychiatric impairments in HD, female SF1 mice were crossed with male BACHD mice to generate mice with a conditional deletion of mutant HTT from SF1-expressing neurons (Figure S1). We first verified the selective expression of Cre in SF1 neurons by crossing SF1 mice with ROSA-EYFP mice and assessed the degree of EYFP expression using immunofluorescence. We confirmed that EYFP-expressing neurons were localized in the VMH (Figure 1A). In addition, the region specificity of Cre recombination resulting in the excision of exon 1 of mutant HTT in BACHD-SF1 mice was validated with PCR analysis. Brain tissue from BACHD-SF1, BACHD, SF1 and WT mice showed the presence of the unrecombined mutant HTT allele (1050 bp) in the BACHD-SF1 and BACHD samples while the recombined mutant HTT allele (600 bp) was only detected in VMH brain samples from the BACHD-SF1 mice (Figure 1B).

The assessment of body weight at 4 months of age showed that female BACHD-SF1 and BACHD mice were significantly different to the two female control groups and that there was no difference between BACHD-SF1 and BACHD mice (Figure 2A). Male BACHD-SF1 and BACHD mice were also significantly different to their WT littermates and there was no difference between male BACHD-SF1 and BACHD mice (Figure 2B). Similarly to previously published data using BACHD mice with FVB/N background, in the current study the body weight gain in BACHD mice was detectable already at 2 months of age in both males and females (data not shown) [14]. Hence, the inactivation of mutant HTT in SF-1 neurons in the BACHD mice does not have an effect on body weight. The percentage body fat as measured by DEXA showed a corresponding increase in body fat in both female BACHD-SF1 and BACHD mice compared to the control groups, whereas there was no difference in body fat percentage in the male groups (Figure 2C and 2D).

To determine if the endocrine abnormalities previously reported in the BACHD mice would be affected by inactivation of mutant HTT in SF1 neurons, serum levels of the pancreatic hormone, insulin and the adipocyte hormone, leptin were measured. In females, insulin levels in BACHD-SF1 and BACHD mice were significantly elevated compared to WT and SF1 controls

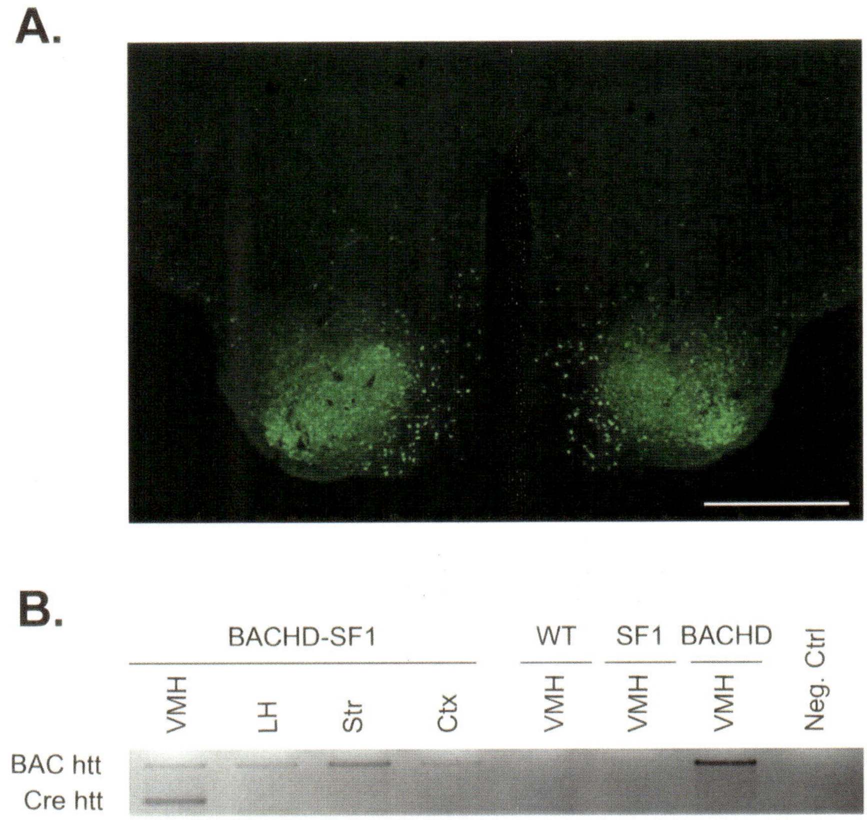

Figure 1. Validation of Cre-excision in SF1-expressing neurons in the VMH. A. SF1 mice were crossed with ROSA-EYFP mice and the expression in SF1 neurons was validated using GFP immunofluorescence. GFP immunoreactive cells were primarily clustered in the VMH. Scale bar represents 500 μm. B. Gel showing Cre recombination as validated by PCR of several brain regions from BACHD-SF1, BACHD, SF1 and WT mice. The presence of the unrecombined mutant HTT allele (1050 bp) was detected in all the BACHD-SF1 and BACHD samples while the recombined mutant HTT allele (600 bp) was only detected in VMH brain samples from the BACHD-SF1 mice.

(Figure 3A). In males, BACHD mice had significantly higher serum insulin levels compared to SF1 controls while insulin levels were not different between BACHD-SF1 and any other groups (Figure 3B). Leptin levels in both female and male mice were significantly higher in BACHD and BACHD-SF1 groups compared to WT and SF1 controls (Figure 3C and 3D). Taken together, the data indicate that inactivation of mutant HTT in SF1 neurons of the VMH has no effect on the metabolic phenotype as assessed by measurements of body weight, body fat and serum insulin and leptin levels in BACHD mice.

Effects of inactivation of mutant HTT in SF1-expressing neurons on the development of anxiety-like behavior in the BACHD mice

We were then interested in examining the effect of inactivation of mutant HTT in SF1 neurons for the development of anxiety-like behavior in the BACHD mouse model. BACHD mice have previously been reported to display anxiety-like behavior already at 2 months of age as assessed using the EPM [15]. However, in this experimental setup, we found no difference in the percentage of time spent on the open arms during the 5 min test period between the different genotypes across both sexes (Figure 4A and B). As anxiety-like behavior has been found previously in 2 month old BACHD mice, a post-hoc power calculation based on the data in the present study was made in order to determine the number of additional animals that would be required to show an increased anxiety-like behavior in the BACHD mice compared to WT mice. This calculation showed that 149 BACHD and 245 WT mice would be required in order to detect a true difference with a probability of 80% (power 0.8). Hence, the lack of anxiety-like behavior in the BACHD mice in this cohort is unlikely to be due to a low number of animals in the different groups.

We also used the NSFT to assess the effect on anxiety-like behavior. We found that female BACHD-SF1 mice had a decreased latency to eat in the novel environment compared to WT mice but there were no differences between BACHD and BACHD-SF1 mice (Figure 5A). In males, there were no differences in the latency to eat in the novel environment across the different genotypes (Figure 5B). As expected, the latency to eat in the home environment was similar across the different genotypes in both females and males (Figure 5C and D). Taken together, in this cohort of mice, we found no effect of the BACHD genotype on anxiety-like behavior and a potential effect of inactivation of mutant HTT in SF1 neurons is therefore difficult to determine.

Effects of inactivation of mutant HTT in SF1-expressing neurons on the development of depressive-like behavior in the BACHD mice

To assess the effect on depressive-like behavior in this study, mice were subjected to the FST. Consistent with previous reports of increased immobility in BACHD mice as an indication of depressive-like behavior [15,32,36], BACHD

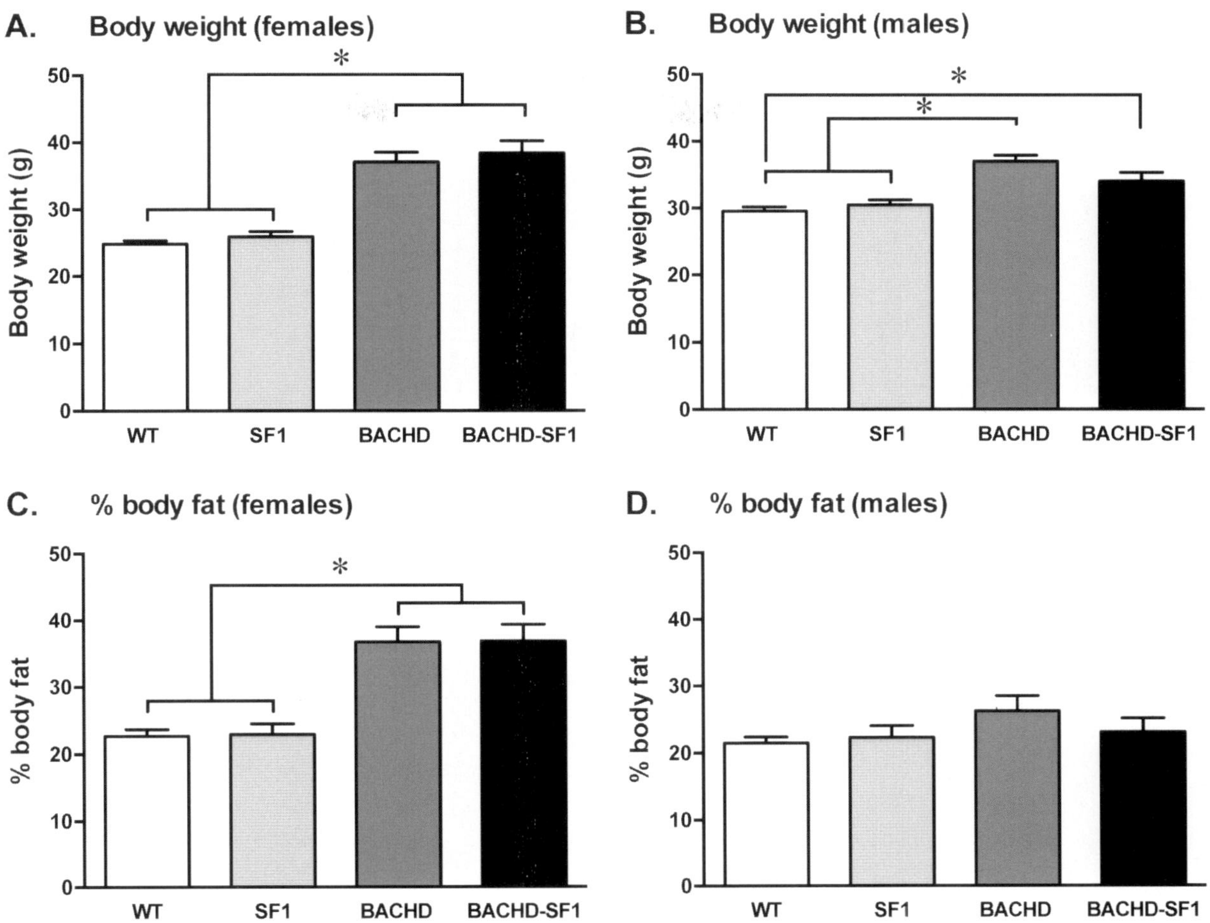

Figure 2. Increased body weight and body fat in 4 months old BACHD and BACHD-SF1 mice. A, B. Body weight were measured in (A) females and (B) males of each genotype. In females, the body weight of BACHD and BACHD-SF1 mice were significantly higher than WT and SF1 control mice. In males, the body weight of BACHD mice were significantly higher than WT and SF1 controls while the body weight of BACHD-SF1 mice were significantly higher than WT mice but not SF1 controls. C, D. The percentage of body fat, as determined by whole body dual energy x-ray absorptiometry (DEXA), revealed a corresponding increased body fat percentage in (C) female BACHD and BACHD-SF1 mice when compared to their WT and SF1 control counterparts but not in (D) males. Data presented as mean ± SEM (A–C, * $p<0.05$, one-way ANOVA with Tukey's multiple comparisons post-hoc test, D, Kruskal-Wallis non-parametric ANOVA with Dunn's multiple comparisons post-hoc test), n = 11–28/genotype/sex in each group. Detailed statistical analyses are outlined in Figure 2 of Statistical Results S1.

females exhibited a significant increase in the percentage of time spent immobile compared to WT and SF1 control littermates (Figure 6A; one-way ANOVA followed by post-hoc Tukey, $p = 0.0004$ BACHD vs WT, $p = 0.014$ BACHD vs SF1). There were no significant differences between BACHD-SF1 and BACHD mice, indicating that SF1 neurons alone are not sufficient for contributing to the depressive-like phenotype (one-way ANOVA, post-hoc Tukey, $p = 0.11$ BACHD vs BACHD-SF1). However, there were also no significant differences between BACHD-SF1 and the control groups. We therefore performed a power calculation to determine the additional number of animals required to prove a potential rescue of the depressive-like behavior and found that 27 BACHD and 27 BACHD-SF1 mice would be required to find a true difference between the two BACHD groups with a probability of 80% (power 0.8). In the present design, 17 female BACHD and 17 BACHD-SF1 mice were included. No differences were detected in the percentage of time spent immobile between the genotypes in males (Figure 6B). Our data suggests that inactivation of mutant HTT in SF1 neurons may have a partial effect on the development of depressive-like behavior in female BACHD mice.

No change in motor activity in mice after conditional deletion of mutant HTT from SF1-expressing neurons in BACHD mice

General locomotor activity was measured with the OF test. No significant differences were detected in the number of line crossings between BACHD-SF1, BACHD, SF1 and WT controls in both sexes, indicating an absence of motor dysfunction at this age in all groups (Figure 7A and B).

Discussion

Non-motor symptoms and signs are common in neurodegenerative HD. As they sometimes manifest before the motor dysfunction, their underlying biological mechanisms may be part of early steps in the pathogenesis of the disease. Identification of the neural substrates responsible for these aspects of the disease may therefore be important in the search for novel targets in the development of potential disease modifying treatments. The

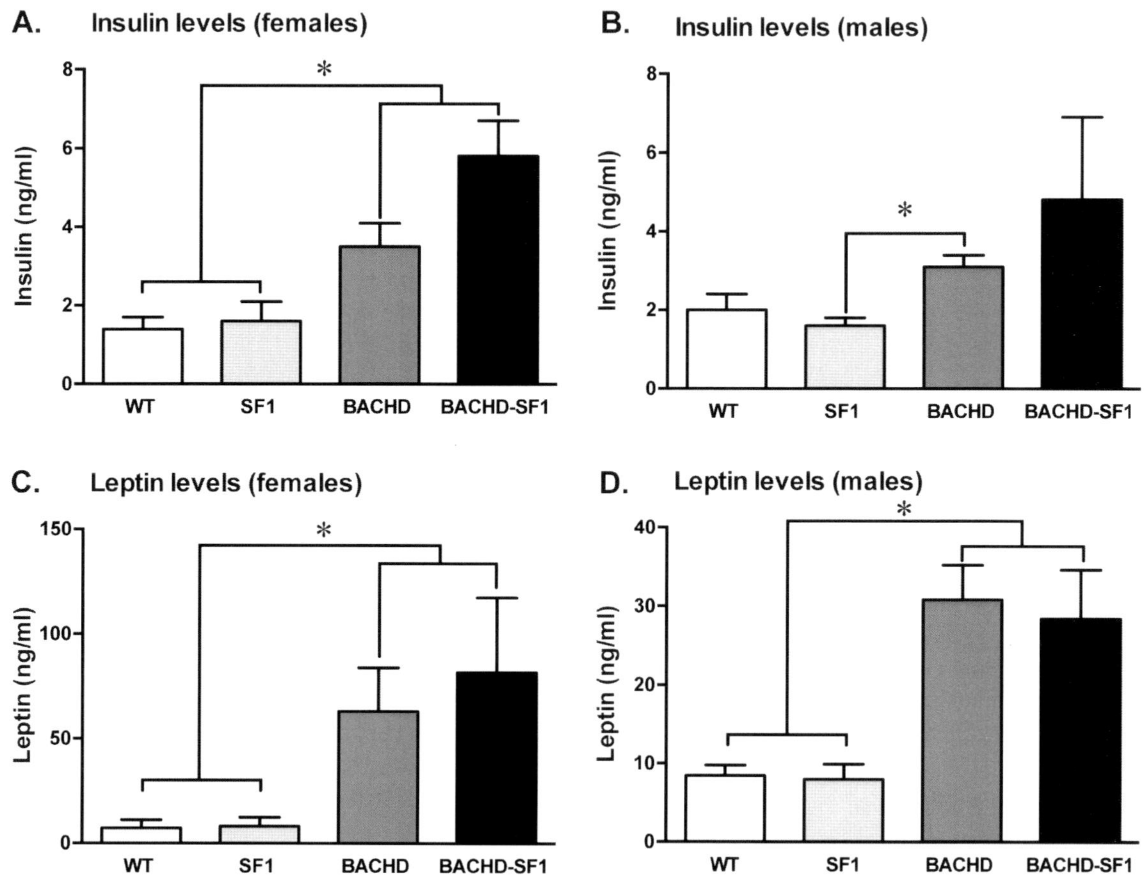

Figure 3. Alterations in serum insulin and leptin levels. A, B. Circulating insulin concentration was measured in blood samples from all genotypes at 4 months of age by ELISA. Serum insulin levels were significantly higher in BACHD and BACHD-SF1 females compared WT and SF1 controls while in males, only the BACHD group had significantly enhanced insulin concentration compared to SF1 controls. C, D. Serum leptin concentration as measured by ELISA was significantly higher in BACHD and BACHD-SF1 mice compared to WT and SF1 controls in both males and females. Data presented as mean ± SEM (A–B, * $p<0.05$, Kruskal-Wallis non-parametric ANOVA with Dunn's multiple comparisons post-hoc test, C–D, * $p<0.05$, one-way ANOVA with Tukey multiple comparisons post-hoc test), n = 11–28/genotype/sex in each group. Detailed statistical analyses are outlined in Figure 3 of Statistical Results S1.

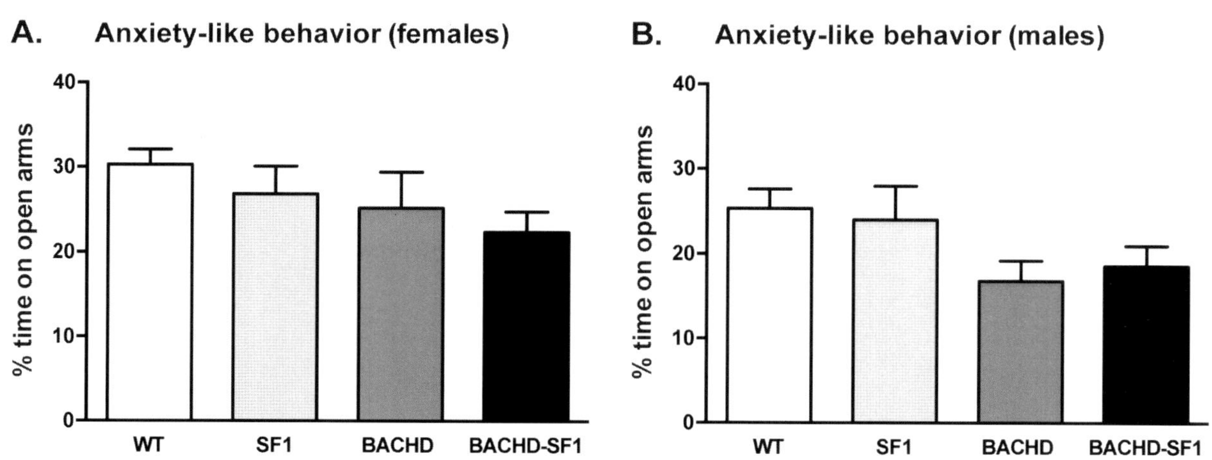

Figure 4. Analysis of anxiety-like behavior in BACHD-SF1 mice. Anxiety-like behavior was assessed using the elevated plus maze test and the percentage time spent on the open arms was recorded for (A) females and (B) males. There were no differences in the percentage time spent on the open arms in BACHD and BACHD-SF1 mice of both sexes compared to WT and SF1 controls. Data presented as mean ± SEM (A, Kruskal-Wallis non-parametric ANOVA with Dunn's multiple comparisons post-hoc test, $p>0.05$ WT vs BACHD, WT vs BACHD-SF1, $p>0.999$ WT vs SF1, SF1 vs BACHD, SF1 vs BACHD-SF1, BACHD vs BACHD-SF1, B, one-way ANOVA with Tukey multiple comparisons post-hoc test), n = 11–28/genotype/sex in each group. Detailed statistical analyses are outlined in Figure 4 of Statistical Results S1.

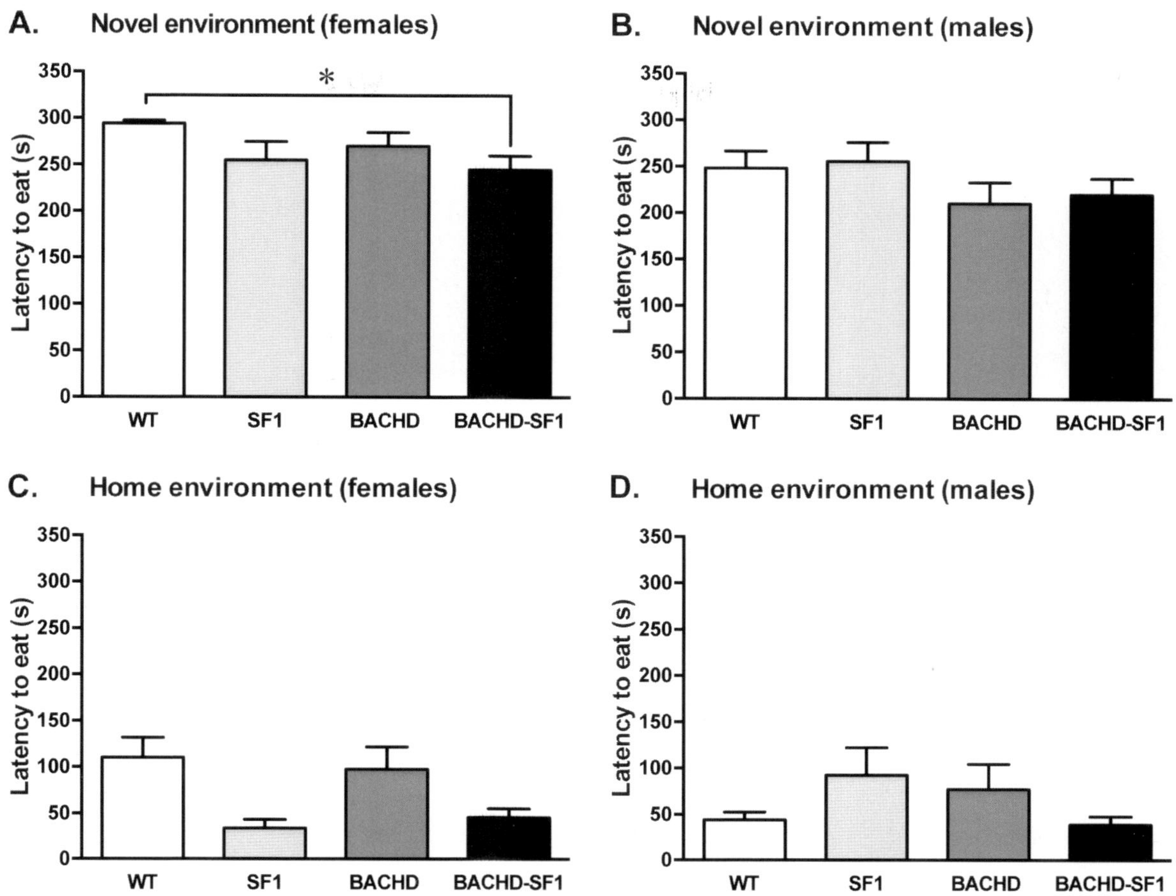

Figure 5. Latency to feed during the novelty-induced suppressed feeding test (NSFT). During the NSFT, the latency to feed in a novel environment as well as in the home cage was assessed. A, B. In females, BACHD-SF1 mice recorded a decreased latency to eat in the novel environment compared to WT controls but there were no differences in the male group across the genotypes. C, D. There were no differences in the latency to feed in the home environment in both sexes across the genotypes. Data presented as mean ± SEM (* $p<0.05$, Kruskal-Wallis non-parametric ANOVA with Dunn's multiple comparisons test), n = 11–28/genotype/sex in each group. Detailed statistical analyses are outlined in Figure 5 of Statistical Results S1.

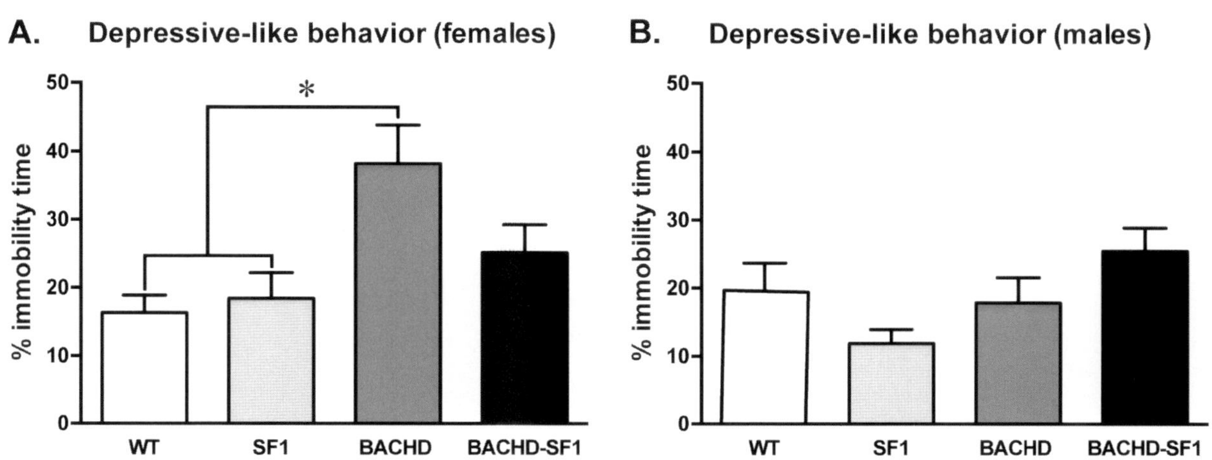

Figure 6. Evaluation of the depressive-like behaviors in BACHD-SF1 mice. Depressive-like behaviors were assessed using the forced swim test (FST) whereby the percentage of time spent immobile was recorded. A. In females, the percentage of time spent immobile was significantly higher in BACHD mice compared to the control groups whereas the result for BACHD-SF1 mice was not significant to any groups, suggesting a partial positive effect of inactivation of mutant HTT in SF1 neurons on this behavior. B. There were no differences in the percentage of time spent immobile across all genotypes in males. Data presented as mean ± SEM (* $p<0.05$, one-way ANOVA with Tukey multiple comparisons post-hoc test), n = 11–28/genotype/sex in each group. Detailed statistical analyses are outlined in Figure 6 of Statistical Results S1.

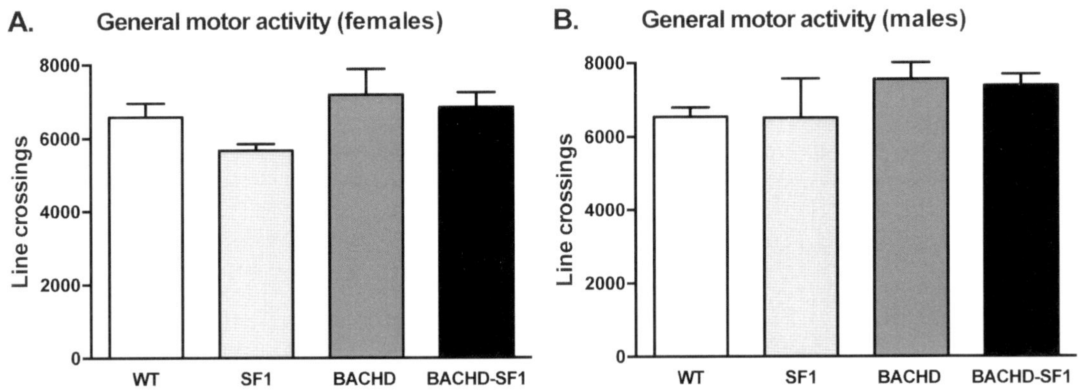

Figure 7. Assessment of motor activity in BACHD-SF1 mice. Motor activity was assessed using the open field test at 4 months of age. Mice were placed in the open field chamber for 1 hour and the total number of line crossings and line crossings in the center were recorded. There were no differences in the number of line crossings (A, B) and in the number of line crossings in the center (C, D) made by BACHD and BACHD-SF1 mice of both sexes compared to their respective WT comparisons. Data presented as mean ± SEM (Kruskal-Wallis non-parametric ANOVA with Dunn's multiple comparisons test), n = 11–28/genotype/sex in each group. Detailed statistical analyses are outlined in Figure 7 of Statistical Results S1.

hypothalamus is an area of the brain involved in the regulation of emotion, metabolism and sleep, functions that are part of non-motor spectra of HD [4]. Imaging studies based on PET and MRI have indeed implicated that the hypothalamus is affected early on in HD gene carriers [12,13]. Recent studies using experimental models of HD have established a link between expression of mutant HTT in the hypothalamus and the development of metabolic dysfunction as well as depressive-like behavior [14,15]. In the present study, we were interested in further dissecting out which specific hypothalamic nuclei/circuitry would be responsible for this effect. We therefore inactivated mutant HTT in SF1-expressing neurons in the VMH, which has been implicated in the regulation of metabolism and emotion [30,37,38]. However, deletion of mutant HTT from these neurons only had a partial positive effect on the depressive-like behavior in female BACHD mice and did not influence other behavioral or metabolic parameters. Hence, dysfunction of neural circuitries involving the VMH is unlikely to be important for the development of the non-motor phenotype in BACHD mice.

Although several models have been developed to study psychiatric disturbances in clinical HD, modelling the full spectrum of symptoms remains a challenge. Several HD mouse models have shown psychiatric abnormalities with the different behavioral tests, thus recapitulating some of the aspects of clinical HD [39,40]. The BACHD model has previously been shown to display depressive-like behavior in the FST as early as 2 months of age and independent of sex [15]. In this cohort of mice, we replicated this finding only in female BACHD mice. Clear sex differences in the psychiatric-like behavior in BACHD mice have not been reported previously but in other HD mouse models such as the R6/1 model, depressive-like behavior has been reported only in female mice [34,41,42]. One possible explanation for this discrepancy and a potential caveat of the study is that the mice used were on a mixed FVB/N and C57BL6/J background and it is well known that strain differences can have major effects on the phenotype in mice [43–45]. It is therefore possible that the depressive-like phenotype in BACHD mice is stronger in female compared to male mice, as it appears more resistant to this potential strain effect. Interestingly, although the FST result in female BACHD-SF1 mice was not different to BACHD mice, it was also no longer different to the result in the control groups, suggesting a partial positive effect of conditional deletion of mutant HTT from SF1-expressing neurons. We therefore performed a power calculation to determine how many additional mice in each group would have been necessary to see a significant difference between BACHD and BACHD-SF1 mice. We find that an additional 10 animals in the BACHD and BACHD-SF1 groups respectively would be required to prove that mutant HTT expression in SF1 neurons is necessary for the depressive-like phenotype with a probability of 80%. Although SF1 neurons and the wider VMH have been implicated in anxiety-like but not depressive-like behaviors [46], this finding suggests that the expression of mutant HTT in SF1 neurons may play a role for the development of the depressive-like phenotype. This is not surprising since the neurons of the VMH project to brain regions and other parts of the limbic system involved with anxiety and affective behaviors [47]. In addition, a recent clinical study from patients with SF1 (Nr5a1) gene mutations show psychiatric symptoms including excessive anxiety and/or depression [48], suggesting that SF1 and the VMH may have roles in both anxiety- and depressive-like behaviors. Nevertheless, we acknowledge that the power calculation is a mathematical estimation and further studies are warranted to determine if mutant HTT expression in SF1 neurons is important for the depressive-like behavior.

SF1-neurons in the VMH have been shown to regulate anxiety-like behaviors as well as genes mediating anxiety [23,46]. Studies with central nervous system-specific SF1 knockout mice displayed an altered expression of genes implicated in anxiety-behavior in the VMH including BDNF, Crhr2, and Ucn 3 [23]. We have demonstrated previously that the BACHD mouse model of HD on the FVB/N strain exhibit anxiety-like behavior already at 2 months of age using the EPM [15]. However, in the present study, we found no evidence for an anxiety-like phenotype in BACHD or BACHD-SF1 mice as assessed using both the EPM and NSFT. Power analysis of the results from the EPM revealed that a very large sample size would be required to substantiate an anxiety-like phenotype in BACHD mice in this cohort, mostly due to a large individual variation within the group. One possible explanation for this discrepancy is again that the mice used were on mixed FVB/N and C57BL6/J background. Several studies including our own have reported anxiety-like behaviors on transgenic models expressing the full-length mutant HTT on the FBV/N strain [15,36]. Phenotypic abnormalities have been associated with strain differences of the YAC128 mice [43], but precisely how these strain differences on a mixed background affect the development of the anxiety-like behaviors in BACHD mice remains unknown.

The VMH has long been regarded to be one of the critical hypothalamic nuclei responsible for the control of energy homeostasis [20,27,37]. Early lesion studies into the VMH described hyperphagic obesity and revealed the importance of this hypothalamic nucleus in regulating food and energy balance [49–51]. There is compelling evidence from studies using various full-length mutant HTT transgenic models such as BACHD and YAC128 demonstrating increased body weight and body fat which is thought to correspond to the increased leptin levels [16,31,52]. Several mechanisms underlying this phenotype have been proposed. Overexpression of the HTT protein independent of the mutation has been suggested as one possibility [52]. However, our previous work have demonstrated that inactivation of mutant HTT in hypothalamic neurons alone prevented the development of the metabolic phenotype of BACHD mice [14]. In undertaking the present study, we sought to determine if the conditional deletion of mutant HTT in SF1-expressing neurons during embryonic development might rescue the metabolic phenotype. However, we found no evidence that mutant HTT expression in SF1 neurons is critical for regulating the increased body weight phenotype or elevated leptin and insulin levels, suggesting that the metabolic phenotype is not attributed to mutant HTT expression in SF1 neurons. Concomitantly, we found that the increased body weight corresponded to a similar increase in body fat assessed in females but not in males. The reason for this discrepancy is unclear since leptin levels remain elevated in BACHD and BACHD-SF1 males. A possible explanation could be the high variability within the group associated with the animals having ad libitum access to food and water. This issue with high group variation can be rectified in future studies by fasting animals prior to blood collection for insulin and leptin measurements.

In conclusion, we find little support for the notion that mutant HTT expression in VMH SF1 neurons is responsible for the development of the psychiatric and metabolic impairments in BACHD mice. However, the deletion of mutant HTT from SF1-expressing neurons occurred from birth and the lack of an effect on the behavioral phenotype may reflect compensatory mechanisms proceeding from the time of mutant HTT deletion during embryonic development. It is possible that the adaptive response in the brain that occurs during embryonic development could lead to the formation of a compensatory circuitry. The degree to which this happens remains unclear. Also, taking into account that the VMH is a heterogeneous nucleus made up of anatomically distinct sub-nuclei and the fact that SF1 itself is not expressed throughout the entire VMH [24,25], the metabolic and psychiatric impairments could however be mediated by non-SF1 neurons also located in the VMH. Further studies using viral vector injections carrying Cre into the VMH in adult mice and/or using SF1 mini promoters may be necessary to determine if the VMH and SF1 neurons are critical for the development of the psychiatric and metabolic impairments in HD without the potential confound from compensatory mechanisms. Overall, these aspects emphasize the complexity of the hypothalamic neuronal system and suggest that it is perhaps too simplistic to consider whole populations of hypothalamic neurons separately in investigations aiming at determining the underlying neural mechanisms of the non-motor aspects of HD.

Supporting Information

Figure S1 Generation of BACHD-SF1 mouse line. Male BACHD mice, expressing human full-length HTT with 97 polyQ and floxed exon1 (Ex1-97Q) were crossed with female mice expressing Cre under the SF1 promoter (SF1). As a result of the crossing four genotypes were obtained: WT animals expressing mouse endogenous WT HTT, SF1 animals expressing Cre, BACHD mice expressing human full-length mutant HTT with 97 polyQ and BACHD-SF1 animals expressing Cre and mutant HTT. In the BACHD-SF1 animals, the presence of Cre induces the recombination of the floxed gene resulting in a conditional deletion of mutant HTT in the SF1 neurons.

Statistical Results S1.

Acknowledgments

We are grateful for the technical assistance provided by Björn Anzelius, Anneli Josefsson, Ulla Samuelsson and Ulrika Sparrhult-Björk at Lund University.

Author Contributions

Conceived and designed the experiments: BB RYC ÅP. Performed the experiments: BB RYC. Analyzed the data: BB RYC. Contributed to the writing of the manuscript: BB RYC ÅP.

References

1. The Huntington's Disease Collaborative Research Group (1993) A novel gene containing a trinucleotide repeat that is expanded and unstable on Huntington's disease chromosomes. Cell 72: 971–983.
2. Ross CA, Aylward EH, Wild EJ, Langbehn DR, Long JD, et al. (2014) Huntington disease: natural history, biomarkers and prospects for therapeutics. Nat Rev Neurol 10: 204–216.
3. Sturrock A, Leavitt BR (2010) The clinical and genetic features of Huntington disease. J Geriatr Psychiatry Neurol 23: 243–259.
4. Petersen A, Gabery S (2012) Hypothalamic and limbic system changes in Huntington's disease. Journal of Huntington's disease 1: 5–16.
5. de la Monte SM, Vonsattel JP, Richardson EP Jr (1988) Morphometric demonstration of atrophic changes in the cerebral cortex, white matter, and neostriatum in Huntington's disease. J Neuropathol Exp Neurol 47: 516–525.
6. Graveland GA, Williams RS, DiFiglia M (1985) Evidence for degenerative and regenerative changes in neostriatal spiny neurons in Huntington's disease. Science 227: 770–773.
7. Swaab DF (2004) Neuropeptides in hypothalamic neuronal disorders. Int Rev Cytol 240: 305–375.
8. Gabery S, Murphy K, Schultz K, Loy CT, McCusker E, et al. (2010) Changes in key hypothalamic neuropeptide populations in Huntington disease revealed by neuropathological analyses. Acta neuropathologica 120: 777–788.
9. Aziz A, Fronczek R, Maat-Schieman M, Unmehopa U, Roelandse F, et al. (2008) Hypocretin and melanin-concentrating hormone in patients with Huntington disease. Brain pathology 18: 474–483.
10. Timmers HJ, Swaab DF, van de Nes JA, Kremer HP (1996) Somatostatin 1–12 immunoreactivity is decreased in the hypothalamic lateral tuberal nucleus of Huntington's disease patients. Brain research 728: 141–148.
11. Petersen A, Gil J, Maat-Schieman ML, Bjorkqvist M, Tanila H, et al. (2005) Orexin loss in Huntington's disease. Human molecular genetics 14: 39–47.
12. Soneson C, Fontes M, Zhou Y, Denisov V, Paulsen JS, et al. (2010) Early changes in the hypothalamic region in prodromal Huntington disease revealed by MRI analysis. Neurobiology of disease 40: 531–543.
13. Politis M, Pavese N, Tai YF, Tabrizi SJ, Barker RA, et al. (2008) Hypothalamic involvement in Huntington's disease: an in vivo PET study. Brain : a journal of neurology 131: 2860–2869.
14. Hult S, Soylu R, Bjorklund T, Belgardt BF, Mauer J, et al. (2011) Mutant huntingtin causes metabolic imbalance by disruption of hypothalamic neurocircuits. Cell metabolism 13: 428–439.
15. Hult Lundh S, Nilsson N, Soylu R, Kirik D, Petersen A (2013) Hypothalamic expression of mutant huntingtin contributes to the development of depressive-like behavior in the BAC transgenic mouse model of Huntington's disease. Hum Mol Genet 22: 3485–3497.
16. Gray M, Shirasaki DI, Cepeda C, Andre VM, Wilburn B, et al. (2008) Full-length human mutant huntingtin with a stable polyglutamine repeat can elicit progressive and selective neuropathogenesis in BACHD mice. J Neurosci 28: 6182–6195.

17. Abada YS, Schreiber R, Ellenbroek B (2013) Motor, emotional and cognitive deficits in adult BACHD mice: a model for Huntington's disease. Behav Brain Res 238: 243–251.
18. Lundh SH, Soylu R, Petersen A (2012) Expression of mutant huntingtin in leptin receptor-expressing neurons does not control the metabolic and psychiatric phenotype of the BACHD mouse. PloS one 7: e51168.
19. Myers MG Jr, Olson DP (2012) Central nervous system control of metabolism. Nature 491: 357–363.
20. Bingham NC, Anderson KK, Reuter AL, Stallings NR, Parker KL (2008) Selective loss of leptin receptors in the ventromedial hypothalamic nucleus results in increased adiposity and a metabolic syndrome. Endocrinology 149: 2138–2148.
21. Budefeld T, Tobet SA, Majdic G (2012) Steroidogenic factor 1 and the central nervous system. J Neuroendocrinol 24: 225–235.
22. Ikeda Y, Takeda Y, Shikayama T, Mukai T, Hisano S, et al. (2001) Comparative localization of Dax-1 and Ad4BP/SF-1 during development of the hypothalamic-pituitary-gonadal axis suggests their closely related and distinct functions. Dev Dyn 220: 363–376.
23. Zhao L, Kim KW, Ikeda Y, Anderson KK, Beck L, et al. (2008) Central nervous system-specific knockout of steroidogenic factor 1 results in increased anxiety-like behavior. Mol Endocrinol 22: 1403–1415.
24. McClellan KM, Parker KL, Tobet S (2006) Development of the ventromedial nucleus of the hypothalamus. Front Neuroendocrinol 27: 193–209.
25. Cheung CC, Kurrasch DM, Liang JK, Ingraham HA (2013) Genetic labeling of steroidogenic factor-1 (SF-1) neurons in mice reveals ventromedial nucleus of the hypothalamus (VMH) circuitry beginning at neurogenesis and development of a separate non-SF-1 neuronal cluster in the ventrolateral VMH. J Comp Neurol 521: 1268–1288.
26. Ikeda Y, Luo X, Abbud R, Nilson JH, Parker KL (1995) The nuclear receptor steroidogenic factor 1 is essential for the formation of the ventromedial hypothalamic nucleus. Mol Endocrinol 9: 478–486.
27. Dhillon H, Zigman JM, Ye C, Lee CE, McGovern RA, et al. (2006) Leptin directly activates SF1 neurons in the VMH, and this action by leptin is required for normal body-weight homeostasis. Neuron 49: 191–203.
28. Kim KW, Zhao L, Donato J Jr, Kohno D, Xu Y, et al. (2011) Steroidogenic factor 1 directs programs regulating diet-induced thermogenesis and leptin action in the ventral medial hypothalamic nucleus. Proc Natl Acad Sci U S A 108: 10673–10678.
29. Kim KW, Jo YH, Zhao L, Stallings NR, Chua SC Jr, et al. (2008) Steroidogenic factor 1 regulates expression of the cannabinoid receptor 1 in the ventromedial hypothalamic nucleus. Mol Endocrinol 22: 1950–1961.
30. Choi YH, Fujikawa T, Lee J, Reuter A, Kim KW (2013) Revisiting the Ventral Medial Nucleus of the Hypothalamus: The Roles of SF-1 Neurons in Energy Homeostasis. Front Neurosci 7: 71.
31. Pouladi MA, Xie Y, Skotte NH, Ehrnhoefer DE, Graham RK, et al. (2010) Full-length huntingtin levels modulate body weight by influencing insulin-like growth factor 1 expression. Hum Mol Genet 19: 1528–1538.
32. Wang N, Gray M, Lu XH, Cantle JP, Holley SM, et al. (2014) Neuronal targets for reducing mutant huntingtin expression to ameliorate disease in a mouse model of Huntington's disease. Nat Med 20: 536–541.
33. Walf AA, Frye CA (2007) The use of the elevated plus maze as an assay of anxiety-related behavior in rodents. Nat Protoc 2: 322–328.
34. Renoir T, Pang TY, Mo C, Chan G, Chevarin C, et al. (2013) Differential effects of early environmental enrichment on emotionality related behaviours in Huntington's disease transgenic mice. J Physiol 591: 41–55.
35. Porsolt RD, Bertin A, Jalfre M (1977) Behavioral despair in mice: a primary screening test for antidepressants. Arch Int Pharmacodyn Ther 229: 327–336.
36. Pouladi MA, Stanek LM, Xie Y, Franciosi S, Southwell AL, et al. (2012) Marked differences in neurochemistry and aggregates despite similar behavioural and neuropathological features of Huntington disease in the full-length BACHD and YAC128 mice. Hum Mol Genet 21: 2219–2232.
37. Parker KL, Rice DA, Lala DS, Ikeda Y, Luo X, et al. (2002) Steroidogenic factor 1: an essential mediator of endocrine development. Recent Prog Horm Res 57: 19–36.
38. Kim KW, Sohn JW, Kohno D, Xu Y, Williams K, et al. (2011) SF-1 in the ventral medial hypothalamic nucleus: a key regulator of homeostasis. Mol Cell Endocrinol 336: 219–223.
39. Pla P, Orvoen S, Saudou F, David DJ, Humbert S (2014) Mood disorders in Huntington's disease: from behavior to cellular and molecular mechanisms. Front Behav Neurosci 8: 135.
40. Pouladi MA, Morton AJ, Hayden MR (2013) Choosing an animal model for the study of Huntington's disease. Nat Rev Neurosci 14: 708–721.
41. Du X, Pang TY, Hannan AJ (2013) A Tale of Two Maladies? Pathogenesis of Depression with and without the Huntington's Disease Gene Mutation. Front Neurol 4: 81.
42. Pang TY, Du X, Zajac MS, Howard ML, Hannan AJ (2009) Altered serotonin receptor expression is associated with depression-related behavior in the R6/1 transgenic mouse model of Huntington's disease. Hum Mol Genet 18: 753–766.
43. Van Raamsdonk JM, Metzler M, Slow E, Pearson J, Schwab C, et al. (2007) Phenotypic abnormalities in the YAC128 mouse model of Huntington disease are penetrant on multiple genetic backgrounds and modulated by strain. Neurobiol Dis 26: 189–200.
44. Lloret A, Dragileva E, Teed A, Espinola J, Fossale E, et al. (2006) Genetic background modifies nuclear mutant huntingtin accumulation and HD CAG repeat instability in Huntington's disease knock-in mice. Hum Mol Genet 15: 2015–2024.
45. Menalled L, El-Khodor BF, Patry M, Suarez-Farinas M, Orenstein SJ, et al. (2009) Systematic behavioral evaluation of Huntington's disease transgenic and knock-in mouse models. Neurobiol Dis 35: 319–336.
46. Bueno CH, Zangrossi H Jr, Viana Mde B (2007) GABA/benzodiazepine receptors in the ventromedial hypothalamic nucleus regulate both anxiety and panic-related defensive responses in the elevated T-maze. Brain Res Bull 74: 134–141.
47. Canteras NS, Simerly RB, Swanson LW (1994) Organization of projections from the ventromedial nucleus of the hypothalamus: a Phaseolus vulgaris-leucoagglutinin study in the rat. J Comp Neurol 348: 41–79.
48. Suwanai AS, Ishii T, Haruna H, Yamataka A, Narumi S, et al. (2013) A report of two novel NR5A1 mutation families: possible clinical phenotype of psychiatric symptoms of anxiety and/or depression. Clin Endocrinol (Oxf) 78: 957–965.
49. Hetherington AW, Ranson SW (1940) Hypothalamic lesions and adiposity in the rat. Anat Rec 78: 149–172.
50. Sakaguchi T, Arase K, Bray GA (1988) Sympathetic activity and food intake of rats with ventromedial hypothalamic lesions. Int J Obes 12: 285–291.
51. Rabin BM (1974) Independence of food intake and obesity following ventromedial hypothalamic lesions in the rat. Physiol Behav 13: 769–772.
52. Van Raamsdonk JM, Gibson WT, Pearson J, Murphy Z, Lu G, et al. (2006) Body weight is modulated by levels of full-length huntingtin. Hum Mol Genet 15: 1513–1523.

18

Outcome of Assisted Reproductive Technology (ART) and Subsequent Self-Reported Life Satisfaction

Paula Kuivasaari-Pirinen[1,2]*, Heli Koivumaa-Honkanen[2,3,4,5,6,7,8,9,10], Maritta Hippeläinen[1,2], Kaisa Raatikainen[1,2], Seppo Heinonen[1,2]

1 Department of Obstetrics and Gynaecology, Kuopio University Hospital, Kuopio, Finland, **2** Institute of Clinical Medicine, University of Eastern Finland, Kuopio, Finland, **3** Clinic of Child Psychiatry, Oulu University Hospital, Oulu, Finland, **4** Department of Psychiatry, Kuopio University Hospital, Kuopio, Finland, **5** Department of Psychiatry, South-Savonia Hospital District, Mikkeli, Finland, **6** Department of Psychiatry, North Karelia Central Hospital, Joensuu, Finland, **7** Department of Psychiatry, SOSTERI, Savonlinna, Finland, **8** Department of Psychiatry, SOTE, Iisalmi, Finland, **9** Department of Psychiatry, Lapland Hospital District, Rovaniemi, Finland, **10** Department of Psychiatry, Institute of Clinical Medicine, University of Oulu, Oulu, Finland

Abstract

Objective: To compare life satisfaction between women with successful or unsuccessful outcome after assisted reproductive treatment (ART) by taking into account the time since the last ART.

Design: Cohort study.

Setting: Tertiary hospital.

Patients: A total of 987 consecutive women who had undergone ART during 1996–2007 were invited and altogether 505 women participated in the study.

Interventions: A postal enquiry with a life satisfaction scale.

Main Outcome Measure: Self-reported life satisfaction in respect to the time since the last ART.

Results: In general, women who achieved a live birth after ART had a significantly higher life satisfaction than those who had unsuccessful ART, especially when compared in the first three years. The difference disappeared in the time period of 6–9 years after ART. The unsuccessfully treated women who had a child by some other means before or after the unsuccessful ART had comparable life satisfaction with successfully treated women even earlier.

Conclusions: Even if unsuccessful ART outcome is associated with subsequent lower level of life satisfaction, it does not seem to threaten the long-term wellbeing.

Editor: James Coyne, University of Pennsylvania, United States of America

Funding: This study was funded by EVO National research funding from Kuopio University Hospital (www.kuh.fi), Finnish Cultural Foundation (www.skr.fi), North Savo Regional fund and The Finnish Society of Obstetrics and Gynaecology (www.gynekologiyhdistys.fi). The funders had no role in study design, data collection and analysis, decision to publish, or preparation of the manuscript.

Competing Interests: The authors have declared that no competing interests exist.

* Email: paula.kuivasaari-pirinen@fimnet.fi

Introduction

Involuntary childlessness is regarded as a major life crisis. The prevalence of infertility has been estimated to range from 417% [1]. In Finland it has been reported to affect one out of five women of childbearing age and over half of them seem to have sought medical help for it [2]. Nevertheless, about 3050% of couples who underwent assisted reproductive technologies (ART) such as in vitro fertilization (IVF) and intra cytoplasmic sperm injection (ICSI) remain childless [3].

The inability to conceive may cause successive disappointments to the couple [4]. Two out of every three women have been reported to remember the time period of infertility as one of the worst and most stressful experiences in their life [5]. Two comprehensive literature reviews on infertility specific distress stated that infertility is associated with distress, which is reflected by higher levels of depression and anxiety among infertile women than fertile counterparts, but still the overall clinical importance is limited in the spectrum of psychiatric disorders [6–7]. Infertility experience is stronger among women than among men and it varies a lot around the world [6–7].

In general, IVF/ICSI treatments are loaded with lots of expectations. Even if the couple may try to be realistic in relation to the treatment, optimism is prone to rise during the ART. Often emotions swing from hopefulness and enthusiasm to sorrow and frustration. High levels of anxiety and depression including suicidal thoughts have been reported to be linked with unsuccessful ART [8–10]. Furthermore, the risk of hospitalizations for psychiatric reasons is higher among unsuccessfully treated women than among those with successful ART [11]. Involuntary childlessness might also lead to other adverse outcomes such as isolation and social estrangement [12]. Infertile couple may avoid social life with families with children to protect the couple from facing uncomfortable situations. Due to differences in the social stigma caused by infertility in different cultures the degree of isolation may vary substantially [7]. Thus, infertility and failure in ART is a matter of quality of life [13] and life satisfaction [14], [15]. For example, Hammaberg et al. have reported that women with unsuccessful infertility treatments have significantly lower life satisfaction [16]. A study from Norway found that 19% of childless infertile women were dissatisfied with their life compared with 14% of fertile women with a child [17]. However, a systematic review of Verhaak et al. (2007) found that most women adjust well to unsuccessful IVF-treatments even if a significant proportion of women suffer from several adverse consequences [18]. So far there is little evidence on how long it takes to adjust to infertility. For example, it has been shown that three years since an unsuccessful IVF, most women still had the grief process unresolved [9]. Furthermore, women who had had unsuccessful ART 5 years earlier and were childless suffered from lower general wellbeing than women with successful ART outcome [19]. Instead, 10 years after infertility treatments the quality of life seems to be comparable in childless women and those who succeeded in the treatments [20].

Subjective wellbeing - indicated by life satisfaction and happiness - is one of the main dimensions of mental health [21]. It can be affected by achievement of one's life goals and personal ability to adjust to a major life setback, e.g. involuntary childlessness. Like in any medical treatment, one of the main goals of infertility treatment is not only to improve somatic outcomes, but also to produce subjective wellbeing. In the management of infertility, it is to help the couple to achieve a resolution to the crisis of childlessness, regardless whether a live birth is achieved or not. Thus, support and improvement of adjustment to childlessness are important in counselling.

The present study was undertaken to compare life satisfaction between women with a live birth after ART and women with unsuccessful ART by taking into account the time since the ART.

Methods

Ethics Statement

The study was approved by the Ethics Committee of Kuopio University Hospital. Written informed consent was given by participants for their clinical data to be used in the study and data of non-responding women were not analyzed, except live birth rate information was obtained anonymously from The Finnish Medical Birth Register.

Study participants

A total of 987 consecutive women underwent an in vitro fertilization (IVF) or intra cytoplasmic sperm injection (ICSI) treatment in Kuopio University Hospital between October 1996 and February 2007. All of them were sent a postal questionnaire in June 2008 with an invitation to the study, a written informed consent and an information sheet on opportunities for professional help if needed due to infertility-related problems. In addition to the questionnaire, data on their IVF/ICSI-treatment (details of ART, i.e. number of treatment cycles, transferred fresh and frozen embryos, outcome of treatments, time of the last ART), women's body mass index and age of the couple were collected from The Fertility Register of the infertility unit in Kuopio University Hospital. The Finnish Medical Birth Register provided a live birth rate of the non-responding women and this information was anonymous.

Altogether, 540 women participated in the study. Consequently, the response rate was 54.7% after one reminder letter. Of these women, 35 had visited private fertility clinics after receiving ART in Kuopio University Hospital. They were excluded due to the inability to obtain detailed information on their treatment in the private sector. This study did not examine the reasons of the clientele to visit private clinics but the most common reasons were that they already have had the maximum number of three publicly funded IVF treatments or that they required a more flexible schedule.

In Finland, ART is offered by both the public and private sectors. ART in public health care is available only to couples who have no more than one common child. The strict age limit is not determined but usually women aged over 40 years are not treated in the public health care, unless the possibility to have success in ART is estimated to be better than 10% (for example sufficient antral follicle count). Principally, the maximum number of IVF treatments is three, and extra stimulation cycles are possible if the next treatment is evaluated to be worthwhile, due to, for instance, miscarriage in the previous cycle. The cost of medications is publicly reimbursed so that a patient has to pay only up to a maximum of about 700€/year.

The questionnaire

The postal questionnaire included several questions about ART (treatment before and during ART, outcome and cessation), couple's decisions after ART, psychosocial support and a four-item life satisfaction scale (LS). The latter has a strong association ($r = 0.6–0.8$) with the 21-item Beck Depression Inventory (BDI) [22], but unlike depression scales it evaluates also the positive pole of mental health, i.e. subjective well-being. Previous studies on LS have proved parallel findings or a statistical significant relationship with other well-established measures such as General Health Questionnaire GHQ-20 and GHQ-12 [23], [24]. LS has been modified from quality of life studies [25–27] and used to measure life satisfaction of the general as well as psychiatric populations [28–30]. Previous studies have documented its usability to predict long-term mortality, morbidity and health habits in the general population [31–35] as well its associations in patient populations with health-related quality of life [36], health habits [24], [37], psychiatric [31] and surgical recovery processes [38] indicated by several well known and widely used scales.

The four items of the LS are following: Do you feel that your life at present is a) very **interesting** (1), fairly interesting (2), fairly boring (4) or very boring (5)? b) very **happy** (1), fairly happy (2), fairly sad (4) or very sad (5)? c) very **easy** (1), fairly easy (2), fairly hard (4) or very hard (5)? d) Do you feel that at the present moment you are very **lonely** (5), fairly lonely (4) or not at all lonely (1)? The scores are presented in the parenthesis. The response "cannot say" or omitting an item is scored as 3. If three or all four questions were omitted, the score was recorded as a missing data. Thus, the total LS score ranges from 4 to 20. As in previous studies the total score was divided to three categories based on the distribution in a general population; the score 4–6 indicated satisfaction, 12–20 dissatisfaction and the intermediate group (LS 7–11) consisted of those subjects within one standard deviation from the mean [25]. All questions were answered by

Table 1. Characteristics of study subjects and the treatments by ART outcome.

Characteristics	Successful ART n = 296	Unsuccessful ART n = 209	*P*-value
Mean age (years ±SD)	31.0±4.3	31.8±4.8	0.045
BMI (kg/m^2)	23.6±4.0	24.8±4.9	0.004
Smoking, daily [n (%)]	32 (10.8)	28 (13.4)	NS
Occupation during ART [n (%)]			
Employed	269 (90.9)	192 (91.9)	NS
Unemployed	9 (3.0)	8 (3.8)	NS
Student or other	18 (6.1)	9 (4.3)	NS
Educational level* [n (%)]			
Basic	20 (6.8)	12 (5.7)	NS
Upper secondary	50 (16.9)	32 (15.3)	NS
Tertiary	226 (76.4)	165 (78.9)	NS
Pregnancies before ART [n (%)]	86 (29.1)	73 (34.9)	NS
Biological child before ART [n (%)]	46 (15.5)	39 (18.7)	NS
Indication of ART [n (%)]			
Female factor	115 (38.9)	87 (41.0)	NS
Endometriosis	59 (19.9)	52 (24.9)	NS
Tubal factor	34 (11.5)	17 (8.1)	NS
Uterine factor	0	6 (2.9)	0.003
Anovulation	22 (7.4)	8 (3.8)	NS
PCOS	21 (7.1)	11 (5.3)	NS
Not specified	16 (5.4)	10 (4.8)	NS
Male factor	43 (14.5)	19 (9.1)	NS
Combined factor	37 (12.5)	17 (8.1)	NS
Unexplained	101 (34.2)	86 (41.1)	NS
Duration of infertility (y ± SD)	3.4±2.2	3.5±2.4	NS
Numbers of (mean ± SD)			
Oocyte retrievals	2.1±1.2	2.5±1.3	0.001
Fresh embryo transfers	2.0±1.1	2.4±1.3	0.001
Frozen embryo transfers	1.6±0.9	1.9±1.3	0.045
Miscarriage or ectopic pregnancy [n (%)]	41 (13.9)	59 (28.2)	0.0001
Time from the last ART (y ± SD)	5.6±3.2	5.5±3.4	NS

ART = assisted reproductive technology.
*In the general Finnish women aged 25–44 years, 11.3% had basic education (i.e. Comprehensive school), 39.9% upper secondary education and 48.8% tertiary level education.

98.4% and at least two questions by 99.4% of responders. Thus, only three subjects (0.6%) were excluded due to incomplete response to LS.

Statistical analyses

The comparison of the two groups, i.e. the women who had a live birth as a result of ART and those who had unsuccessful outcome, was performed using SPSS version 17.0 (SPSS Inc., Chicago, IL, USA). When time was taken into consideration, the comparisons were conducted between three groups: i) women with a live birth after ART, ii) women with unsuccessful ART but with a biological child either before or after ART, and iii) childless women with unsuccessful ART. The statistical significance of continuous variables was analysed using a two-tailed pooled t tests, and Mann-Whitney U-test when appropriate, and displayed as mean ± standard deviation (SD). Frequencies were compared by the χ^2-test or by Fisher's exact test, as appropriate. A value of $p < 0.05$ was considered statistically significant. The risk ratios for being satisfied (LS 4–6) were calculated by using unadjusted relative risk ratios comparing successfully treated women with unsuccessfully treated women with or without children.

Results

Background

The final study group (n = 505) consisted of 296 women with successful and 209 women with unsuccessful ART. Their background data were comparable, with the exception that the latter group was somewhat older and had a slightly higher body mass index (Table 1). The mean age (33.4±5.9 vs. 34.1±5.9) of spouses and their current smoking (28.0% vs. 30.6%) were also similar in these two groups.

Table 2. Life satisfaction by ART outcome and offspring status.

	Successful ART	Unsuccessful ART					
	ALL	ALL	*P*-value	CHILD+	*P*-value	CHILD–	*P*-value
	n = 296	n = 209		n = 78		n = 131	
Life satisfaction score							
(range 4–20)							
mean LS ± SD	6.8±2.4	7.6±3.0	0.003	7.3±2.9	NS	7.7±3.1	0.003
Satisfied, n (%)	154 (52.0)	91 (43.5)	NS	37 (47.4)	NS	54 (41.2)	0.04
(score 4–6)							
Intermediate, n (%)	125 (42.2)	92 (44.0)	NS	34 (43.6)	NS	58 (44.3)	NS
(score 7–11)							
Dissatisfied, n (%)	17 (5.7)	26 (12.4)	0.008	7 (9.0)	NS	19 (14.5)	0.003
(score 12–20)							

ART = assisted reproductive technology.
CHILD +/– = women with/without a biological child.
Successfully treated women displayed as a control group.

Indications for the ART were similar in both ART outcome groups (Table 1). If one includes frozen embryo transfers, 55.0% of women had 1–2 transfers, and 40.6% had three or more transfers. The rest of the women had undergone oocyte retrieval without a transfer due to an unsuccessful stimulation. The time since the last ART ranged between 1.3 and 11.7 years (mean: 5.6 y; median: 5.2 y).

Women with unsuccessful ART had had significantly more miscarriages, ectopic pregnancies and ART trials than those with successful ART (Table 1). Duration of infertility, time since last ART and indications for the ART were similar in these two ART outcome groups (Table 1). However, no cases with uterine factor as an indication for ART were found among women with successful ART compared to six cases among women with unsuccessful ART.

In the successful ART group 46 women had a biological child before the treatment. In the unsuccessful ART group, as many as 78 women (37.3%; 78/209) had a biological child either before (n = 39, 18.7%) or after the treatment (n = 47, 22.5%) with altogether eight of women having a child both before and after an unsuccessful treatment.

ART outcome and life satisfaction

Women with successful ART were significantly more satisfied with their lives in 2008 than the women with unsuccessful ART (mean LS 6.8±2.4 vs. 7.6±3.0, p = 0.003), this was also seen in the proportion of dissatisfied women in these two groups (Table 2). In the intermediate category, instead, there were no differences between the groups. When women with unsuccessful treatment were categorized into two groups according their motherhood status (without a child or with a child without ART either before or after unsuccessful ART treatment), there were no differences when the latter group was compared to the women with successful ART.

When the time since last ART was taken into account, the relationship between LS-score and outcome of ART displayed more variation (Table 3 and Fig. 1). If less than three years have gone after the ART, women with unsuccessful ART with or without a biological child had similar LS scores. Both of these groups were statistically significantly more dissatisfied than successfully treated women. However, if 3–6 years had elapsed since the last treatment, only the childless women with unsuccessful ART were still more dissatisfied compared to successfully treated women. If over 6 years has gone after ART, no statistically significant differences in life satisfaction were found between any of these three groups.

According to The Finnish Medical Birth Register the live birth rate of the non-responding women (n = 447) was comparable with that of our final study group (n = 540) i.e. 57.5% vs. 58.6%. The mean age of the non-responding women was higher than in the responding women (40.1 *vs.* 38.8 y).

Discussion

The present study investigated how the outcome of ART is associated with women's life satisfaction and how time since last ART is relevant to it. Women who had given birth through ART had higher life satisfaction than the women who did not conceive, especially if the time lag was less than three years. However, passing of time (i.e. more than 6 years) and having a biological child by some other means before or after ART seemed to buffer between unsuccessful ART and life satisfaction.

There is little evidence on how the duration of time from the last ART is associated with life satisfaction. Previously, Leiblum et al.

Table 3. Life Satisfaction score (mean ±SD) by time since last previous ART and risk ratios in respect to life satisfaction between successfully treated women with unsuccessfully treated women with (Child+) or without (Child-) a biological child.

Women with	Time since the last ART				
	<3 years	3–6 years	6–9 years	>9 years	All
Successful ART					
n	82	86	75	53	296
mean ±SD	6.2±2.0[a,b]	7.2±2.4[b]	6.9±2.5	6.9±2.6	6.8±2.4[b]
RR, 95% CI	1	1	1	1	1
Unsuccessful ART, Child+					
n	17	22	24	15	78
mean ±SD	8.0±3.4	7.1±2.3	6.8±3.0	7.3±3.2	7.3±2.9
RR, 95% CI	0.6 (0.3–1.1)	1.1 (0.6–1.8)	1.2 (0.8–1.8)	1.0 (0.6–1.7)	0.9 (0.7–1.2)
Unsuccessful ART, Child–					
n	50	26	26	29	131
mean ±SD	8.1±3.3	8.5±2.9	7.12±2.6	6.9±3.0	7.7±3.1
RR, 95% CI	0.6 (0.4–0.9)	0.5 (0.3–1.1)	0.8 (0.5–1.4)	1.1 (0.8–1.7)	0.8 (0.6–1.0)

ART = assisted reproductive technology; RR = Risk ratio; CI = Confidence interval.
CHILD +/− = women with/without a biological child.
[a]Statistically significant different (*P-value*<0.05), the comparison between successfully treated women with unsuccessfully treated women who had a biological child.
[b]Statistically significant different (*P-value*<0.05), the comparison between successfully treated women with unsuccessfully treated women who remained childless.

(1998) found no association between time since the last treatment (2 to 13 years ago) and life satisfaction in their cross-sectional study [15]. Still, findings supporting our results can be found. According to Verhaak et al. (2005) adjustment to unsuccessful IVF did not occur after six months from IVF in over 20% of their patients [39]. Hammarberg et al. (2001) reported that lower life satisfaction was found after 2–3 years of treatment cessation among women who failed to conceive than among women who succeeded [40]. In a Swedish study, after 5 years since ART, a group with successful IVF had significantly higher general wellbeing than participants in unsuccessful IVF group [19]. Recently, Wischmann (2012) found that three out of four childless women had no further desire for a child after ten years from the first treatment contact [20]. When combining these findings with ours, the adjustment to involuntary childlessness may take place by five to ten years, at least in the majority of the women. Nevertheless, this result does not take into

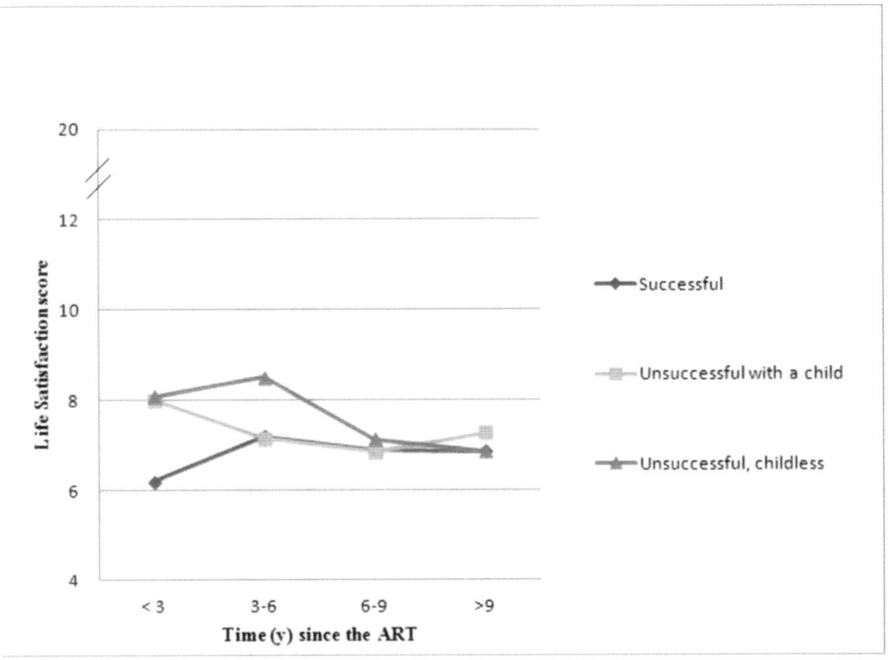

Figure 1. The association of time since the last ART with life satisfaction. The score 4–6 indicates satisfaction, 1220 dissatisfaction and the intermediate group (LS 7–11) consisted of those subjects within one standard deviation from the mean.

account that some women may have had psychological support to relieve the grief of childlessness.

The present study found positive messages. Firstly, great majority of women with previous ART were satisfied with their life. Only 5.7% of the successfully treated women and 14.5% of women who remained childless were subsequently dissatisfied according the LS scale. The group difference was significant also in the category of satisfied women, but in the intermediate group the proportions of women in the successful and unsuccessful group were equal. The categories of satisfied and unsatisfied represent responses' extremities while in the intermediate group other factors in life may have diluted the responses. The mean LS score among women undergoing ART was lower (i.e. indicating better life satisfaction) in adult women aged somewhat the same, but the latter data was collected decades ago [30] without taking into account marital status.

In a previous study, the level of psychosocial stress among involuntarily childless women was in the normal range, even if it was higher than in women with successful infertility treatments [41]. Selection may partly explain this. Our participants had higher educational level than women of the same age group in the general Finnish population which may reflect better life management and consequently better adjustment to the possibility of infertility [42]. Moreover, couples willing to attend ART treatment might have better life management than childless couples not capable or willing to the stressful fertility treatment [4]. Furthermore, in a recent Danish study, women who attended ART had lower rate of depression diagnosis than the age-matched general population and the risk of depression decreased within few years after ART [43]. On the one hand, women who do not participate to infertility treatments might have lower desire for a child [44]. Still, both life dissatisfaction [22] as well as unsuccessful IVF has been repeatedly associated with depression [2], [14], [45–47]. Recurrent failures in ART can increase the risk of depression, but also miscarriages or ectopic pregnancies, which are more common among women with unsuccessful ART, play a role. This should be taken into consideration in counseling infertile couples, especially at the time of decisions after unsuccessful attempts.

The second positive message was that women with unsuccessful ART were, in general, adjusted to their infertility after few years. However, further longitudinal follow-up studies are needed, especially those including also childless women who do not attempt ART at all.

Overall, one strength in this cross sectional study was the comparable background data of both groups, i.e. those with successful or unsuccessful outcome as for educational level, occupation during ART, motherhood status and duration of infertility. We used the valid self-assessment scales and register based information of the actual time since last ART was reliable. The life satisfaction scale we have chosen has a strong correlation with Beck Depression Inventory (BDI) [22], which is a widely used instrument for depression. BDI, however, does not measure positive aspects of life in contrast to the life satisfaction scale. Our survey focused on women who were public health care clients. Thus, access to ART and treatment procedures was equal for all, regardless of the social status. All women were treated in the same clinic by the same physicians and were living in the same district.

Despite the strengths mentioned above this study has some limitations, such as a relatively low response rate (55%) but it is in line with other infertility related surveys [40]. According to non-responder analysis, the non-responders were statistically significantly somewhat older (1.3years) than women in the study groups. However, its clinical significance was unlikely crucial in this setting. One can speculate also that women with advancing age may have somewhat diluted significance of infertility. Live birth rate, on the contrary, was equal among the responders and non-responders (59% vs. 58%, respectively). Still, women with decreased ability to process their infertility, might respond less willingly to a questionnaire about infertility. If they had responded, it might have increased the life satisfaction differences between ART outcome groups. Thus, our results may be a conservative.

In the present study the group of women who did not consider ART as a possible treatment option could not be assessed. Only about every second woman with infertility will seek help and two thirds of them have been reported to discontinue fertility care before attempting IVF [48]. A limitation was also that the spouses were not included, even if infertility affects also men or couples as a whole. Still, according to previous studies, infertility has a greater emotional effect on women than on men [15], [49–51].

In a cross sectional study design it is not possible to show causalities. Thus, we do not claim that the success in ART will cause higher life satisfaction, but we were able to point the association between ART outcome, life satisfaction and time passing. Still, we did not have potential to take into account other life occurrences such as adoption, divorce or severe illness. Previously, it has been shown that mothers through adoption have higher general wellbeing than women with non-successful IVF or mothers through spontaneous pregnancy [19]. In a longitudinal setting there is a problem of declining response rate over time and selection bias in the study subjects. In our study, the distribution of the responders was equal at the different time points. They also filled in the questionnaire at the same time point. Thus, environmental factors such as economic highs and lows in the society did not affect the responses in the present study.

This study was conducted in Finland, where it is, like in other developed countries, socially acceptable to be voluntarily childless. In low-income settings, on the contrary, involuntary childless women may feel themselves as a society's outcast [52]. By taking into consideration these circumstances, including that in Finland ART is available for all social classes, the results of the current study can be generalized to women living in developed countries with a similar structure of the society and to women who have a chance to attend ART.

In conclusion, even if infertility is a source of grief and a risk for poor well-being it can be a life crisis which seems not to have a tendency to jeopardize the long-term well-being of a woman in developed countries. Nevertheless, the current study does not allege that the grief will disappear, but it is possible to learn, after obtaining help from professionals or family if necessary, to live alongside with it.

Acknowledgments

Great thanks must go to Mika Gissler, Professor in National Institute of Health and Welfare, who provided the information of Finnish Medical Birth Register.

Author Contributions

Conceived and designed the experiments: PK MH KR HK SH. Performed the experiments: PK MH KR HK SH. Analyzed the data: PK MH KR HK SH. Contributed reagents/materials/analysis tools: PK MH KR HK SH. Contributed to the writing of the manuscript: PK MH KR HK SH.

References

1. Boivin J, Bunting L, Collins JA, Nygren KG (2007) International estimates of infertility prevalence and treatment-seeking: Potential need and demand for infertility medical care. Hum Reprod 22: 1506–1512.
2. Klemetti R, Raitanen J, Sihvo S, Saarni S, Koponen P (2010) Infertility, mental disorders and well-being a nationwide survey. Acta Obstet Gynecol Scand 89: 677–682.
3. Malizia BA, Hacker MR, Penzias AS (2009) Cumulative live-birth rates after in vitro fertilization. N Engl J Med 360: 236–243.
4. Cousineau TM, Domar AD (2007) Psychological impact of infertility. Best Pract Res Clin Obstet Gynaecol 21: 293–308.
5. Sundby J, Schmidt L, Heldaas K, Bugge S, Tanbo T (2007) Consequences of IVF among women: 10 years post-treatment. J Psychosom Obstet Gynaecol 28: 115–120.
6. Greil AL (1997) Infertility and psychological distress: A critical review of the literature. Soc Sci Med 45: 1679–1704.
7. Greil AL, Slauson-Blevins K, McQuillan J (2010) The experience of infertility: A review of recent literature. Sociol Health Illn 32: 140–162.
8. Verhaak CM, Smeenk JM, Nahuis MJ, Kremer JA, Braat DD (2007) Long-term psychological adjustment to IVF/ICSI treatment in women. Hum Reprod 22: 305–308.
9. Volgsten H, Svanberg AS, Olsson P (2010) Unresolved grief in women and men in sweden three years after undergoing unsuccessful in vitro fertilization treatment. Acta Obstet Gynecol Scand 89: 1290–1297.
10. Volgsten H, Skoog Svanberg A, Ekselius L, Lundkvist O, Sundstrom Poromaa I (2010) Risk factors for psychiatric disorders in infertile women and men undergoing in vitro fertilization treatment. Fertil Steril 93: 1088–1096.
11. Yli-Kuha AN, Gissler M, Klemetti R, Luoto R, Koivisto E, et al. (2010) Psychiatric disorders leading to hospitalization before and after infertility treatments. Hum Reprod 25: 2018–2023.
12. Schmidt L, Holstein BE, Christensen U, Boivin J (2005) Communication and coping as predictors of fertility problem stress: Cohort study of 816 participants who did not achieve a delivery after 12 months of fertility treatment. Hum Reprod 20: 3248–3256.
13. Chachamovich JR, Chachamovich E, Ezer H, Fleck MP, Knauth D, et al. (2010) Investigating quality of life and health-related quality of life in infertility: A systematic review. J Psychosom Obstet Gynaecol 31: 101–110.
14. Weaver SM, Clifford E, Hay DM, Robinson J (1997) Psychosocial adjustment to unsuccessful IVF and GIFT treatment. Patient Educ Couns 31: 7–18.
15. Leiblum SR, Aviv A, Hamer R (1998) Life after infertility treatment: A long-term investigation of marital and sexual function. Hum Reprod 13: 3569–3574.
16. Hammarberg K, Astbury J, Baker H (2001) Women's experience of IVF: A follow-up study. Hum Reprod 16: 374–383.
17. Rostad B, Schmidt L, Sundby J, Schei B (2014) Infertility experience and health differentials - a population-based comparative study on infertile and non-infertile women (the HUNT study). Acta Obstet Gynecol Scand 93: 757–764.
18. Verhaak CM, Smeenk JM, Evers AW, Kremer JA, Kraaimaat FW, et al. (2007) Women's emotional adjustment to IVF: A systematic review of 25 years of research. Hum Reprod Update 13: 27–36.
19. Högstrom L, Johansson M, Janson PO, Berg M, Francis J, et al. (2012) Quality of life after adopting compared with childbirth with or without assisted reproduction. Acta Obstet Gynecol Scand 91: 1077–1085.
20. Wischmann T, Korge K, Scherg H, Strowitzki T, Verres R (2012) A 10-year follow-up study of psychosocial factors affecting couples after infertility treatment. Hum Reprod 27: 3226–3232.
21. Vaillant GE (2003) Mental health. Am J Psychiatry 160: 1373–1384.
22. Koivumaa-Honkanen H, Kaprio J, Honkanen R, Viinamäki H, Koskenvuo M (2004) Life satisfaction and depression in a 15-year follow-up of healthy adults. Soc Psychiatry Psychiatr Epidemiol 39: 994–999.
23. Linna MS, Kaprio J, Raevuori A, Sihvola E, Keski-Rahkonen A, et al. (2013) Body mass index and subjective well-being in young adults: A twin population study. BMC Public Health 13: 231-2458-13-231.
24. Rissanen T, Viinamäki H, Honkalampi K, Lehto SM, Hintikka J, et al. (2011) Long term life dissatisfaction and subsequent major depressive disorder and poor mental health. BMC Psychiatry 11: 140-244X-11-140.
25. Allardt E (1973) About dimension of welfare: An explanatory analysis of the comparative scandinavian survey. University of Helsinki reseach group of comparative sociology reseach report 1. Helsinki, Finland; University of Helsinki.
26. Andrews F, Withey S (1976) Social indicators of well-being: Americans' perception of life quality. New York: Plenum Press.
27. Campbell A, Converse P, Rodgers W (1976) The quality of American life. New York: Russell Stage Foundation.
28. Koivumaa-Honkanen HT, Viinamäki H, Honkanen R, Tanskanen A, Antikainen R, et al. (1996) Correlates of life satisfaction among psychiatric patients. Acta Psychiatr Scand 94: 372–378.
29. Koivumaa-Honkanen H, Honkanen R, Antikainen R, Hintikka J, Laukkanen E, et al. (2001) Self-reported life satisfaction and recovery from depression in a 1-year prospective study. Acta Psychiatr Scand 103: 38–44.
30. Koivumaa-Honkanen H, Kaprio J, Honkanen RJ, Viinamäki H, Koskenvuo M (2005) The stability of life satisfaction in a 15-year follow-up of adult finns healthy at baseline. BMC Psychiatry 5: 4.
31. Koivumaa-Honkanen H, Honkanen R, Viinamäki H, Heikkila K, Kaprio J, et al. (2000) Self-reported life satisfaction and 20-year mortality in healthy finnish adults. Am J Epidemiol 152: 983–991.
32. Koivumaa-Honkanen H, Honkanen R, Viinamäki H, Heikkilä K, Kaprio J, et al. (2001) Life satisfaction and suicide: A 20-year follow-up study. Am J Psychiatry 158: 433–439.
33. Koivumaa-Honkanen H, Honkanen R, Koskenvuo M, Viinamäki H, Kaprio J (2002) Life dissatisfaction as a predictor of fatal injury in a 20-year follow-up. Acta Psychiatr Scand 105: 444–450.
34. Koivumaa-Honkanen H, Koskenvuo M, Honkanen RJ, Viinamäki H, Heikkilä K, et al. (2004) Life dissatisfaction and subsequent work disability in an 11-year follow-up. Psychol Med 34: 221–228.
35. Koivumaa-Honkanen H, Kaprio J, Korhonen T, Honkanen RJ, Heikkilä K, et al. (2012) Self-reported life satisfaction and alcohol use: A 15-year follow-up of healthy adult twins. Alcohol Alcohol 47: 160–168.
36. Saharinen T, Koivumaa-Honkanen H, Hintikka J, Kylmä J, Lehto SM, et al. (2013) The effect of long-term life dissatisfaction on health-related quality of life among general population subjects. J Psychiatr Ment Health Nurs.
37. Koivumaa-Honkanen H, Kaprio J, Korhonen T, Honkanen RJ, Heikkilä K, et al. (2012) Self-reported life satisfaction and alcohol use: A 15-year follow-up of healthy adult twins. Alcohol Alcohol 47: 160–168.
38. Pakarinen M, Koivumaa-Honkanen H, Sinikallio S, Lehto SM, Aalto T, et al. (2014) Life dissatisfaction burden is associated with a poor surgical outcome among lumbar spinal stenosis patients: A 5-year follow-up study. Int J Rehabil Res 37: 80–85.
39. Verhaak CM, Smeenk JM, van Minnen A, Kremer JA, Kraaimaat FW (2005) A longitudinal, prospective study on emotional adjustment before, during and after consecutive fertility treatment cycles. Hum Reprod 20: 2253–2260.
40. Hammarberg K, Astbury J, Baker H (2001) Women's experience of IVF: A follow-up study. Hum Reprod 16: 374–383.
41. Bryson CA, Sykes DH, Traub AI (2000) In vitro fertilization: A long-term follow-up after treatment failure. Hum Fertil (Camb) 3: 214–220.
42. Educational structure of population. Helsinki: Official Statistics of Finland (OSF); 2010. Available: http://www.stat.fi/til/vkour/index_en.html. Accessed 2010 Dec 3.
43. Sejbaek CS, Hageman I, Pinborg A, Hougaard CO, Schmidt L (2013) Incidence of depression and influence of depression on the number of treatment cycles and births in a national cohort of 42,880 women treated with ART. Hum Reprod 28: 1100–1109.
44. Greil AL, Shreffler KM, Schmidt L, McQuillan J (2011) Variation in distress among women with infertility: Evidence from a population-based sample. Hum Reprod 26: 2101–2112.
45. Slade P, Emery J, Lieberman BA (1997) A prospective, longitudinal study of emotions and relationships in in-vitro fertilization treatment. Hum Reprod 12: 183–190.
46. Kee BS, Jung BJ, Lee SH (2000) A study on psychological strain in IVF patients. J Assist Reprod Genet 17: 445–448.
47. Johansson M, Adolfsson A, Berg M, Francis J, Hogstrom L, et al. (2010) Gender perspective on quality of life, comparisons between groups 4–5.5 years after unsuccessful or successful IVF treatment. Acta Obstet Gynecol Scand 89: 683–691.
48. Brandes M, van der Steen JO, Bokdam SB, Hamilton CJ, de Bruin JP, et al. (2009) When and why do subfertile couples discontinue their fertility care? A longitudinal cohort study in a secondary care subfertility population. Hum Reprod 24: 3127–3135.
49. Hjelmstedt A, Andersson L, Skoog-Svanberg A, Bergh T, Boivin J, et al. (1999) Gender differences in psychological reactions to infertility among couples seeking IVF- and ICSI-treatment. Acta Obstet Gynecol Scand 78: 42–48.
50. Newton CR, Sherrard W, Glavac I (1999) The fertility problem inventory: Measuring perceived infertility-related stress. Fertil Steril 72: 54–62.
51. Wichman CL, Ehlers SL, Wichman SE, Weaver AL, Coddington C (2011) Comparison of multiple psychological distress measures between men and women preparing for in vitro fertilization. Fertil Steril 95: 717–721.
52. Cui W (2010) Mother or nothing: The agony of infertility. Bull World Health Organ 88: 881–882.

Prevalence of Suicidal Ideation in Chinese College Students

Zhan-Zhan Li[1], Ya-Ming Li[2,3], Xian-Yang Lei[3], Dan Zhang[2], Li Liu[2], Si-Yuan Tang[2], Lizhang Chen[1]*

1 Department of Epidemiology and Health Statistics, School of Public Health, Central South University, Changsha, China, **2** Department of Nursing, Central South University, Changsha, Hunan Province, China, **3** The Second Affiliated Hospital, Xiangya Medical School, Central South University, Changsha, Hunan Province, China

Abstract

Background: About 1 million people worldwide commit suicide each year, and college students with suicidal ideation are at high risk of suicide. The prevalence of suicidal ideation in college students has been estimated extensively, but quantitative syntheses of overall prevalence are scarce, especially in China. Accurate estimates of prevalence are important for making public policy. In this paper, we aimed to determine the prevalence of suicidal ideation in Chinese college students.

Objective and Methods: Databases including PubMed, Web of Knowledge, Chinese Web of Knowledge, Wangfang (Chinese database) and Weipu (Chinese database) were systematically reviewed to identify articles published between 2004 to July 2013, in either English or Chinese, reporting prevalence estimates of suicidal ideation among Chinese college students. The strategy also included a secondary search of reference lists of records retrieved from databases. Then the prevalence estimates were summarized using a random effects model. The effects of moderator variables on the prevalence estimates were assessed using a meta-regression model.

Results: A total of 41 studies involving 160339 college students were identified, and the prevalence ranged from 1.24% to 26.00%. The overall pooled prevalence of suicidal ideation among Chinese college students was 10.72% (95%CI: 8.41% to 13.28%). We noted substantial heterogeneity in prevalence estimates. Subgroup analyses showed that prevalence of suicidal ideation in females is higher than in males.

Conclusions: The prevalence of suicidal ideation in Chinese college students is relatively high, although the suicide rate is lower compared with the entire society, suggesting the need for local surveys to inform the development of health services for college students.

Editor: Martin Voracek, University of Vienna, Austria

Funding: This study was supported by Hunan Province Science and Technology Project (2014FJ3093). The funder had no role in study design, data collection and analysis, decision to publish, or preparation of the manuscript.

Competing Interests: The authors have declared that no competing interests exist.

* Email: liche4005@126.com

Introduction

Suicide is usually not an isolated event, but a sequence of processes starting from death wishes, suicidal ideation, suicidal contemplation, suicide attempt, to suicide completion [1–2]. Suicidal ideation, which is defined as thoughts of self-harming or -killing [3] is a significant marker not only for mental-health problems but also for the suicide attempt and completed suicide among youths. Various suicidal cognitions (death wish, suicidal ideation, and suicide plan) and behaviors (suicide attempt, and commit suicide) are determined by common factors, such as personality characteristics, psychopathology, parenting style, family function, and substance [4–5]. Thus, it is imperative to identify the characteristics of suicidal ideation and to develop effective prevention and intervention programs.

Currently, suicide is the leading cause of death among 15- to 34-year-old in China, accounting for 19% of deaths in this age group [6]. Suicide has become an important public health issue. A tough challenge placed on top of China's higher education institutions is how to prevent college students from committing suicide and to early detect individuals at high risk of suicide. Given that about 30% of those with suicidal ideation (those who are seriously considering suicide) will attempt suicide, the first step is to determine the overall prevalence of suicidal ideation among college students [7].

Most college students in China are born after post-1980s when the "One-Child" policy switched from a promotive to a mandatory status. Consequently, the majority of them are from single-child families [8]. Hence, it has been becoming a primary argument regarding their relative impulsiveness and inability to withstand negative life events, compared with young adults with siblings. Despite many investigations into the prevalence of suicidal ideation in college students, quantitative syntheses of overall prevalence are scarce, especially in China. Primary prevention as the best and most important strategy requires a sensible plan of action for prevention and improving current policies against suicidal ideation in college students. Therefore, summarizing the prevalence of suicidal ideation in college students is the first step in developing research priorities. We performed a systematic review and meta-analysis of studies on suicidal ideation in Chinese college students with the aim to explore the prevalence of suicidal ideation in this area.

Materials and Methods

Literature Search Strategy

Databases including PubMed, Web of Knowledge, Chinese Web of Knowledge, Wangfang (Chinese database) and Weipu (Chinese database) were systematically reviewed to identify articles published between 2004 to July 2013, in either English or Chinese, reporting the estimates of suicidal ideation prevalence in Chinese college students. Articles were identified with search strategy "suicide" OR "suicidal ideation" OR "suicidal tendency" AND ("college student" OR "undergraduate"). The strategy also included a secondary search of reference lists of records retrieved from databases. Two authors screened the titles and abstracts and reviewed the full-text of the eligible articles.

Inclusion Criteria

The included studies met the following criteria: 1) an original epidemiological study aimed at Chinese college students; 2) with definition of criteria for screening methods and/or screening tools for suicidal ideation and with the provision of description of screening methods; 3) providing information about sample size and prevalence estimation for college students during the prior 12 months; 4) a cross-sectional study or a baseline survey of longitudinal study; 5) a sample size >500. 6) Language is limited to English and Chinese.

Data Extraction

Information was extracted from all selected publications by two investigators separately. Any disagreement was discussed and resolved by a third investigator. After the duplicates were removed, the following information was extracted from each article: first author, year of publication, region, area (South or North China), age range and mean age if possible, percent of males, major (medical student or not), screening method, screening tool, sample size, response rate, number of people with suicidal ideation, prevalence estimation, and sex-specific prevalence if possible.

Statistical Analysis

We first transformed proportions into a quantity (the Freeman-Tukey variant of the arcsine square root transformed proportion [9] suitable for the usual fixed and random effects summaries [10]), because the inverse variance weight in fixed-effects meta-analyses is suboptimum when dealing with binary data with low prevalence. Additionally, the transformed prevalence is weighted very slightly towards 50% and thus studies with prevalence of 0 can be included in the analysis. The pooled proportion is calculated as the back-transform of the weighted mean of the transformed proportions, using inverse arcsine variance weights for the fixed effect's model and DerSimonian-Laird weights for the random effect's model.

According to the expected heterogeneity across studies, a random-effects model was used to calculate pooled prevalence and 95% confidence interval (CIs). Between-study heterogeneity was evaluated with the Cochran chi-square (χ^2) and quantified with the I^2 statistic, which will be used to estimate total variation across studies due to heterogeneity rather than chance (<25% is considered as low heterogeneity, 25%–50% as moderate, and > 50% as high) [11,12]. In order to understand the prevalence of suicidal ideation in different sex, mean age, study year, sample, area and major and also explore the potential heterogeneity between studies, dummy-coding is used for three or more categories variables. We conducted subgroups analysis. Then the effects of these covariates on the logit prevalence of the outcome were estimated using meta-regression. Each covariate was included separately in univariate analyses, and then a multivariable meta-regression model was constructed including all covariates. Publication bias was evaluated Begg's test, the modified Egger's linear regression test and Trim-and-fill approach. Significance was set at $P<0.05$. All statistical calculations were made using Stata 11.0 (College Station, Texas) and Statsdirect 2.7.9 (http://www.statsdirect.com).

Results

Study flow and characteristics

A total of 1908 studies were identified after initial search. After removal of duplicates and an initial screening, we reviewed 177 papers in full. After exclusion of ineligible reports, 41 studies [13–53] published between January 2004 and July 20, 2013 were finally included. The flow diagram of the search process is exhibited in Figure 1. The characteristics of studies on the prevalence of suicidal ideation among college students are shown in Table 1. The sample size of the reviewed studies ranged from 610 to 21072 (median 2374), with a total of 160339 college students. Among them, 28 (68.3%) reports reported data on male ($n = 69701$), 28 (68.3%) reports on female ($n = 55140$), and 13 (31.7%) reports included mixed sex population size ($n = 35228$). In the surveys with samples, more than 54% of the individuals were men. The age ranged from 16 to 25 years old. Among them, 29 (70.7%) reports were aimed at South China ($n = 112706$), 12 reports at North China ($n = 47633$), 16 (39.0%) at medical universities ($n = 51645$), and 25 (61.0%) at non-medical students ($n = 108694$). Table 1 shows details from the 41 selected studies. Questionnaire is used to collect the information in the most of studies. 18 use the self-made scale, 9 for beck scale for suicide ideation-Chinese version, 7 for university personality inventory, and the left use other scales.

Pooled analysis in different category

Overall prevalence. The point prevalence of suicidal ideation with the 41 individual study populations ranged between 1.24% and 26.00%, with an overall meta-analysis prevalence of 10.72% (95%CI: 8.41%–13.28%, Figure 2) and evident high-level heterogeneity between studies ($I^2 = 99.6\%$, $P<0.0001$).

Sex. Pooled prevalence of all subgroups of study year, population size, male percent, area, major and sex are presented in Table 2. The summarized prevalence of females (10.32%, 95%CI: 7.17%–13.97%, Figure 3) was higher than that of males (8.84%, 95%CI: 6.45%–11.57%, Figure 4). The prevalence estimates for studies with more than 50% males were lower than estimates of groups with less than 50% males (8.84%, 95%CI: 6.45%–11.57%).

Periods. The pooled prevalence estimate decreased over time. Between 2004 and 2007, the pooled prevalence estimate was 12.10% (*95%CI:* 6.97%–18.44%), which decreased to 10.73% (95%CI: 6.16%–16.39%) between 2008 and 2009. The estimate was 10.77% (95%CI: 8.30%–13.53%) in 2010 to 2011, and 9.35% (95%CI: 5.13%–14.68%) in 2012 to 2013.

Major and area. The prevalence for the non-medical group (9.61%, 95%CI: 6.97%–12.62%) was smaller than medical group (12.58 95%CI: 10.09%–15.30%). Prevalence among college students from South and North China were 11.95% (95%CI: 9.09%–15.14%) and 8.00% (95%CI: 4.67%–12.14%) respectively.

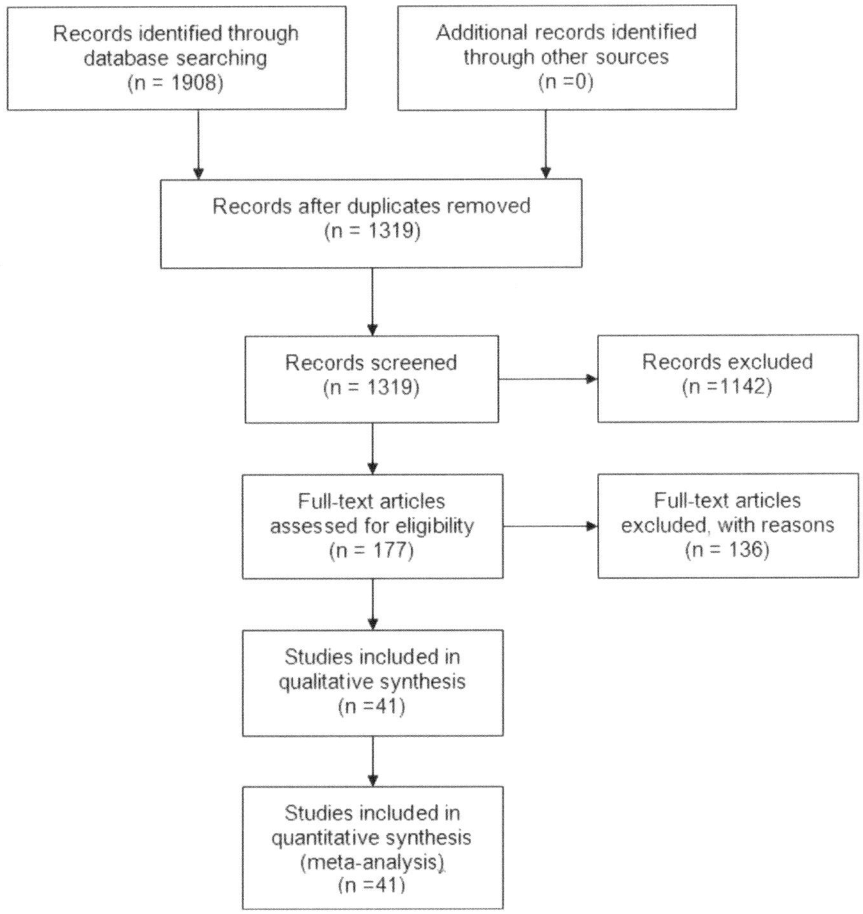

Figure 1. Flow diagram of included/excluded studies.

Population size and response rate. Regarding population size, the pooled prevalence was 11.40% (95%CI: 8.89%–14.19%) for population size <2000, 12.22% (95%CI: 9.30%–15.49%) and 7.70% (95%CI: 3.77%–12.85%) for population size >4000. Table 2 shows information about heterogeneity and publication bias. The pooled prevalence for response rate ≤90% was 12.81% (95%CI: 9.30–17.32) and 10.93 (95%CI: 9.72–12.13) for response rate >90%.

Meta-regression analysis, assessment of publication bias

We noted significant heterogeneity within studies and subgroups ($P<0.001$, $I^2=97.9\%–99.0\%$). In the univariate meta-regression analyses (Table 3), year of publication, male percent and major used to define suicidal ideation did not modify the estimate of prevalence. In three population size groups (<2000, 2000–4000, >4000), the prevalence estimates in population size >4000 were significantly lower compared with the other two groups. Mean age ($P=0.017$) and response rates ($P=0.012$) were significantly associated with the prevalence estimates. A meta-regression model was constructed including male ratio, response rate and population size (2000–4000). This model explained much of the heterogeneity between studies ($R^2=52.85\%$, $P=0.016$, Table 3). We noted the prevalence of suicidal ideation decrease with response rate and male rate increase in the proportion and increase with the sample size increase. Then bias of publication was assessed using Begg's funnel plot and Egger's test. Significant publication bias was indicated by Begg's test ($P=0.008$), but not by the modified Egger's linear regression test ($P=0.258$). The funnel plot an apparent asymmetry that suggested the presence of a potential publication bias (Figure 5). Trim-and-Fill analyses was also used to assess publication bias. The pooled estimations for fixed and random models were −2.10 (95%CI: −2.17 to −2.02) and −2.21 (95%CI: −2.45 to −1.97). After estimated missing study was included into the meta-analysis, the pooled estimations for fixed and random models were −2.40 (95%CI: −2.47 to −2.33) and −2.43 (95%CI: −2.68 to −2.17). The estimated missing number of study is eight, which suggested the presence of publication bias.

Discussion

There is a lack of nationwide data regarding prevalence of suicidal ideation in Chinese college students at present. This is the first report attempting to synthesize the prevalence estimations of suicidal ideation among Chinese college students using meta-analysis. This comprehensive systematic review with meta-analysis of observational studies done in China in the last decade included 41 reports and more than 160 thousand college students. Therefore, it was possible to provide a reliable estimate of prevalence. This meta-analysis indicates that the prevalence of suicidal ideation in Chinese college students is 10.72% (95%CI: 8.41%–13.28%), which was close to previously reported rates [31] and fell in the range of 6%–39.2% reported in other countries [54–56].

Table 1. Characteristic of Studies on the Prevalence of Suicidal Ideation among College Students.

NO.	First author	Publication year	Region	Province	Area	Age (mean years)	Male Percent (%)	Medical student	Screening method	Screening tools	Response Rate (%)	Suicidal ideation	Sample size	Prevalence (%)
1	Wang [13]	2012	Mainland	Henan	Northern	17–22	44.2	No	Q	UPI	97.10	162	3850	4.21
2	Chen [14]	2010	Mainland	Chongqing	Southern	20.0	56.6	Yes	Q	SMQ	81.0	1279	9808	13.0
3	Xu [15]	2004	Mainland	Hunan	Southern	-	53.4	Yes	Q	SMQ	97.9	89	610	14.6
4	Chen [16]	2008	Mainland	Jilin	Northern	21.3	67.1	Yes	QI	CIDI	98.9	97	1822	5.3
5	Liu [17]	2007	Mainland	Yunnan	Southern	21.2	50.4	No	Q	SMQ	97.4	437	3313	13.2
6	Chao [18]	2008	Mainland	Jiangxi	Southern	-	51.8	No	Q	SMQ	84.2	113	1010	11.2
7	Shang [19]	2008	Mainland	Gansu	Northern	20.5	35.8	Yes	Q	SMQ	92.3	411	2678	15.4
8	Qian [20]	2008	Mainland	Beijing	Northern	-	35.4	Yes	Q	SMQ	88.2	122	2199	5.6
9	Yang [21]	2013	Mainland	Henan	Southern	20.7	33.5	Yes	Q	UPI	92.2	110	1372	8.0
10	Zhang [22]	2007	Mainland	Guangdong	Southern	-	52.8	Yes	Q	EPQ	99.3	1763	7189	24.5
11	Wang [23]	2011	Mainland	Yunnan	Southern	18.9	35.5	Yes	Q	SMQ	99.84	409	1850	22.1
12	Jiang [24]	2006	Mainland	Fujian	Southern	-	56.3	Yes	Q	SMQ	90.4	171	1254	13.6
13	Li [25]	2009	Mainland	Beijing	Northern	25.1	64.4	No	Q	UPI	97.6	380	21072	1.8
14	Li [26]	2007	Mainland	Zhejiang	Southern	18.6	40.1	No	Q	SCL-90	95.0	800	8160	9.8
15	Bao [27]	2009	Mainland	Anhui	Southern	20.1	61.0	Yes	Q	BSSI	92.7	217	1529	14.2
16	Huang [28]	2007	Mainland	Zhejiang	Southern	18.85	64.0	No	QI	SCL-90	94.2	219	3564	6.1
17	Wang [29]	2011	Mainland	Shanxi	Northern	19.2	44.9	Yes	Q	SDSS	98.3	74	1177	6.3
18	Kong [30]	2012	Mainland	Anhui	Southern	20.4	42.9	Yes	Q	SMQ	91.8	444	3030	14.7
19	Song [31]	2010	Mainland	Anhui	Southern	21.8	55.9	Yes	Q	BSSI	95.9	210	2062	10.2
20	Sun [32]	2010	Mainland	Shandong	Northern	20.4	42.4	No	Q	BSSI	94.3	228	1886	12.1
21	Yang [33]	2010	Mainland	Harbin	Northern	21.3	51.1	No	Q	SMQ	87.8	479	5240	9.1
22	Yan [34]	2009	Mainland	Guangdong	Southern	21.2	46.8	No	Q	SMQ	87.2	57	772	7.4
23	Shi [35]	2007	Mainland	Guangdong	Southern	20.6	49.8	No	Q	SMQ	98.0	297	2564	11.6
24	Shi [36]	2013	Mainland	Guangxi	Southern	20.4	52.7	No	Q	BSSI	91.0	434	2730	15.9
25	Ran [37]	2006	Mainland	Sichuan	Southern	-	70.6	No	Q	UPI	100.0	229	8850	2.6
26	Kan [38]	2013	Mainland	Zhejiang	Southern	-	46.1	No	Q	UPI	99.9	263	10138	2.6
27	Zhao [39]	2011	Mainland	Guangdong	Southern	21.7	56.6	No	Q	SMQ	96.35	98	1450	6.8
28	Yin [40]	2009	Mainland	Jiangsu	Southern	21.3	36.4	No	QI	SMQ	95.7	90	670	13.4
29	Yang [41]	2007	Mainland	Henan	Northern	16–24	74.6	No	Q	SCL-90	93.9	705	3568	19.8
30	Liu [42]	2013	Mainland	Guangdong	Southern	14–25	58.5	No	Q	SPS	100.0	585	6154	9.5
31	Tu [43]	2013	Mainland	Guangdong	Southern	21.0	60.0	No	Q	UPI	100.0	144	11603	1.24
32	Liu [44]	2008	Mainland	Beijing	Northern	-	42.5	Yes	Q	SMQ	91.4	125	1204	10.4
33	Li [45]	2008	Mainland	Beijing	Northern	20.0	55.6	No	Q	BSSI	97.6	166	2055	8.1
34	Cao [46]	2009	Mainland	Anhui	Southern	19.3	46.2	Yes	QI	BSSI	91.8	1669	10344	16.4

Table 1. Cont.

NO.	First author	Publication year	Region	Province	Area	Age (mean years)	Male Percent (%)	Medical student	Screening method	Screening tools	Response Rate (%)	Suicidal ideation	Sample size	Prevalence (%)
35	Fan [47]	2008	Mainland	Anhui	Southern	20.3	53.5	Yes	Q	BSSI	94.4	496	3517	14.1
36	Tang [48]	2011	Mainland	Hubei	Southern	10–24	54.7	No	Q	SMQ	100.0	178	2013	8.8
37	Zhang [49]	2012	Mainland	Guangdong	Southern	21.8	48.6	No	Q	SMQ	87.2	137	689	19.9
38	Zhu [50]	2011	Mainland	Jiangsu	Southern	19.6	47.1	No	Q	BSSI	98.1	430	2374	18.1
39	Zhao [51]	2012	Mainland	Guangdong	Southern	19.5	46.4	No	Q	BSSI	84.0	225	1168	19.3
40	Wang [52]	2010	Mainland	Shanxi	Northern	19.0	46.9	No	Q	UPI	93.0	46	882	5.6
41	Gau [53]	2008	Taiwan	Taiwan	Southern	19.4	48.5	No	Q	SMQ	79.2	759	2919	26.0

Screen methods: Q, questionnaire distribution; QI, questionnaire-based interview. Screening tools: UPI, University Personality Inventory, SMQ, Self-made scale; CIDI, Composite International Diagnostic Interview; BSSI, Beck Scale for Suicide Ideation-Chinese Version.

Suicidal ideation among college students is associated with various factors, which can be categorized into several domains, including physiology, suicide attitude, psychological health status, stress, and social support.

Sex may significantly affect the prevalence of suicidal ideation. A national representative population-based study from Korea found the prevalence of suicidal ideation was significantly higher among females: about 19% of females and 11% of males reported suicidal ideation [57]. In Kampala (Uganda), the prevalence of suicidal ideation was significantly higher in girls (34%) than boys (23.2%) [58]. However, other studies did not report the sex difference for suicidal ideation [59]. This meta-analysis showed that 8.84% of males and 10.32% of females had suicidal ideation, and this difference can be partially explained by the following reasons. According to the gender role socialization theory, males are expected to be independent and decisive, and display masculinity (e.g. engagement in risky behaviors). In contrast, females are expected to be dependent and indecisive, and express their stress via rumination. So females have a higher rate of suicide attempts than males, while males have a higher rate of mortality from suicide than females [60]. In China, fatal suicide rate for male was higher than females. But fatal suicide rate for females was still higher than males among population aged 15 to 34 (including college student) [61]. Suicidal ideation pattern in this meta-analysis may be similar to the pattern of fatal suicide.

Psychological health status exerts an implicit, deep and fundamental influence on suicidal ideation. About 50%–75% of children and adolescents who have suicidal ideation suffered from emotional disturbance, especially severe depression; about 1/4–2/3 of adolescents with suicidal ideation have a history of drug dependence and abuse [62]. Personality disorder in adults with suicidal ideation is more common than adolescents, indicating that adolescents with personality disorder are easily addicted to drug abuse and more likely to develop suicidal ideation [63]. Sexual orientation will greatly affect the suicidal ideation and suicidal behaviors of the youths, which is regulated by depression, hopelessness and drug abuse [64–65].

Negative life events that are a direct source of stimulation inducing suicidal ideation. College students who experience more negative life events are at increased risk for suicidal ideation. Associations between suicidal ideation and failure in love, financial problems, and divorce/separation of parents have been reported [71]. Findings also suggest that negative life events may be associated with suicidal ideation among adolescent, depressive symptoms were associated with suicidality and depressive symptoms may mediate the association of minor negative life events with suicidality [66].

Higher levels of family cohesion and family support were associated with lower levels of suicidal ideation and depression [67]. Living alone increased the risk for suicidal ideation among college students [68], suggesting that facilitating access to support resources might reduce the risk for suicidal behavior among college students. In addition, friends are also an important source of support and may be an even greater resource than the family [69]. Therefore, evaluating the support system of friends may provide further information that can help prevent suicide.

There are other factors of suicidal ideation such as cultural orientation [70], religious belief [51], history of family suicide [36], and social-economic status [46]. The factors affecting suicidal ideation in college students are not single, but multifaceted. Depression fully mediated the relationship between physical illness, interpersonal conflict and suicidal ideation, but not the relationship between financial problem and suicidal ideation [71]. Another study confirmed the hypothesis that family cohesion and

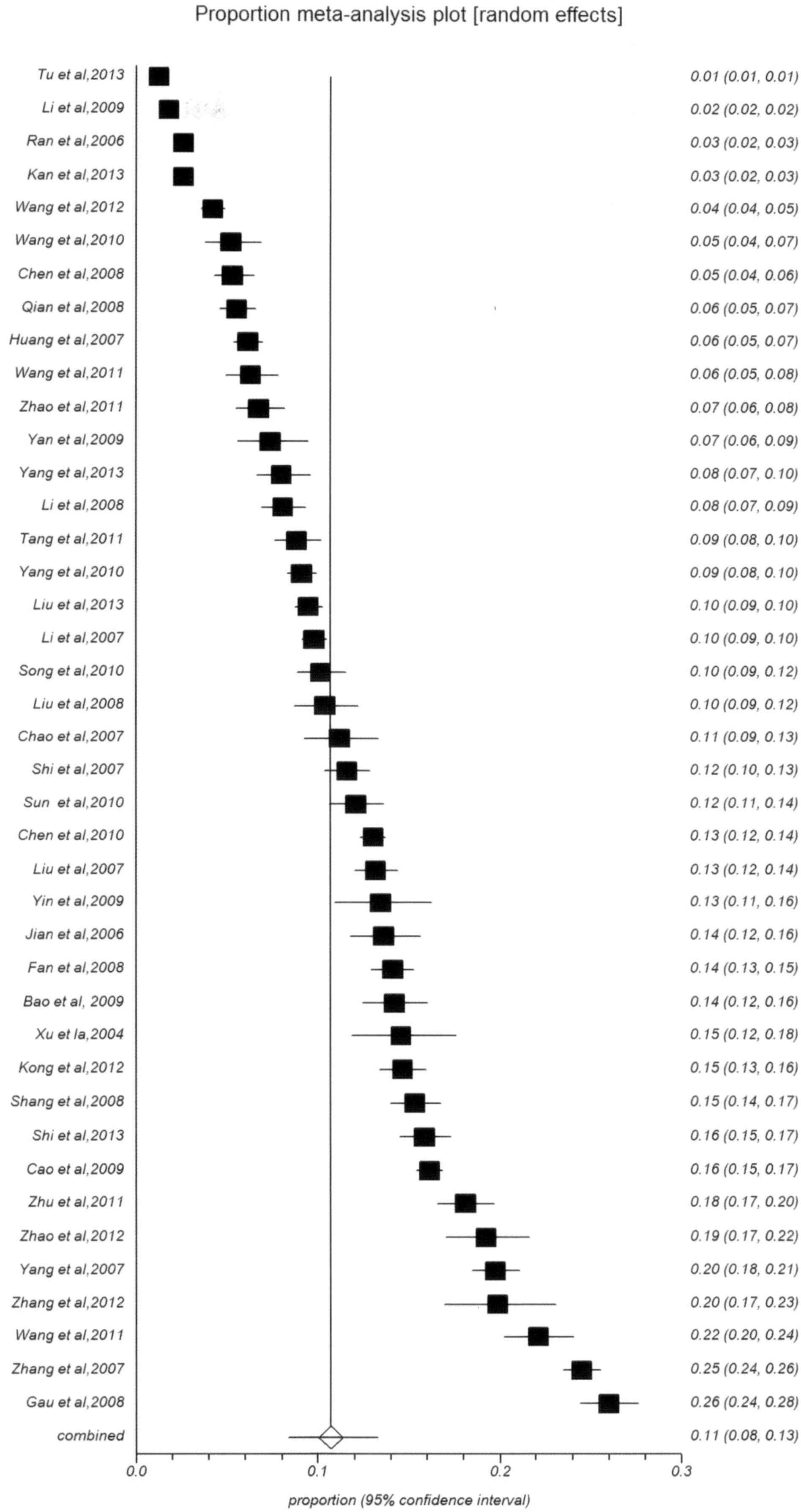

Figure 2. Forest plot of prevalence of suicidal ideation for total people.

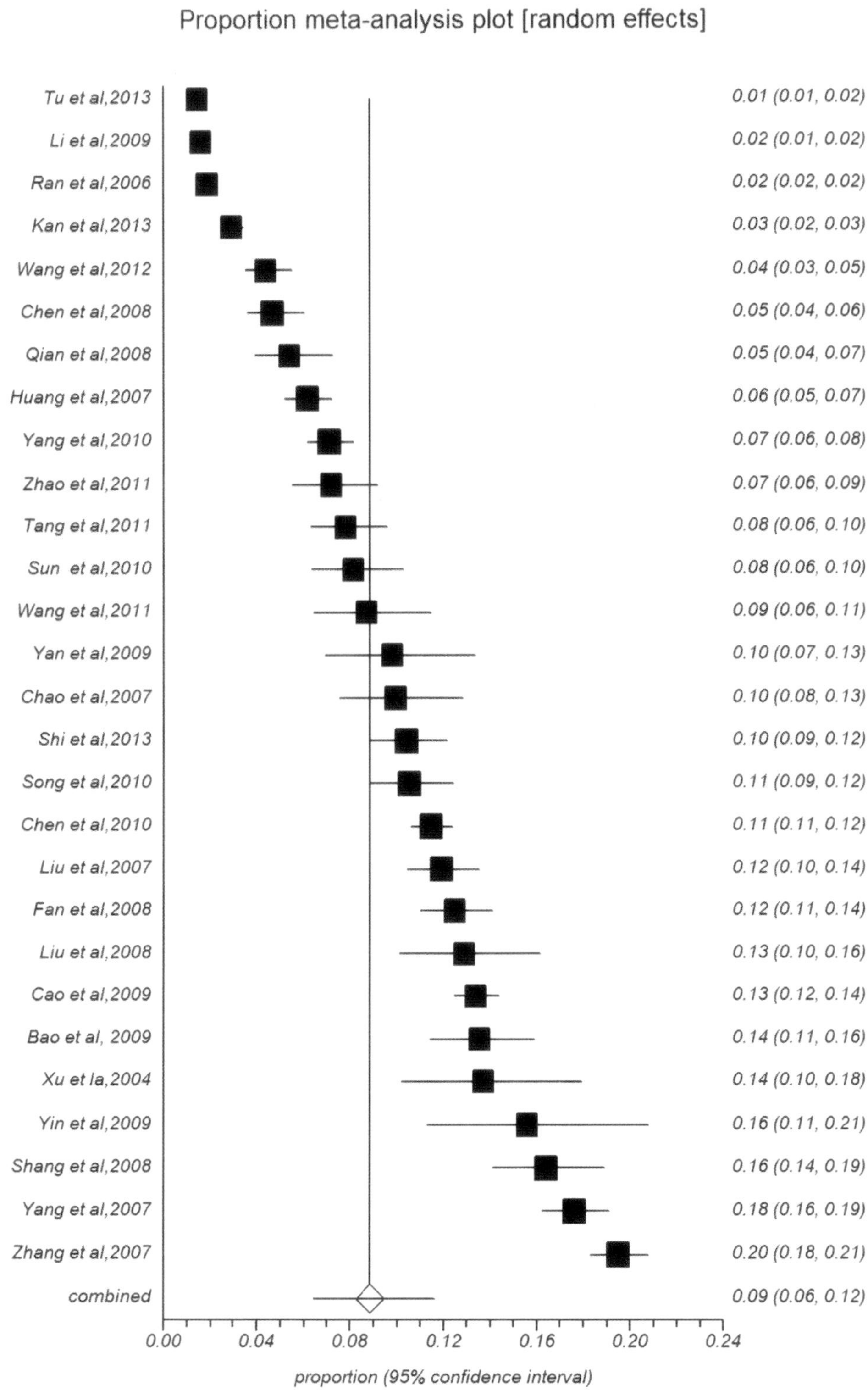

Figure 3. Forest plot of prevalence of suicidal ideation for male.

social self-concept were significant moderators for children and adolescents [70]. In sum, on an individual basis, one or all three factors could work, and even accidental factors may also contribute to suicidal ideation.

For the reasons given above, some effective measures should be taken. It is suggested that the experience of violence had a significant negative direct effect and peer support had a significant positive direct effect on their happiness. Happiness had a significant negative effect and the experience of violence had a significant positive effect on suicidal ideation. These findings demonstrate the fundamental importance of reducing exposure of violence to the youth, and that increasing peer support and their

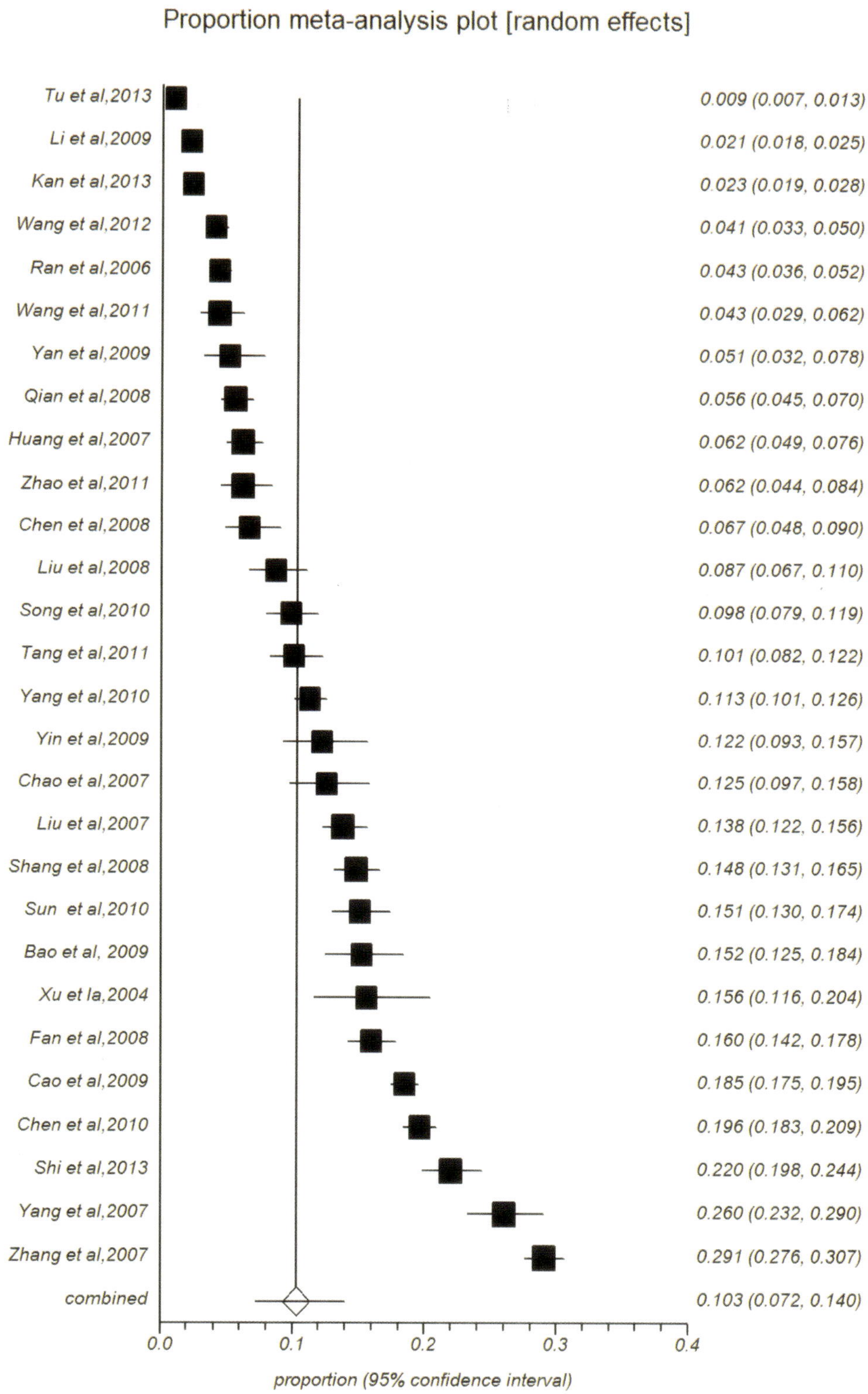

Figure 4. Forest plot of prevalence of suicidal ideation for female.

happiness may be the key to adolescent suicidal ideation prevention [72]. Sakamoto et al found that watching the video had substantial psych educational effects, which could be considered as prevention measures [73]. What is more, the lack of mental health services is an urgent problem of campus populations in China. More mental health counselors are needed [74]. College students would benefit greatly by attention to this measures.

Although this meta-analysis includes 41 studies encompassing a larger sample size than individual studies, there are still some limitations. First, the heterogeneity of both total population and subgroup was high. Most of the included studies had large sample

Table 2. Prevalence of Suicidal Ideation among College Students According to Different Category.

Category	Subgroup	NO. of Studies	Prevalence (*95%CI*)(%)	*N*	I^2 (%)	*P*	Publication Bias Test	
							P(Begg's Test)	*P*(Egger's Test)
	Total	41	10.72[8.41–13.28]	160339	99.6	<0.0001	0.258	0.008
Study year	2004–2007	9	12.10[6.97–18.44]	39072	99.7	<0.0001	0.915	0.704
	2008–2009	13	10.73[6.16–16.39]	51791	99.7	<0.0001	0.858	0.183
	2010–2011	10	10.77[8.30–13.53]	28742	97.9	<0.0001	0.600	0.942
	2012–2013	9	9.35[5.13–14.68]	47034	99.6	<0.0001	0.119	0.009
Sample size	<2000	16	11.40[8.89–14.19]	19345	97.5	<0.0001	0.003	0.001
	2000–4000	15	12.22[9.30–15.49]	42436	99.0	<0.0001	0.0001	0.0001
	>4000	10	7.70[3.77–12.85]	98558	99.9	<0.0001	0.009	0.0001
Male percent	<50%	20	11.67[8.63–15.10]	59926	99.3	<0.0001	0.186	0.388
	≥50%	21	9.85[6.68–13.57]	100413	99.7	<0.0001	0.492	0.069
Area	Northern	12	8.00[4.67–12.14]	47633	99.5	<0.0001	0.381	0.065
	Southern	29	11.95[9.09–15.14]	112706	99.6	<0.0001	0.838	0.119
Medical students	Yes	16	12.58[10.09–15.30]	51645	98.7	<0.0001	0.757	0.792
	No	25	9.61[6.97–12.62]	108694	99.6	<0.0001	0.083	0.008
Sex	Male	28	8.84 [6.45–11.57]	69701	99.3	<0.0001	0.570	0.0001
	Female	28	10.32[7.17–13.97]	55140	99.4	<0.0001	0.101	0.422
Response rate	90%≤	9	12.81[9.30–17.32]	25059	98.7	<0.0001	0.531	0.589
	<90%	32	10.93[9.72–12.13]	135280	99.5	<0.0001	0.023	0.004

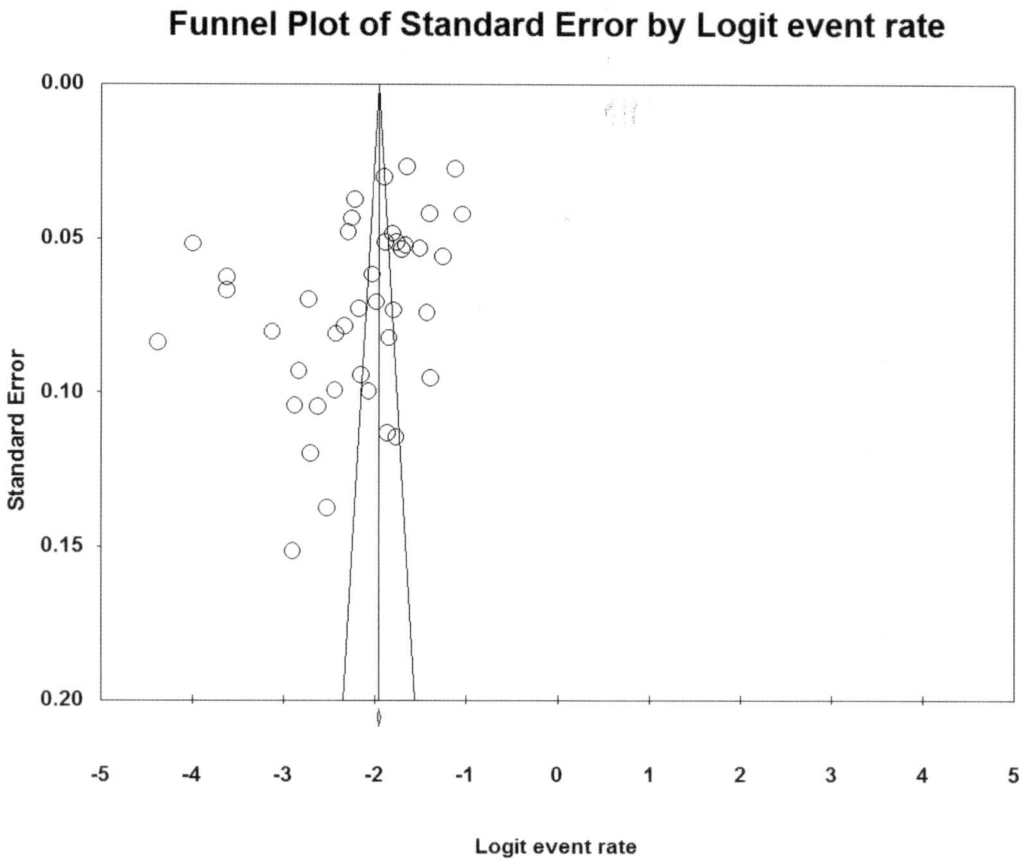

Figure 5. Funnel plot of studies included in the synthesis.

Table 3. Results of Meta-regression for Prevalence among Chinese College Students.

Covariate	Meta-regression coefficient	*95%CI*	*P* value	Variance explained (%)
Univariate analyses				
Year of publication				
2004–2007	0.176	−0.356 to 0.709	0.507	−1.40
2008–2009	0.015	−0.460 to 0.492	0.946	−2.55
2010–2011	0.078	−0.437 to 0.594	0.759	−2.31
2012–2013	−0.281	−0.809 to 0.246	0.288	0.41
Male percent	−0.235	−0.672 to 0.202	0.283	0.46
Sample size				
<2000	0.192	−0.258 to 0.642	0.394	−0.64
2000–4000	0.283	−0.168 to 0.734	0.212	1.51
>4000	−0.604	−1.082 to −0.126	0.015	12.16
Area	0.392	−0.077 to 0.863	0.099	4.43
Mean age	−0.230	−0.417 to −0.044	0.017	16.2
Screening tool	−0.435	−0.859 to −0.010	0.045	7.26
Response rate	−0.050	−0.088 to −0.011	0.012	13.01
Medical student	0.359	−0.080 to 0.799	0.106	4.16
Multivariable analyses			0.016	52.85
Response rate	−0.057	−0.10 to −0.014	0.011	
Male rate	−0.030	−0.055 to −0.004	0.024	
Sample size(2000–4000)	0.778	0.210 to 1.346	0.010	

sizes that produced very precise estimates. Meta-regression analysis showed that male ratio, sample size and response rate may be associated with the prevalence of suicidal ideation, which explained about the half of the heterogeneity between studies. But non-theory-guided selection of predictors based on an algorithm may lead to replication difficulties in future studies. We noted the prevalence of suicidal ideation decrease with response rate and male rate increase in the proportion and increase with the sample size increase. The difference of screening methods may have an influence on the heterogeneity. But this result should be carefully explained. Because some variable are associated with outcome variables in a single, and not associated with outcome variable after being combined. We call this aggregation bias, ecological bias, ecological confounding or ecological fallacy. It is acknowledged that there must be some factors affecting the heterogeneity. According to the present data, we cannot further identify the source of heterogeneity. Second, results from Begg's funnel plot and Egger's test are different but the funnel plot and Trim and Fill methods suggested the presence of a potential publication bias, a language bias, and inflated estimates by a flawed methodological design in smaller studies. The available studies had important methodological limitations, particularly related to college students with suicidal ideation selection and recruitment, which may have led to subjects included in studies differing in important ways from those excluded or ineligible for analyses, and that may have unpredictably affected prevalence estimates. Finally, the studies with a sample size less than 500 subjects were not included on the basis of the sake of representativeness of survey samples. The information bias may still affect the pooled results, although we restricted sampling methods in inclusion criteria.

In conclusion, the prevalence of suicidal ideation in Chinese college students is relatively high, although the suicide rate is lower than that of the entire society. Considering the policy of enrollment expansion of higher education in China is implemented, It is sincerely hoped that this meta-analysis synthesized within the past decade will serve as a "wake-up" call to university administration alike. The results should encourage not only more needed research in terms of the college student group as a distinct population unto itself, but also prompt colleges, society and family to develop and implement programs to address, educate and prevent those college students who are most at risk for suicidal ideation.

Author Contributions

Conceived and designed the experiments: ZZL YML SYT. Performed the experiments: LZC ZZL. Analyzed the data: DZ LL ZZL. Contributed reagents/materials/analysis tools: XYL ZZL LZC. Wrote the paper: ZZL YML LZC. Revised the manuscript: ZZL LZC.

References

1. Jiang M, Hu Z, Cao Y (2007) Suicide deaths concentrated in Beijing universities. Am J Psychiatry 164: 1758.
2. Perez WV (2005) The relationship between seriously considering, planning, and attempting suicide in the youth risk behavior survey. Suicide and Life-threatening Behavior 35: 35–49.
3. National Research Council (2002) Reducing Suicide: A National Imperative. Washington, DC: The National Academies Press.
4. Beautrais AL (2000) Risk factors for suicide and attempted suicide among young people. Aust N Z J Psychiatry 34: 420–436.
5. Kuo PH, Yang HJ, Soong WT, Chen WJ (2002) Substance use among adolescents in Taiwan: associated personality traits, incompetence, and behavioral/emotional problems. Drug Alcohol Depend 67:27–39.
6. Phillips MR, Li X, Zhang Y (2002) Suicide rates in China, 1995–99. Lancet 359: 835–840.
7. Kirmayer LJ, Fraser SL, Faurus V, Heather Clarke, M.A.Saucier Jean-François, et al. (2009) Cultural and Mental Health Research Unit working paper 14. Montreal, Quebec: 2009. Current approaches to Aboriginal youth suicide prevention.
8. Luo MY (2010) Social Assessment and Subdividing of After-1980s. China Youth Study 11: 32–35.
9. Stuart A, Ord JK (1994) Kendall's Advanced Theory of Statistics (6th edition). London: Edward Arnold.
10. DerSimonian R, Laird N (1986) Meta-analysis in Clinical Trials. Controlled Clinical Trials 7: 177–188.
11. Brittain EH, Fay MP, Follmann DA (2012) A valid formulation of the analysis of noninferiority trials under random effects meta-analysis. Biostatistics 13: 637–649.
12. Chootrakool H, Shi JQ, Yue R (2011) Meta-analysis and sensitivity analysis for multi-arm trials with selection bias. Stat Med 30: 1183–1198.
13. Wang BW (2012) Psychological health condition and its influence factors among freshmen with suicidal ideation. Chin J Public Health 28: 1086–1088.
14. Chen JM, Ai M, Kuang L, Wang MJ, Shen Y, et al. (2010) Suicide ideation among college students in Chongqing. Chin J Epidemiol 31: 290–293.
15. Xu HL, Xiao SY, Feng SS, Chen XX (2004) Risk factors for suicide attempt among college students at Central South University. Chin J Epidemiol 25: 288–291.
16. Chen YF, Kou CG, Zhang D, Xie B, Yu YQ, et al. (2008) Analysis on suicide tendency and its risk factors of undergraduate students[J]. Chin J Dis Control Prev 12: 450–453.
17. Liu QQ, Li H, Fang XY (2007) An investigation of suicidal ideation and suicide attempts of undergraduate in Yunnan province with their self-esteem and mental health status. China Journal of Health Psychology 15: 57–58.
18. Chao XC (2008) Different personality of undergraduate students with and without suicide ideation [J]. Health Medicine Research and Practice 5: 42–44.
19. Shang YX, Dong GQ, Liu T (2008) Analysis on prevalence of suicidal ideation and depression and its influence factors among undergraduate students in Yinchuan. Chin J Public Health 24: 934–936.
20. Qian WC, Liu BH, Huang YQ, Hao WL, Li WYTN (2008) Study on risk factors for suicidal ideation among undergraduate of medical college. Chin J Public Health 24: 1285–1286.
21. Yang CW, Shi SC, Liu JX, Jia RR, Chui WW, et al. (2013) Analysis on suicide ideation and its risk factors among medical college students. Chin J Social Medicine 30: 193–195.
22. Zhang XY, Yu SY, Zhao JB (2007) Correlation between suicidal ideation and personality, internal-external locus of control, self-esteem in medical college students. J Fourth Mil Med Univ 28: 747–749.
23. Wang T, Jiang RS, Zhou M, Huang YY, Di YX (2011) A study on influencing factors of the undergraduate suicide ideation. Journal of Kunming Medical University 12:44–47.
24. Wang XL, Xu NF, Xue HT, Jiang DW, Yang DH (2006) Analysis on suicide ideation and its factors among medical undergraduate students. Chin J Public Health 22: 653–655.
25. Li H, Huang YQ (2009) Study on the related factors of suicide ideation among graduate students in national research institutions. China Journal of Health Psychology 17: 963–966.
26. Li FH, Dai WL (2007) Analysis on suicide ideation and its factors among college students in Wenzhou. Chin J School Doctor 21: 290–291.
27. Bao DX, Fan YG, Ye DQ (2009) Correlation between suicidal ideation and Life events and social support among medical college students of Wanxi. Chin J Sch Health 30: 939–941.
28. Huang QR, Liu B, Feng TL (2007) The relationship between life event and suicide attempts among college students. China J Health Psychology 15: 210–213.
29. Wang H, Wang MX, Chu XP (2011) Study on the factors of suicidal ideation and its influences among undergraduates in Shanxi province. Foreign medical science section of med geography 32: 188–191.
30. Kong G, Sun YH, Yang LS, Zhou CX (2012) Investigation of psychosocial factors of suicide attitude among the students in a medical college. J Bengbu Med Coll 37: 1240–1243.
31. Song YM, Wan YH, Pan FM, Ye DQ (2010) Analysis on suicide ideation and its risk factors among medical college students. Chinese Journal of Health Statistics 27: 178–179.
32. Sun AY, Sun YM, Xu HL (2010) Analysis on suicide ideation and its risk factors among college students in Liao cheng. Journal of Qilu Nursing 16: 55–56.
33. Yang YJ, Qiu XH, Yang XX, Qiao ZX, Han D, et al. (2010) Study on the influencing factors of suicidal ideation among university students in Harbin. Chin J Epidemiology 31: 1103–1106.

34. Yan HH, Liu ZM, Wang SY, Yang G, Chen LF, et al. (2009) Study on the relationship between life events and suicidal ideation among undergraduates in Guangzhou. Modern Preventive Medicine 36: 476–479.
35. Shi WJ, Ma SB, Wang SY (2007) Study on prevalence of suicidal ideation and its related factors in college students in Guangzhou. Chin J Sch Health 28: 999–1000.
36. Shi XL, Liu YY, Liu SY, Zhao WS, Jiang CL (2013) Analysis of suicidal ideation and relationship with depressive disorder of Guangxi college students countermeasures research. Popular science and technology 15: 114–117.
37. Ran CF, Zhang YQ, Wang W, Tian S, Wei J, et al. (2006) Suicide-preventive and suicide-intervening mechanism for vocational college students. J Prev MedInf 22: 548–552.
38. Kan SY, Zheng XF (2013) Relationship between suicide ideation and family environment among university students. Chin J Public Health 29: 167–168.
39. Zhao GX, Jin CX, Wang SY, Chen QS, Liu GN et al. (2011) Analysis on influencing factors of suicide ideation among college students: a structural equation model study. Chin J Behv Med Brain Sci 20: 357–359.
40. Yi L (2009) Analysis on influencing factors of suicide ideation among college students. Chin J School Doctor 23: 388–390.
41. Yang XH, Zhou H, Wang SM (2007) Epidemiological investigation of suicidal ideation in college students. Chin J Sch Health 28: 527–528.
42. Liu GH, Zhang GY (2013) The relationship between personality factors and suicide ideation of undergraduates. China Journal of Health Psychology 21: 456–457.
43. Tu YM, Zhang QJ (2013) The relationship between life events, coping style and suicide ideation of undergraduates. Educational circles, 15: 60.
44. Liu BH, Huang YQ, Niu WY, Lv ZZ, Wang PY, et al. (2008) Study on the factors influencing suicidal ideation among medical students in Beijing. Chin J Epidemiol 29: 128–131.
45. Li XN, Liu HY, Liu ZR, Guo Q, Huang YQ (2008) A cross-sectional study on related factors of suicidal ideation among college students. Chinese Mental Health Journal 22: 806–815.
46. Cao HY, Sun YH, Yao YS, Zhou CX, Yang LS (2009) Suicide behavior and its factors among medical undergraduates in Anhui province. Chin J Sch Health, 30: 38–39.
47. Fan YG (2008) Study on the influencing factors of suicide ideation among underrates in Anhui Provinces. Anhui: Anhui Medical University, 2008.
48. Tang J, Yu Y, Wu Y, Du YK, Ma Y, et al. (2011) Association between non-suicidal self-injuries and suicide attempts in Chinese adolescents and college students: a cross-section study. PLoS One 6: e17977.
49. Zhang X, Wang H, Xia Y (2012) Stress, coping and suicide ideation in Chinese college students. J Adolesc 35: 683–690.
50. Zhu XH, Wang CD, Zhou Q, Zhaou HF, Yang YJ, et al. (2011) Study on the factors influencing suicidal ideation among 2374 college students. Chin J Behav and Brain Sci 20: 461–462.
51. Zhao J, Yang X, Xiao R, Zhang X, Aguilera D, et al. (2012) Belief system, meaningfulness, and psychopathology associated with suicidal among Chinese college students: a cross-sectional survey. BMC Public Health 12:668.
52. Wang Y, Guo XL (2010) Survey and analysis of psychological health in 882 higher vocational freshmen. Chin J Sch Doctor 24: 202–204.
53. Gau S S, Chen YY, Tsai FJ, Li MB, Qiu YN, et al. (2008) Risk factors for suicide in Taiwanese college students. J Am Coll Health 57: 135–142.
54. Arria AM, O'Grady KE, Caldeira KM, Vincent KB, Wilcox HC, et al.(2009) Suicide ideation among college students: a multivariate analysis [J]. Arch Suicide Res 13: 230–46.
55. Garlow SJ, Rosenberg J, Moore JD, Haas AP, Koestner B, et al. (2008) Depression, desperation, and suicidal ideation in college students: results from the American Foundation for Suicide Prevention College Screening Project at Emory University. Depress Anxiety 25: 482–488.
56. Mackenzie S, Wiegel JR, Mundt M, Brown D, Saewyc E, et al. (20111) Depression and suicide ideation among students accessing campus health care. Am J Orthopsychiatry 81: 101–108.
57. Park S (2013) Gender-specific factors of suicide ideation among adolescents in the Republic of Korea: a nationally representative population-based study. Arch Psychiatr Nurs 27:253–262.
58. Swahn MS, Palmier JB, Kasirye R, Yao H (2012) Correlates of Suicide Ideation and Attempt among Youth Living in the Slums of Kampala. Int J Environ Res Public Health 9: 596–609.
59. Ellis JB, Lamis DA (2007) Adaptive characteristics and suicidal behavior: a gender comparison of young adults. Death Stud 31:845–854.
60. Canetto SS, Sakinofsky I (1998) The gender paradox in suicide. Suicide Life Threat Behav 14:1–23.
61. Cai Y, Hu N, Liu WN, Wang LJ (2012) Current situation of suicide deaths among Chinese population in 2010. Chin Pre Med 13:480–482.
62. Gunn JR, Lester D, Mcswain S (2011) Testing the warning signs of suicidal behavior among suicide ideators using the 2009 National survey on drug abuse and health. Int J Emerg Ment Health 13: 147–154.
63. Sharp C1, Green KL, Yaroslavsky I, Venta A, Zanarini MC, et al. (2012) The incremental validity of borderline personality disorder relative to major depressive disorder for suicidal ideation and deliberate self-harm in adolescents. J Pers Disord 26: 927–938.
64. Hiramura H, Shono M, Tanaka N, Nagata T, Kotamura T, et al. (2008) Prospective study on suicidal ideation among Japanese undergraduate students: correlation with stressful life events, depression, and depress genic cognitive patterns. Arch Suicide Res 12: 238–250.
65. Silenzio VM, Pena JB, Duberstein PR, Cerel J, Kerry L, et al. (2007) Sexual orientation and risk factors for suicidal ideation and suicide attempts among adolescents and young adults. Am J Public Health 97: 2017–2019.
66. Hardt J, Johnson JG (2010) Suicidality, depression, major and minor negative life events: a mediator model. Psychosoc Med 7: c5.
67. Harris TL, Molock SD (2000) Cultural orientation, family cohesion, and family support in suicide ideation and depression among African American college students. Suicide Life Threat Behav 30:341–53.
68. Lee HS, Kim S, Choi I, Lee KU (2008) Prevalence and Risk Factors Associated with Suicide Ideation and Attempts in Korean College Students. Psychiatry Investig 5: 86–93.
69. Dubow EF, Tisak J, Causey D, Hryshko A, Reid G (1991) A two-year longitudinal study of stressful life events, social support, and social problem-solving skills: contributions to children's behavioral and academic adjustment. Child Dev 62:583–599.
70. Au AC, Lau S, Lee MT (2009) Suicide ideation and depression: the moderation effects of family cohesion and social self-concept. Adolescence 44: 851–868.
71. Wu J, Wu YT, Feng SX, Meng H, Chen H (2012) Mediating effects on depression regarding the relationship between negative life events and suicide ideation among college students. Chin J Epidem 33:1111–1115.
72. Choi JH, Yu M, Kim KE (2014) Suicidal ideation in adolescents: A structural equation modeling approach. Nurs Health Sci. doi: 10.1111/nhs.12142.
73. Sakamoto S, Tanaka E, Kameyama A, Takizawa T, Takizawa S, et al. (2014) The effects of suicide prevention measures reported through a psychoeducational video: A practice in Japan. Int J Soc Psychiatry Epub ahead of print.
74. Iang M, Hu Z, Cao Y (2007) Suicide deaths concentrated in Beijing universities. Am J Psychiatry 164: 1758.

Pro-Inflammatory Cytokines Reduce the Proliferation of NG2 Cells and Increase Shedding of NG2 *In Vivo* and *In Vitro*

Malin Wennström[1]*, Shorena Janelidze[1], Cecilie Bay-Richter[2], Lennart Minthon[1], Lena Brundin[3,4]

1 Lund University, Department of Clinical Sciences, Clinical Memory Research Unit, Wallenberg Laboratory, Malmö, Sweden, **2** Aarhus University, Department of Clinical Medicine, Translational Neuropsychiatry Unit, Risskov, Denmark, **3** Michigan State University, College of Human Medicine, Department of Psychiatry and Behavioral Medicine, Grand Rapids, Michigan, United States of America, **4** Van Andel Research Institute, Laboratory of Behavioral Medicine, Grand Rapids, Michigan, United States of America

Abstract

Neuron glial 2 (NG2) cells become strongly activated in injured brain areas. The activation is characterized by increased proliferation as well as increased expression and shedding of the proteoglycan NG2 expressed on their cell surface. It is currently not known how these cells respond to low-grade neuroinflammation provoked by systemic inflammation. To investigate this, we analyzed NG2 cell proliferation as well as soluble NG2 (sNG2) in cerebrospinal fluid (CSF) from rats treated with an acute intraperitoneal (i.p) injection of lipopolysaccharides (LPS) or saline and sacrificed after 2 or 24 hours. The systemically induced neuroinflammation was confirmed as elevated levels of cytokines, including interleukin (IL)-6 and IL-1β, and MHCII expressing microglia were found 24 h after LPS treatment. At this time point NG2 cell proliferation was significantly decreased in both amygdala and hippocampus and sNG2 levels in CSF were increased twofold. We also exposed human NG2 cells in culture to IL-6 and IL-1β for 24 h and found, in line with our *in vivo* study, a direct impact of these cytokines reducing cell proliferation and increasing shedding of NG2. We conclude that LPS induced systemic inflammation significantly affects NG2 cell proliferation and shedding and that these two events at least in in part are mediated by IL-6 and IL-1β.

Editor: Javier Vitorica, Universidad de Sevilla, Spain

Funding: This work was financed by the Swedish Brain Foundation, Magnus Bergvall Foundation, regional state grants (ALF), the Swedish Research Council (No. K2009-61X-21524-01-1), and the Royal Fysiografiska Society. LB was supported by start-up grants from Michigan State University and Van Andel Research Institute, Grand Rapids, Michigan. The funders had no role in study design, data collection and analysis, decision to publish, or preparation of the manuscript.

Competing Interests: The authors have declared that no competing interests exist.

* Email: malin.wennstrom@med.lu.se

Introduction

The neuron glial 2 (NG2) cell is a glial cell type representing the majority of proliferating cells in the central nervous system (CNS)[1,2,3,4]. The cell population is primarily known to serve as an oligodendrocyte progenitor pool, but many of the NG2 cells, particularly in the gray matter, remain undifferentiated for a significant time. As such, they become well integrated into the cellular network, displaying several interesting properties including forming direct synapses with neurons (for review see[5,6]). Although an increasing number of studies have started to chart the function and properties of NG2 cells, little is known about their role in pathological conditions. Interestingly, rodent studies have shown robust changes in the NG2 cell population in brain areas subjected to focal injury. After stab wound injury or kainite induced lesions, NG2 cells become activated, a state characterized by altered morphology, enhanced proliferation and increased expression of its cell characteristic surface bound proteoglycan NG2 [7,8]. Also stereotactic microinjection of cytokines and lipopolysaccharide (LPS) into the rat brain robustly activates NG2 cells [9]. In addition, damage and neuroinflammatory processes affect the metabolism of surface bound NG2 proteoglycan, as studies have demonstrated an increased amount of soluble (i.e shedded) proteoglycan NG2 (sNG2) in stab-wounded rat cortex [10] and experimental autoimmune encephalomyelitis lesions[11].

The studies mentioned above provide evidence that severe focal injury greatly affects the NG2 cell population, which is of interest when investigating clinical conditions linked to direct brain damage such as stroke, wounds or concussions. However, milder or chronic alterations in the cellular environment may also provoke pathological conditions in the brain. Although the brain long was considered to be an immuno-privileged site [12] it has become clear that systemic inflammation can induce specific immunological mechanisms within the brain. The underlying mechanisms are not completely understood, but both direct transmission of peripherally derived cytokines across the blood-brain-barrier (BBB) and indirect effects on afferent nerves, such as the vagus nerve, have been described (for review see [13]). Studies using LPS to induce systemic inflammation show a marked increase of microglial activity. These alterations include enhanced MHC II expression [14], up-regulation of ED-1 (indicative of lysosomal activity) [15], morphological changes [14,16,17] and increased levels of the microglial derived proinflammatory cytokines, such as tumor necrosis factor alpha (TNF- α) [18] and interleukin 1β (IL-1β)[19]. Furthermore, post-mortem studies on brain tissue from patients with sepsis show increased microglia expression of ED-1 and MHC II [20] and patients with invasive meningococcal disease (IMD) are known to display elevated levels of several cytokines in the cerebrospinal fluid (CSF)[21].

Although there are several studies demonstrating microglial activity in response to systemic inflammation, there are to our knowledge few (if any) reports describing how the NG2 cell population reacts upon these pathological events. In the current study we therefore investigate whether systemically induced neuroinflammation, induced by intraperitoneal injection of LPS, affects the NG2 cell population in regard to proliferation and morphological changes. We also analyzed the sNG2 levels in CSF of the LPS treated rats to establish whether changes in sNG2 levels correlate to NG2 cell population alterations in the brain. Finally, in order to determine whether cytokines have a direct impact on proliferation of NG2 cells and sNG2 shedding, we stimulated human NG2-expressing oligodendrocyte progenitor cells (further referred to as human NG2 cells in this text) with the cytokines IL-8, IL-6, IL-4 and IL-1β.

Materials and Methods

Animals

Adult male Wistar rats (Harlan Laboratories, Holland) weighing 250–300 g were used. Experimental procedures were approved by the Swedish Board of Agriculture (Jordbruksverket) and carried out according to the guidelines set by the Ethical Committee for Use of Laboratory Animals in the Lund/Malmö region. Three rats were housed in each cage on a 12 hours light/dark cycle with access to food and water ad libitum. Since previous studies have shown that microglia and NG2 cells become reactive within 8–24 h after injury [8,22] we conducted two studies with different survival time points, before and during glial activation i) LPS2h: 2 h survival after LPS (n = 9) and saline treatment (n = 9) and ii) LPS24h: 24 h survival after LPS (n = 8) and saline treatment (n = 9).

Administration of lipopolysaccaride

Rats received a single intraperitoneal injection of 5 mg/kg of bacterial LPS (Escherichia coli serotype 055:B5; SIGMA, St Louis, MO) in sterile physiological saline. This dose is adequate to induce inflammation in the brain, but not lethal sepsis [18]. Control groups received sterile physiological saline.

Sample collection

Rats were anesthetized with sodium pentobarbital 60 mg/ml and after the disappearance of nociceptive reflexes, the cerebrospinal fluid from the cisterna magna was collected according to procedure described previously [23]. Briefly, a stereotaxic instrument horizontally fixed the rat head, whereas the rest of the body was lying vertically. A needle connected to a syringe was inserted vertically between the occipital protuberance and the spine of the atlas and the CSF was collected with a gentle aspiration.

Blood samples were collected by cardiac puncture and kept at room temperature (RT) for 1 h, followed by centrifugation at 4°C, 1300 × g for 10 minutes and serum collection. CSF and serum samples were stored in −80°C. Finally, after the CSF and blood collection, the rats were transcardially perfused with 0.9% saline (50 ml), followed by 4% ice-cold paraformaldehyde (250 ml). Brains were postfixed in 4% paraformaldehyde at 4°C for 4 hours and thereafter in 30% sucrose in PBS until they sank. Coronal sections (40 μm) of the entire brain were cut on a freezing microtome and stored in antifreeze cryoprotectant solution at − 20°C.

Cytokine analysis

Multiplex ultra-sensitive electrochemiluminescence immunoassay (Meso Scale Discovery, UK) was used for quantification of the following cytokines in rat CSF and blood samples: interferon gamma (IFN- γ), interleukine-13 (IL-13), interleukin-1 beta (IL-1ß), interleukin-4 (IL-4), interleukin-5 (IL-5), interleukin-6 (IL-6), tumor necrosis factor alpha (TNF- α) and chemokine growth-related oncogeneCXCL1 (rGro/KC), as previously described [24]. Standards and samples were analyzed in duplicates. Detection limits for the different cytokines in serum were as follows: IFN- γ: 9.65 pg/ml, IL-13: 17 pg/ml, IL-1ß: 26.8 pg/ml, IL-4: 12.3 pg/ml, IL-5: 27.5 pg/ml,rGro/KC:132 pg/ml and TNF- α: 23.1 pg/ml. The detections limits for cytokines in CSF were: IFN- γ: 33.2 pg/ml, IL-13: 146 pg/ml, IL-1ß: 34.8 pg/ml, IL-4: 9.86 pg/ml, IL-5: 49.2 pg/ml, TNF- α: 131 pg/ml and rGro/KC:645 pg/ml. The detection limits for IL-6 in serum and CSF were17.7 and 35.2 pg/ml, respectively. Samples with zero cytokine levels were assigned the value of the respective detection limit.

Immunohistological staining procedures

Reactive microglia and proliferating NG2 cells were investigated by double immunofluorescence stainings. The following primary antibodies were used: rabbit anti-NG2 (1:500, Millipore, Temecula, USA), rabbit anti-Iba-1 (1:200; Wako, Neuss, Germany) mouse-anti- RT1B against MHC II (1:500, AbDSerotec, Oxford, UK) and rabbit anti Ki67 (1:200, Abcam, Cambridge, UK). The latter antibody is directed against the endogenous proliferation marker Ki67 [25] and stain cells dividing at the time point of perfusion, which is of importance when assessing alteration in ongoing cell proliferation at different time points [26]. Sections were incubated with the primary antibodies (Iba-1/MHCII and NG2/ki67) overnight at 4°C and were the following day incubated with Alexa 488 conjugated goat anti-rabbit (1:200; Vector BA-1000, Vector Laboratories Inc., Burlingame, CA, USA) and Cy3 conjugated horse anti-mouse (1:200; Jackson Immunoresearch, West Grove, PA, USA) for 2 hours in room temperature (RT). Thereafter the sections were mounted in Vectashield anti-fading mounting medium with DAPI (Vector Laboratories, Burlingame, CA).

Alterations in NG2 immunoreactivity were investigated using immunohistochemistry (IHC).

Data analysis of immunohistological stainings

Number of proliferating NG2-cells (NG2+/Ki67+) and MHCII expressing microglia were analyzed in the medial prefrontal cortex (mPFC), the basolateral nucleus (BL) of amygdala and the granular cell layer (GCL), the dentate hilus and the molecular layer (ML) of hippocampus. Analysis of the number of Ki67+ cells in the GCL was confined to the subgranular zone (SGZ) and cells extending into the dentate hilus, but being part of clusters of Ki67+ cells in the SGZ, were included. Cells were counted bilaterally through the mid-dorsal part of hippocampus (−2.8 mm to −4.52 mm relative to the bregma, 5 sections per animal). Amygdala was analyzed, according to previously described guidelines [27,28], through the mid-part of the rostrocaudal extension of the basolateral nucleus (−2.65 mm to −3.40 mm relative to the bregma, 3 section per animal). Medial prefrontal cortex (−2.65 mm to −3.40 mm relative to the bregma, 3 section per animal) was analyzed according to previously described guidelines [29]. The chosen coordinates give a maximal cross-sectional diameter of the analyzed regions and a minimum change in counted area size per section. To further ensure that the sizes of the analyzed regions did not differ between treatment groups, we quantified the cross-sectional areas of the NG2-stained sections using CellSense dimension software (Olympus Optical Co., Ltd., Tokyo, Japan). None of the regions analyzed differed in size between treatment groups (Table S1). All Iba-1+, MHCII+ and NG2+/Ki67+ cells were counted using an Olympus BX41 epifluorescence microscope with a 40× objective (Olympus Optical Co., Ltd., Tokyo, Japan). When counting MHCII +cells, we differentiated between dendritic MHCII, indicative of activated microglia, and non-dendritic MHCII+ cells. Since NG2 is expressed on both pericytes and glial cells in the rat brain, we only counted NG2+ cells with the specific morphological features of NG2 expressing glial cells (i.e. dendritic NG2 cells). Before counting double-labeled cells in the epifluorescencemicroscope, we confirmed that our judgment of a double-labeled cell was correct using a confocal laser-scanning microscope (Leica TCS SL, Heidelberg, Germany). Number of cells per section and region was determined and the values were averaged and presented as the mean cell number per section and region.

Cell culture studies

Primary fetal human brain oligodendrocyte progenitors bought from the commercial company ScienCell Research Laboratories (Carlsbad, USA) were cultured in OPC medium (ScienCell Research Laboratories, Carlsbad, USA). The cells were grown as monolayers in poly-L-lysine (PLL) coated culture flasks in humified air with 5% CO_2 at 37°C until 80–90 % confluent. The cells were thereafter harvested by gentle scraping and plated in poly-L-lysine coated 96 well ViewPlates (Perkin Elmer, Waltham, MA USA) and grown until 70% confluent. For cell experiment the culture media was removed and replaced by OPC medium containing either 0.3 ng/ml human recombinant IL-1β, 150 pg/ml human recombinant IL-4, 1.5 ng/ml human recombinant IL-6 or 20 ng/ml human recombinant IL-8. The cytokine concentration chosen were based on the concentrations found in the rat CSF 2 h after LPS treatment. Cells exposed to normal OPC medium were used as controls cells. Labeling of proliferating cells was performed using Click-iT EdU Alexa Fluor 488 Imaging Kit (Life technologies, Waltham, MA USA) according to the suppliers instructions. The thymidine analog EdU was added to the cell cultures directly after cytokine supplementation. The cells were thereafter incubated for 24 h at 37°C in 5% CO_2. The experiment was independently repeated 6 times in duplicates. After treatment the cell culture supernatants were collected, centrifuged (275× g, 5 min, 4°C), aliquoted and stored at −80°C until used. Cell culture purity was analyzed by immunocytoflourenscence staining against NG2 and PDGFR-AA. Cells were fixed with 2% formaldehyde and unspecific binding was blocked by PBS containing 1% BSA (Boehringer Mannheim, Kircheim, Germany) and 5% goat serum (Jackson immunoresearch, West Grove, USA). The cells were thereafter incubated with either mouse anti-human NG2 (1:200 Millipore, Darmstadt, Germany) or rabbit anti-PDGF-AAR in blocking solution (1:200 Abcam, Cambridge, UK followed by an incubation with the secondary antibodies (dylight549-conjugated anti-rabbit Igs (1:500 Molecular probes) or Cy3-conjugated anti-mouse Igs (1:500, Jackson Immunoresearch, West Grove, USA). Analysis of DAPI staining (n = 200) showed that the majority of DAPI positive cells (>97%) expressed NG2 and PDGFR-AA. Proliferation of cells was measured by analyzing the ratio of EdU positive cell area to DAPI positive cell area. The number of DAPI positive cells for each assessment was more than 200. The area of EdU positive cells and DAPI positive cells was determined using CellSense dimension software (Olympus Optical Co., Ltd., Tokyo, Japan).

NG2 quantification assay

Levels of soluble NG2 in rat CSF and in supernatants from cultured human NG2 cells were analyzed with an in-house assay using the Mesoscale Discovery (MSD) electrochemiluminescence (ECL) technology employing immunoassay conversion kits (MSD, Rockville, USA) as described previously[30]. In brief, samples were diluted in PBS and coated onto MSD multi array plates in duplicate wells (25μl) and allowed to adhere overnight at 4°C. The following day wells were rinsed and incubated with blocking solution (1% BSA containing 1% milk in PBS-T) for 1 h at RT followed by another rinse and incubation with mouse anti NG2 antibody (1:100, clone B5, ATCC kind gift from Dr William Stallcup) for 2 h at RT on an orbital shaker. Wells were then rinsed and incubated with sulfo-Tag goat-anti mouse antibody (MSD, Rockville, USA) for 1 h in RT on an orbital shaker. Recombinant rat NG2 (kind gift from Dr William Stallcup) or recombinant human NG2 (Origene technologies) was used as standard. Resulting ECL signal was quantified using an MSD SECTOR Imager 6000. Readings of the duplicate standards and samples were averaged and NG2 concentrations determined by interpolation of a 4 parametric curve fit. Detection limit of the rat NG2 analysis was determined to be 33.40ng/ml, whereas detection limit of the human NG2 analysis was 2.28 pg/ml.

Statistical analysis

Statistical analysis was performed using the SPSS software (version 20.0 for Windows, SPSS Inc., Chicago, IL, USA). Cytokine data was analyzed with Mann-Whitney Test due to a non normal distribution. The *in vivo* cell counting studies as well as the NG2 fraction study and fibrinogen area study were analyzed with student t-test. Differences in rat CSF NG2 concentrations were assessed by Student t-test. Data are presented as mean ± SEM with a statistical significance set to $p<0.05$. The sNG2 levels and ratio of EdU+ cell area to DAPI + cell area assessed in the *in vitro* study was analyzed using Paired T-test.

Results

Blood and CNS cytokine changes after systemically administered LPS

In order to confirm systemic inflammation after LPS treatment we analyzed cytokine and chemokine levels in serum 2 h and 24 h after treatment. Levels of IL-13, IL-1β, IL-4, TNF-α, IL-6 and rGro/KCwere significantly increased in rats treated with LPS compared to controls 2 hours after treatment (Table 1). After 24 hours, the IL-13, IL-4 and TNF-α levels in LPS treated rats were reduced back to baseline levels and they no longer differed significantly from controls. Although the levels of IL-1β, IL-6 and rGro/KC were still significantly elevated 24 hours after LPS treatment (Table 1), we noted a drastic decline also in theses cytokines (18- fold ($p<0.001$), 63- fold ($p<0.001$) and 150-fold ($p<0.001$), respectively).

To verify that the systemic inflammation led to inflammation in the CNS compartment, we moreover analyzed cytokine and chemokine levels in CSF 2 h and 24 h after LPS treatment. Analysis of CSF showed a significant increase in IL-1β, IL-4, TNF-α and IL-6, rGro/KC levels 2 hours after the LPS treatment (Table 2). In contrast to the transient cytokine elevations in blood, IL-1β and IL-6 continued to increase in CSF 24 hours after the

Table 1. Serum cytokine levels (pg/ml) 2 h and 24 h after LPS and saline treatment.

	Saline2h	LPS2h	Saline24h	LPS24h
IFN-γ	9.65 ± 0.00[a]	19.05 ± 3.80	9.65 ± 0.00 [a]	9.65 ± 0.00 [a]
IL-13	17.00 ± 0.00 [a]	*44.63 ± 8.73	17.00 ± 0.00 [a]	17.00 ± 0.00 [a]
IL-1β	34.57 ± 7.77	***612.81 ± 101.98	26.80 ± 0.00 [a]	*33.7 ± 3.55
IL-4	12.3 ± 0.00 [a]	***22.63 ± 2.13	12.30 ± 0.00 [a]	19.32 ± 7.02
IL-5	27.50 ± 0.00 [a]	49.98 ± 9.59	27.50 ± 0.00 [a]	27.50 ± 0.00
TNF-α	23.63 ± 0.53	***17058.92 ± 6145.95	23.10 ± 0.00 [a]	23.10 ± 0.00 [a]
IL-6	35.61 ±2.53	***10920.36 ± 1522.67	35.09 ± 2.36	***76.06 ± 8.95
rGro/KC	145.43 ± 13.05	***19115.55 ± 684.37	135.73 ± 3.73	**306.19 ± 50.36

Values represent means ± SEM * $p = 0.01$, ** $p = 0.001$ and *** $p = 0.001$ indicates a significant difference compared to controls. [a]indicate values set that were to detection limit.

LPS treatment (Table 2). IL-4 and rGro/KC levels, although still significantly higher compared to control, declined somewhat after 24 hours. Levels of TNF-α in LPS treated rats were no longer significantly increased compared to controls 24 hours after the LPS treatment (Table 2). Cerebrospinal fluid levels of IFN-γ, IL-13 and IL-5 were below detection limit both 2 and 24 hours after LPS treatment.

Microglial activity in response to systemic LPS administration

Immunohistochemical analysis of microglial activation showed that the number of dendritic MHC II expressing cells did not differ in any of the examined areas when comparing LPS treated rats with controls 2 h after treatment (Table S2). However, enhanced numbers of MHCII expressing microglia were found in all examined brain areas (i.e. BL of amygdala, ML, hilus and GCL of hippocampus and mPFC) 24 hours after the LPS treatment (figure 1).

Alterations in the NG2 cell population after systemically administered LPS

To evaluate the impact of systemically administered LPS on NG2 cells we investigated changes in NG2 cell proliferation and NG2 shedding. Staining against Ki67 together with NG2 (figure 2) showed no significant difference in NG2+/Ki67+ cell number in any of the examined areas when comparing LPS treated rats to controls 2 h after treatment (figure 2). However, a significant reduction in the number of NG2+/Ki67+ cells was found in BL ($p = 0.028$), Hilus ($p = 0.002$) and ML ($p < 0.0001$) of LPS treated rats compared to controls at the later time-point at 24 h after treatment. No reduction in NG2 cell proliferation was detected in the mPFC at the 24 h survival time point (figure 2).

Less than 1% of the NG2 cells displayed morphological changes in all the groups. A decline in number of Ki67+ cells in the subgranular zone (SGZ) was also detected 24 hours after LPS treatment (figure 2). Finally, no significant changes in CSF sNG2 levels were detected at 2 h, while at 24 h after treatment sNG2 levels were significantly increased in rats treated with LPS compared to controls (figure 3).

Altered proliferation and NG2 shedding of human NG2 cells after cytokine exposure

Human NG2 cells were treated with IL-1β, IL-4, IL-6 and IL-8 in concentrations correlating to the CSF concentrations found at 2 hours, and left in culture for 24 hours. Analysis of the cell culture supernatant showed that IL-1β ($p = 0.016$), IL-4 ($p = 0.038$) and IL-6 $p = 0.005$, but not IL-8, significantly increased the levels of sNG2 (figure 4). Moreover, the proliferation analysis, where fraction of EdU positive cell area/DAPI positive cell area was used as a measure of proliferation, revealed a significant decreased proliferation of NG2 cells stimulated with IL-1β ($p = 0.039$), and IL-6 ($p = 0.009$), but not IL-4 or IL-8 (figure 4).

Table 2. CSF cytokine levels (pg/ml) 2 h and 24 h after LPS and saline treatment.

	Saline2h	LPS2h	Saline24h	LPS24h
IFN-γ	33.20 ± 0.00 [a]	33.20 ± 0.00 [a]	33.20 ± 0.00 [a]	33.20 ± 0.00 [a]
IL-13	146 ± 0.00 [a]	146 ± 0.00 [a]	146.00 ± 0.00[a]	146.00 ± 0.00 [a]
IL-1β	34.80 ± 0.00 [a]	*58.96 ± 10.81	34.80 ± 0.00	***294.54 ± 40.18
IL-4	9.86 ± 0.00 [a]	**33.81 ± 10.94	9.86 ± 0.00	**15.11 ± 1.97
IL-5	49.20 ± 0.00 [a]	49.20 ± 0.00	49.20 ± 0.00	49.20 ± 0.00 [a]
TNF-α	131.00 ± 0.00 [a]	*202.44 ± 30.59	131.00 ± 0.00 [a]	131.00 ±0.00 [a]
IL-6	35.20 ± 0.00 [a]	***296.90 ± 112.17	35.20 ± 0.00 [a]	***975. 23 ± 197.47
rGro/KC	645.00 ± 0.00 [a]	***4605.36 ± 1213.70	645.00 ± 0.00 [a]	***3250.62 ± 280.10

Values represent means ± SEM * $p = 0.01$, ** $p = 0.001$ and *** $p = 0.001$ indicates a significant difference compared to controls. [a] indicate values set that were to detection limit.

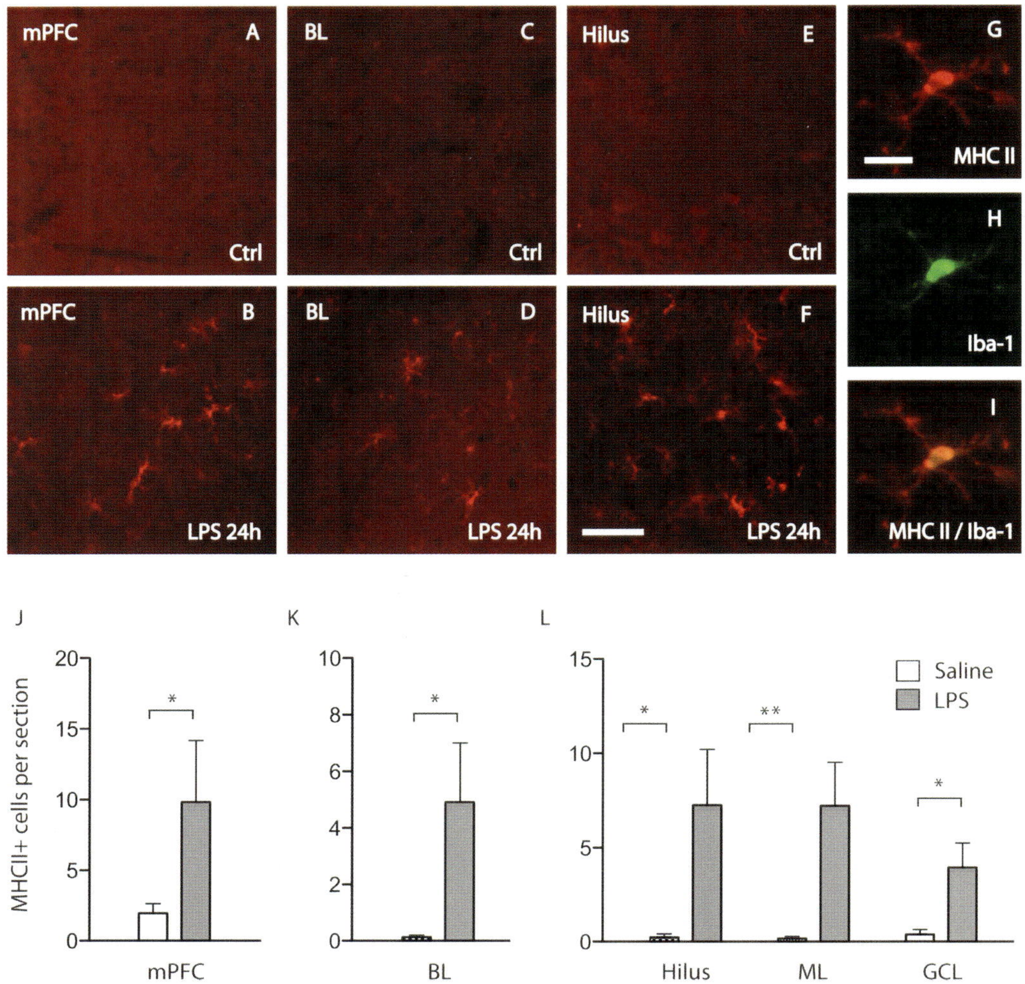

Figure 1. Microglial activity in response to systemic lipopolysaccharide treatment. Images in (A–L) demonstrate immunoflourescence stainings of dendritic MHCII+ cells in the medial prefrontal cortex (mPFC), basolateral nucleus of amygdala (BL) and hippocampus (Hilus) 24 hours after LPS treatment (LPS) (B, D, F) and saline treatment (Ctrl) (A, C, E). Scale bar = 80μm. Images to the right show a microglia double-labeled with antibodies directed towards MHC II (G) and Iba-1 (H). Images (G) and (H) are superimposed in (I). Scale bar = 10 μm. Bar graphs in (J-L) show a significant increase in number of dendritic MHCII+ cells per section of mPFC (J), BL (K) and Hilus, molecular layer (ML) and granular cell layer (GCL) (L) 24 h after LPS treatment (LPS) compared to saline treatment (Saline). ** indicates a significant difference at $p<0.01$ level. * indicates a significant difference at $p<0.05$ level.

Discussion

We here demonstrate significantly decreased numbers of newly formed NG2 cells in the rat amygdala and hippocampus and an almost 2-fold increase of soluble NG2 in CSF 24 h after systemic LPS treatment. At this time-point the systemic inflammation had ceased, although the CSF cytokines remained elevated which was paralleled by increased numbers of MHC II expressing microglia. Our *in vitro* experiment on human NG2 cells confirmed a direct impact of the cytokines IL-1β and IL-6 decreasing proliferation and increasing NG2 shedding.

Our results show that low-grade neuroinflammation has an inhibitory effect on NG2 cell proliferation. This result stands in contrast with previous studies demonstrating increased proliferation of NG2 cells in brain areas with severe focal brain injury [7,8]. Nevertheless, it should be emphasized that milder neuroinflammation induced by peripherally derived cytokines does not affect proliferation of brain cells in the same way as a direct brain injury. This is exemplified by the fact that stereotactic intracranial injections with LPS increase hippocampal neurogenesis [31], whereas systemically administered LPS instead has been shown to decrease neurogenesis [32,33,34]. In line with these findings, also our study showed decreased number of Ki67+ cells in the SGZ (the hippocampal area were neurogenesis occurs) 24 h after LPS stimulation. Supporting our in vivo results, the culture experiment, where we stimulated human NG2 cells for 24 h with IL-4, IL-6, IL-1β or IL-8 (the latter is the human homologue for rGro/KC), further showed that the cytokines IL-6 and IL-1β specifically inhibit proliferation of NG2 cells. Both IL-1β and IL-6 are produced by activated microglia [35,36,37] and interestingly, an impact on NG2 cell proliferation by microglial-derived factors, but not by factors derived from astrocytes and perineuronal macrophages [38], has been observed before. Whole medium from LPS stimulated microglial cultures has previously shown to inhibit NG2 cell renewal [39]. These results suggests an intimate link between microglial activity and NG2 cell proliferation, an idea supported by the number of studies showing a simultaneously activation of NG2 cells and microglia in response to external stimuli[27,40]. Microglia and NG2 cells are moreover commonly found spatially

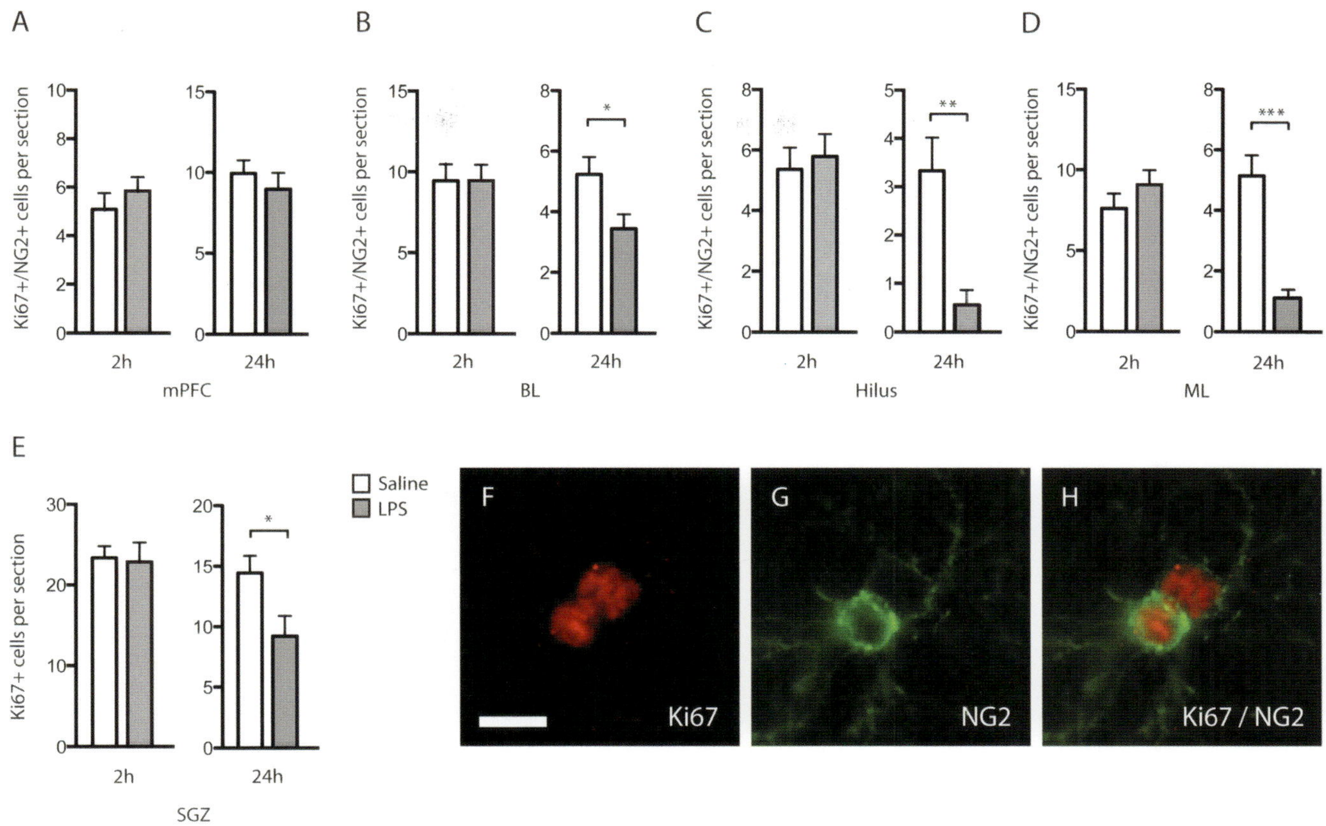

Figure 2. Proliferation of NG2+ cells in response to systemic lipopolysaccharide treatment. Unaltered number of NG2+/ki67+ cell numbers was found in the medial prefrontal cortex (mPFC) (A), the basolateral nucleus (BL) (B), the dentate hilus (Hilus) (C) and the molecular layer (ML) (D) 2 h after lipopolysaccharides (LPS) treatment compared to saline treatment (Saline). In contrast, a significant decreased number of NG2+/ki67+ cells were detected in the BL (B), the Hilus (C) and the ML (D), but not in the mPFC (A), 24 h after LPS treatment compared to saline treatment. The number of Ki67+ cell in the subgranular zone (SGZ) of the hippocampal granular cell layer (E) was also unaltered after 2 h, but significantly reduced 24 h after LPS compared to saline treatment. *** indicates a significant difference at $p<0.001$ level. ** indicates a significant difference at $p<0.01$ level. * indicates a significant difference at $p<0.05$ level. Images in (F–H) demonstrate a double immunoflourescence staining with antibodies directed against the endogenous proliferation marker Ki67 (F) and NG2 (G). Images (F) and (G) are superimposed in (H). Scale bar = 10 μm.

close to each other in the brain parenchyma [40]. Our own study demonstrating decreased NG2 cell proliferation at the same time point as the expression of MHC II is increased in microglia further support the notion of an interdependent relation between these cell types.

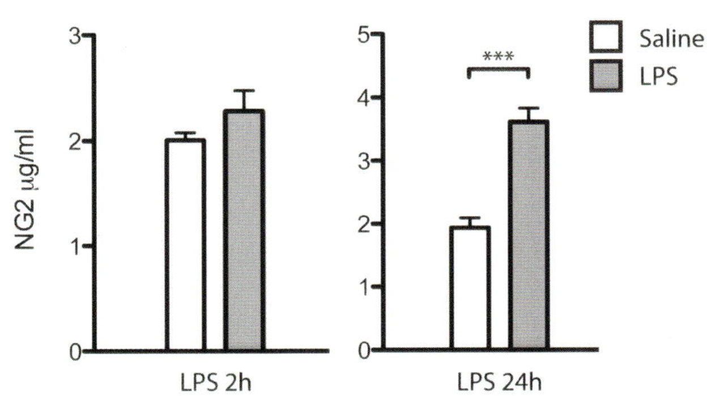

Figure 3. Levels of sNG2 in CSF from rats 2 h and 24 h after LPS treatment. Levels of CSF sNG2 were not significantly altered 2 h after LPS treatment compared to saline treatment (Saline), but 24 h after LPS treatment CSF sNG2 levels were significantly increased compared to saline treatment.*** indicates a significant difference at $p<0.001$ level.

Microglia has been shown to express NG2 in response to systemically administered LPS [41], an event that could potentially confound our findings on NG2 cell proliferation. However, the NG2 expressing microglia cells are hypertrophic and amoebic in shape, displaying features of strongly activated microglia. In our study, we found very few NG2 cells with amoebic morphology and when counting NG2+/Ki67+ cells we only included cells that displayed the well-characterized NG2 cell ramified morphology. Hence, we found that the risk of including any potential NG2 expressing microglia in our analysis was extremely low. In addition, any confounding effects would be expected to be in the opposite direction (increased proliferation) in case microglial cells would have been included.

As mentioned in the introduction, previous studies have shown an increased amount of shedded NG2 in brain areas exposed to damage. The specific function of the shedded form of the transmembrane proteoglycan NG2 is still mainly unrevealed, but several studies indicate a role for the surface bound proteoglycan in NG2 cell proliferation. Decreased proliferation is found in the presence of antibodies directed against NG2[42,43] and NG2 null mice pups show a delayed generation of new NG2 cells in developing white matter [44]. Moreover, renewal of NG2 cells in demyelinating lesions in the brain of NG2 null mice is decreased compared to wild type mice[45]. The proteoglycan has been

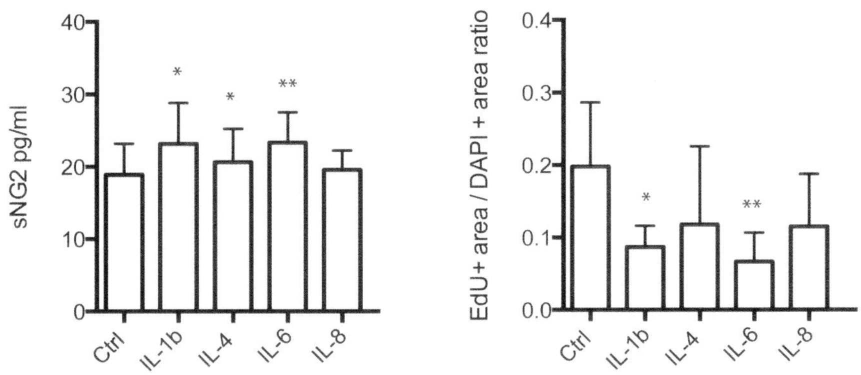

Figure 4. Proliferation and supernatant sNG2 levels of cultured human NG2 cells after exposure cytokines. The left bar graph shown the significantly increased sNG2 levels found in cell culture supernatant after 24 h stimulation with interleukin (IL)-1β (0.3 ng/ml), IL-6 (1.5 ng/ml) and IL-4 (150 pg/ml). The sNG2 levels were not altered in response to 20 ng/ml IL-8. The right bar graph demonstrates the significantly decreased EdU + cell area to DAPI cell area ratio after exposure to IL-1b and IL-6, but not after IL-8 or IL-4. * indicates a significant difference at $p<0.05$ level, ** indicates a significant difference at $p<0.01$ level.

suggested to affect proliferation via its ability to bind directly to the two NG2 cell mitogens, platelet derived growth factor AA (PDGF-AA) and basic fibroblast growth factor (bFGF) [46], enhancing the binding of these growth factors to their receptors[47]. It may thus be suggested that an increased shedding of NG2 leaves less NG2 on the cell surface, which in turn reduce the possibility to anchor the mitogens, consequently causing a reduced proliferation. Such a hypothesis would explain the opposing effect on NG2 cell proliferation (decreased) and sNG2 levels (increased) found in our *in vitro* and *in vivo* study. The fact that we detected increased levels of the shedded NG2 in CSF raises the possibility that it might function as a biomarker for pathological states involving NG2 cells. However it should be pointed out that NG2 cells are not the only brain cell type expressing NG2. Pericytes [48] also express NG2, something that must be kept in mind when interpreting the result of changes of sNG2 levels in CSF.

The reduced NG2 cell proliferation in response to systemic inflammation, as seen in our LPS treated rats, should be viewed from the fact that NG2 cells over the years have been shown to possess important and unique properties. Besides functioning as oligodendrocyte progenitors, they form multiple contacts with surrounding astrocytes and neurons (for review see [49]), contact nodes of Ranvier [50], stabilize neuronal synapses (for review see [51]) and promote axonal outgrowth [52], all properties dependent on the NG2 proteoglycan. Given this recognized role for NG2 cells in the neuronal network, it is reasonable to hypothesize that an inhibition of renewal of these cells and a loss of the surface bound NG2 could have an important impact on brain function and behavior. From this perspective it is interesting that downregulation of NG2 cells proliferation have been observed in rats chronically treated with corticosterone [1,53], in rats exposed to chronic social stress [54] as well as in rats exposed to chronic mild stress [55], all treatments known to induce depressive-like behavior[54,56]. Moreover, the down-regulation of NG2 cells proliferation in these rat models of depression were reversed by antidepressant treatments [53,54,55]. Also clinical studies indicate a link between depression and cells of the oligodendrocyte linage, as studies on postmortem brain tissue from depressive patients have revealed decreased number of oligodendrocytes in amygdala and prefrontal cortex [57,58] as well as white matter changes and downregulation of oligodendrocytes genes (for review see [59]).

The reduced renewal of NG2 cells in neuroinflammation is particularly interesting given the increasing amount of clinical studies demonstrating a strong link between systemic inflammation and depressive behavior. For example, in humans certain infections induce a condition known as sickness behaviour, characterized by depressive symptoms [60]. Patients undergoing cytokine therapy often develop symptoms of depression [61] and elevated levels of cytokines (including IL-6 and IL-1β) are found in both blood and CSF from depressed patients [62,63,64,65]. Finally, rats exposed to systemically administered LPS and IL-1β show depressive-like behaviour [66,67,68] and increased microglial activation in several depression associated brain regions (including hippocampus, amygdala and prefrontal cortex)[17,69].

Conclusions

Our results show that systemically administered LPS induces neuroinflammation and reduces NG2 cell proliferation in the rat brain, which can be monitored by analysis of shedded NG2 levels in CSF. These results add to a growing body of evidence that systemic inflammation might have profound effects on both the extra cellular milieu and distinct cell populations in the CNS; findings likely to be of importance for symptoms in depression and sickness behaviour.

Supporting Information

Table S1 Cross-sectional areas of NG2-stained brain sections from lipopolysaccharide and saline treated rats. mPFC = medial prefrontal cortex, BL = basolateral nuclei, ML = molecular layer, Hilus = dentate hilus, GCL = granular cell layer, LPS = lipopolysaccharide. Values are presented as mean ± SEM and analyzed using student t-test. All p-value>0.05 when 2 h and 24 h groups were compared to respective saline group.

Table S2 Number of MHC II expressing microglia 2 h after saline and lipopolysaccharide treatment. mPFC = medial prefrontal cortex, BL = basolateral nuclei, ML = molecular layer, Hilus = dentate hilus, GCL = granular cell layer, LPS = lipopolysaccharide. Values are presented as mean ± SEM and analyzed using student t-test. All p-value>0.05 when 2 h and 24 h groups were compared to respective saline group.

Acknowledgments

We thank Ludvig Hallberg (Lund University, Lund, Sweden) for assistance during the collection of rat CSF. We also thank Dr William Stallcup (Burnham Institute, La Jolla, CA) for the B5 antibody and the rat NG2 recombinant protein used in the NG2 quantification assay.

Author Contributions

Conceived and designed the experiments: MW LB. Performed the experiments: MW SJ CBR. Analyzed the data: MW SJ. Contributed reagents/materials/analysis tools: MW LM LB. Wrote the paper: MW SJ CBR LM LB.

References

1. Alonso G (2000) Prolonged corticosterone treatment of adult rats inhibits the proliferation of oligodendrocyte progenitors present throughout white and gray matter regions of the brain. Glia 31: 219–231.
2. Dawson MR, Polito A, Levine JM, Reynolds R (2003) NG2-expressing glial progenitor cells: an abundant and widespread population of cycling cells in the adult rat CNS. Molecular and Cellular Neurosciences 24: 476–488.
3. Geha S, Pallud J, Junier MP, Devaux B, Leonard N, et al. (2010) NG2+/Olig2+ cells are the major cycle-related cell population of the adult human normal brain. Brain Pathology 20: 399–411.
4. Tamura Y, Kataoka Y, Cui Y, Takamori Y, Watanabe Y, et al. (2007) Multi-directional differentiation of doublecortin- and NG2-immunopositive progenitor cells in the adult rat neocortex in vivo. The European journal of neuroscience 25: 3489-3498.
5. Trotter J, Karram K, Nishiyama A (2010) NG2 cells: Properties, progeny and origin. Brain Res Rev 63: 72–82.
6. Wang A, He BP (2009) Characteristics and functions of NG2 cells in normal brain and neuropathology. Neurological Research 31: 144–150.
7. Hampton DW, Rhodes KE, Zhao C, Franklin RJ, Fawcett JW (2004) The responses of oligodendrocyte precursor cells, astrocytes and microglia to a cortical stab injury, in the brain. Neuroscience 127: 813–820.
8. Ong WY, Levine JM (1999) A light and electron microscopic study of NG2 chondroitin sulfate proteoglycan-positive oligodendrocyte precursor cells in the normal and kainate-lesioned rat hippocampus. Neuroscience 92: 83–95.
9. Rhodes KE, Raivich G, Fawcett JW (2006) The injury response of oligodendrocyte precursor cells is induced by platelets, macrophages and inflammation-associated cytokines. Neuroscience 140: 87–100.
10. Asher RA, Morgenstern DA, Properzi F, Nishiyama A, Levine JM, et al. (2005) Two separate metalloproteinase activities are responsible for the shedding and processing of the NG2 proteoglycan in vitro. Molecular and cellular neurosciences 29: 82–96.
11. Moransard M, Dann A, Staszewski O, Fontana A, Prinz M, et al. (2011) NG2 expressed by macrophages and oligodendrocyte precursor cells is dispensable in experimental autoimmune encephalomyelitis. Brain: a journal of neurology 134: 1315–1330.
12. Larsson LC, Widner H (2000) Neural tissue xenografting. Scandinavian journal of immunology 52: 249–256.
13. Dantzer R (2009) Cytokine, sickness behavior, and depression. Immunol Allergy Clin North Am 29: 247–264.
14. Buttini M, Limonta S, Boddeke HW (1996) Peripheral administration of lipopolysaccharide induces activation of microglial cells in rat brain. Neurochem Int 29: 25–35.
15. Semmler A, Okulla T, Sastre M, Dumitrescu-Ozimek L, Heneka MT (2005) Systemic inflammation induces apoptosis with variable vulnerability of different brain regions. J Chem Neuroanat 30: 144–157.
16. Nishioku T, Dohgu S, Takata F, Eto T, Ishikawa N, et al. (2009) Detachment of brain pericytes from the basal lamina is involved in disruption of the blood-brain barrier caused by lipopolysaccharide-induced sepsis in mice. Cell Mol Neurobiol 29: 309–316.
17. Sugama S, Takenouchi T, Fujita M, Conti B, Hashimoto M (2009) Differential microglial activation between acute stress and lipopolysaccharide treatment. J Neuroimmunol 207: 24–31.
18. Qin L, Wu X, Block ML, Liu Y, Breese GR, et al. (2007) Systemic LPS causes chronic neuroinflammation and progressive neurodegeneration. Glia 55: 453–462.
19. Quan N, Sundar SK, Weiss JM (1994) Induction of interleukin-1 in various brain regions after peripheral and central injections of lipopolysaccharide. Journal of Neuroimmunology 49: 125–134.
20. Lemstra AW, Groen in't Woud JC, Hoozemans JJ, van Haastert ES, Rozemuller AJ, et al. (2007) Microglia activation in sepsis: a case-control study. J Neuroinflammation 4: 4.
21. Beran O, Lawrence DA, Andersen N, Dzupova O, Kalmusova J, et al. (2009) Sequential analysis of biomarkers in cerebrospinal fluid and serum during invasive meningococcal disease. European journal of clinical microbiology & infectious diseases: official publication of the European Society of Clinical Microbiology 28: 793–799.
22. Streit WJ, Walter SA, Pennell NA (1999) Reactive microgliosis. Prog Neurobiol 57: 563–581.
23. Erhardt S, Engberg G (2002) Increased phasic activity of dopaminergic neurones in the rat ventral tegmental area following pharmacologically elevated levels of endogenous kynurenic acid. Acta Physiol Scand 175: 45–53.
24. Bay-Richter C, Hallberg L, Ventorp F, Janelidze S, Brundin L (2012) Aldosterone synergizes with peripheral inflammation to induce brain IL-1beta expression and depressive-like effects. Cytokine 60: 749–754.
25. Scholzen T, Gerdes J (2000) The Ki-67 protein: from the known and the unknown. Journal of Cellular Physiology 182: 311–322.
26. Kee N, Sivalingam S, Boonstra R, Wojtowicz JM (2002) The utility of Ki-67 and BrdU as proliferative markers of adult neurogenesis. Journal of Neuroscience Methods 115: 97–105.
27. Jansson L, Wennstrom M, Johanson A, Tingstrom A (2009) Glial cell activation in response to electroconvulsive seizures. Prog Neuropsychopharmacol Biol Psychiatry 33: 1119–1128.
28. Wennstrom M, Hellsten J, Tingstrom A (2004) Electroconvulsive seizures induce proliferation of NG2-expressing glial cells in adult rat amygdala. Biol Psychiatry 55: 464–471.
29. Madsen TM, Yeh DD, Valentine GW, Duman RS (2005) Electroconvulsive seizure treatment increases cell proliferation in rat frontal cortex. Neuropsychopharmacology 30: 27–34.
30. Nielsen H, Ek D, Avdic U, Orbjorn C, Hansson O, et al. (2013) NG2 cells, a new trail for Alzheimer's disease mechanisms? Acta Neuropathologica Communications 1: 7.
31. Kim SE, Ko IG, Park CY, Shin MS, Kim CJ, et al. (2013) Treadmill and wheel exercise alleviate lipopolysaccharide-induced short-term memory impairment by enhancing neuronal maturation in rats. Molecular medicine reports 7: 31–36.
32. Monje ML, Toda H, Palmer TD (2003) Inflammatory blockade restores adult hippocampal neurogenesis. Science 302: 1760–1765.
33. Fujioka H, Akema T (2010) Lipopolysaccharide acutely inhibits proliferation of neural precursor cells in the dentate gyrus in adult rats. Brain Research 1352: 35–42.
34. Russo I, Amornphimoltham P, Weigert R, Barlati S, Bosetti F (2011) Cyclooxygenase-1 is involved in the inhibition of hippocampal neurogenesis after lipopolysaccharide-induced neuroinflammation. Cell Cycle 10: 2568–2573.
35. Woodroofe MN, Sarna GS, Wadhwa M, Hayes GM, Loughlin AJ, et al. (1991) Detection of interleukin-1 and interleukin-6 in adult rat brain, following mechanical injury, by in vivo microdialysis: evidence of a role for microglia in cytokine production. Journal of Neuroimmunology 33: 227–236.
36. Yao J, Keri JE, Taffs RE, Colton CA (1992) Characterization of interleukin-1 production by microglia in culture. Brain Research 591: 88–93.
37. Pinteaux E, Parker LC, Rothwell NJ, Luheshi GN (2002) Expression of interleukin-1 receptors and their role in interleukin-1 actions in murine microglial cells. Journal of Neurochemistry 83: 754–763.
38. Wu J, Yoo S, Wilcock D, Lytle JM, Leung PY, et al. (2010) Interaction of NG2 (+) glial progenitors and microglia/macrophages from the injured spinal cord. Glia 58: 410–422.
39. Paintlia MK, Paintlia AS, Khan M, Singh I, Singh AK (2008) Modulation of peroxisome proliferator-activated receptor-alpha activity by N-acetyl cysteine attenuates inhibition of oligodendrocyte development in lipopolysaccharide stimulated mixed glial cultures. J Neurochem 105: 956–970.
40. Nishiyama A, Yu M, Drazba JA, Tuohy VK (1997) Normal and reactive NG2+ glial cells are distinct from resting and activated microglia. J Neurosci Res 48: 299–312.
41. Gao Q, Lu J, Huo Y, Baby N, Ling EA, et al. (2010) NG2, a member of chondroitin sulfate proteoglycans family mediates the inflammatory response of activated microglia. Neuroscience 165: 386–394.
42. Grako KA, Ochiya T, Barritt D, Nishiyama A, Stallcup WB (1999) PDGF (alpha)-receptor is unresponsive to PDGF-AA in aortic smooth muscle cells from the NG2 knockout mouse. J Cell Sci 112 (Pt 6): 905–915.
43. Nishiyama A, Lin XH, Giese N, Heldin CH, Stallcup WB (1996) Interaction between NG2 proteoglycan and PDGF alpha-receptor on O2A progenitor cells is required for optimal response to PDGF. Journal of Neuroscience Research 43: 315–330.
44. Kucharova K, Stallcup WB (2010) The NG2 proteoglycan promotes oligodendrocyte progenitor proliferation and developmental myelination. Neuroscience 166: 185–194.
45. Kucharova K, Chang Y, Boor A, Yong VW, Stallcup WB (2011) Reduced inflammation accompanies diminished myelin damage and repair in the NG2 null mouse spinal cord. Journal of neuroinflammation 8: 158.
46. Goretzki L, Burg MA, Grako KA, Stallcup WB (1999) High-affinity binding of basic fibroblast growth factor and platelet-derived growth factor-AA to the core protein of the NG2 proteoglycan. The Journal of biological chemistry 274: 16831–16837.
47. Grako KA, Ochiya T, Barritt D, Nishiyama A, Stallcup WB (1999) PDGF (alpha)-receptor is unresponsive to PDGF-AA in aortic smooth muscle cells from the NG2 knockout mouse. Journal of Cell Science 112 (Pt 6): 905–915.
48. Ozerdem U, Monosov E, Stallcup WB (2002) NG2 proteoglycan expression by pericytes in pathological microvasculature. Microvascular research 63: 129–134.
49. Butt AM, Hamilton N, Hubbard P, Pugh M, Ibrahim M (2005) Synantocytes: the fifth element. J Anat 207: 695–706.

50. Butt AM, Duncan A, Hornby MF, Kirvell SL, Hunter A, et al. (1999) Cells expressing the NG2 antigen contact nodes of Ranvier in adult CNS white matter. Glia 26: 84–91.
51. Gallo V, Mangin JM, Kukley M, Dietrich D (2008) Synapses on NG2-expressing progenitors in the brain: multiple functions? The Journal of physiology 586: 3767–3781.
52. Yang Z, Suzuki R, Daniels SB, Brunquell CB, Sala CJ, et al. (2006) NG2 glial cells provide a favorable substrate for growing axons. The Journal of neuroscience: the official journal of the Society for Neuroscience 26: 3829–3839.
53. Wennstrom M, Hellsten J, Ekstrand J, Lindgren H, Tingstrom A (2006) Corticosterone-induced inhibition of gliogenesis in rat hippocampus is counteracted by electroconvulsive seizures. Biol Psychiatry 59: 178–186.
54. Czeh B, Muller-Keuker JI, Rygula R, Abumaria N, Hiemke C, et al. (2007) Chronic social stress inhibits cell proliferation in the adult medial prefrontal cortex: hemispheric asymmetry and reversal by fluoxetine treatment. Neuropsychopharmacology: official publication of the American College of Neuropsychopharmacology 32: 1490–1503.
55. Banasr M, Valentine GW, Li XY, Gourley SL, Taylor JR, et al. (2007) Chronic unpredictable stress decreases cell proliferation in the cerebral cortex of the adult rat. Biological Psychiatry 62: 496–504.
56. Gregus A, Wintink AJ, Davis AC, Kalynchuk LE (2005) Effect of repeated corticosterone injections and restraint stress on anxiety and depression-like behavior in male rats. Behav Brain Res 156: 105–114.
57. Hamidi M, Drevets WC, Price JL (2004) Glial reduction in amygdala in major depressive disorder is due to oligodendrocytes. Biol Psychiatry 55: 563–569.
58. Uranova NA, Vostrikov VM, Orlovskaya DD, Rachmanova VI (2004) Oligodendroglial density in the prefrontal cortex in schizophrenia and mood disorders: a study from the Stanley Neuropathology Consortium. Schizophrenia Research 67: 269–275.
59. Edgar N, Sibille E (2012) A putative functional role for oligodendrocytes in mood regulation. Translational psychiatry 2: e109.
60. Dantzer R, O'Connor JC, Lawson MA, Kelley KW (2011) Inflammation-associated depression: From serotonin to kynurenine. Psychoneuroendocrinology 36(3): 426–36.
61. Raison CL, Borisov AS, Majer M, Drake DF, Pagnoni G, et al. (2009) Activation of central nervous system inflammatory pathways by interferon-alpha: relationship to monoamines and depression. Biol Psychiatry 65: 296–303.
62. Dowlati Y, Herrmann N, Swardfager W, Liu H, Sham L, et al. (2010) A meta-analysis of cytokines in major depression. Biol Psychiatry 67: 446–457.
63. Levine J, Barak Y, Chengappa KN, Rapoport A, Rebey M, et al. (1999) Cerebrospinal cytokine levels in patients with acute depression. Neuropsychobiology 40: 171–176.
64. Lindqvist D, Janelidze S, Hagell P, Erhardt S, Samuelsson M, et al. (2009) Interleukin-6 is elevated in the cerebrospinal fluid of suicide attempters and related to symptom severity. Biol Psychiatry 66: 287–292.
65. Thomas AJ, Davis S, Morris C, Jackson E, Harrison R, et al. (2005) Increase in interleukin-1beta in late-life depression. The American journal of psychiatry 162: 175–177.
66. Bay-Richter C, Janelidze S, Hallberg L, Brundin L (2011) Changes in behaviour and cytokine expression upon a peripheral immune challenge. Behavioural brain research 222: 193–199.
67. Dunn AJ, Swiergiel AH (2005) Effects of interleukin-1 and endotoxin in the forced swim and tail suspension tests in mice. Pharmacol Biochem Behav 81: 688–693.
68. Yang C, Shen J, Hong T, Hu TT, Li ZJ, et al. (2013) Effects of ketamine on lipopolysaccharide-induced depressive-like behavior and the expression of inflammatory cytokines in the rat prefrontal cortex. Molecular medicine reports 8: 887–890.
69. Tynan RJ, Naicker S, Hinwood M, Nalivaiko E, Buller KM, et al. (2010) Chronic stress alters the density and morphology of microglia in a subset of stress-responsive brain regions. Brain Behav Immun 24: 1058–1068.

Heterogeneity in Patient-Reported Outcomes following Low-Intensity Mental Health Interventions: A Multilevel Analysis

Shehzad Ali[1,2*], Elizabeth Littlewood[1], Dean McMillan[1], Jaime Delgadillo[3], Alfonso Miranda[4], Tim Croudace[1], Simon Gilbody[1]

1 Department of Health Sciences, University of York, York, United Kingdom, **2** Centre for Health Economics, University of York, York, United Kingdom, **3** Primary Care Mental Health Service, Leeds Community Healthcare NHS Trust, Leeds, United Kingdom, **4** Centro de Investigación y Docencia Económicas, Mexico City, Mexico

Abstract

Background: Variability in patient-reported outcomes of psychological treatments has been partly attributed to therapists – a phenomenon commonly known as therapist effects. Meta-analytic reviews reveal wide variation in therapist-attributable variability in psychotherapy outcomes, with most studies reporting therapist effects in the region of 5% to 10% and some finding minimal to no therapist effects. However, all except one study to date have been conducted in high-intensity or mixed intervention groups; therefore, there is scarcity of evidence on therapist effects in brief low-intensity psychological interventions.

Objective: To examine therapist effects in low-intensity interventions for depression and anxiety in a naturalistic setting.

Data and Analysis: Session-by-session data on patient-reported outcome measures were available for a cohort of 1,376 primary care psychotherapy patients treated by 38 therapists. Outcome measures included PHQ-9 (sensitive to depression) and GAD-7 (sensitive to general anxiety disorder) measures. Three-level hierarchical linear modelling was employed to estimate therapist-attributable proportion of variance in clinical outcomes. Therapist effects were evaluated using the intra-cluster correlation coefficient (ICC) and Bayesian empirical predictions of therapist random effects. Three sensitivity analyses were conducted: 1) using both treatment completers and non-completers; 2) a sub-sample of cases with baseline scores above the conventional clinical thresholds for PHQ-9 and GAD-7; and 3) a two-level model (using patient-level pre- and post-treatment scores nested within therapists).

Results: The ICC estimates for all outcome measures were very small, ranging between 0% and 1.3%, although most were statistically significant. The Bayesian empirical predictions showed that therapist random effects were not statistically significantly different from each other. Between patient variability explained most of the variance in outcomes.

Conclusion: Consistent with the only other study to date in low intensity interventions, evidence was found to suggest minimal to no therapist effects in patient-reported outcomes. This draws attention to the more prominent source of variability which is found at the between-patient level.

Editor: Jerson Laks, Federal University of Rio de Janeiro, Brazil

Funding: The authors have no support or funding to report.

Competing Interests: The authors have declared that no competing interests exist.

* Email: shehzad.ali@york.ac.uk

Introduction

Variability in outcomes of psychological treatments has been partly attributed to therapists – a phenomenon commonly known as therapist effects (TE). However, despite a wealth of research over more than 20 years, the extent to which TE determine psychotherapy outcomes remains a widely debated topic [1–10]. TE may be an important factor to consider when evaluating observed differences between psychotherapy treatments which may be partly explained by differences in the mix of therapists [6,11]. For example, in a sample of severely depressed patients in the National Institute of Mental Health Treatment of Depression Collaborative Research Program (NIMH TDCRP), Kim et al. (2006) found that observed treatment differences between two psychotherapy interventions disappeared once therapists effects were taken into account [6]. These observations have led some researchers to conclude that ignoring TE in clinical outcome studies may lead to inaccurate effect size estimates and hence result in misleading conclusions [12,13]. Therapist effects are also be important in understanding the variability in patient-reported outcomes that can partly be explained by heterogeneity of therapists (4, 5).

A prominent source of debate is the wide variation in TE estimates across studies. Some studies report strong evidence of TE (e.g. [4,6,9,14,15], whilst other studies demonstrate negligible or statistically non-significant TE (e.g. [2,7,10,16,17]. A meta-analysis of 15 studies involving a heterogeneous mix of patient groups, psychological treatments, therapist numbers and patient sample sizes found that TE accounted for an estimated 8.6% (range 0% to almost 50%) of the variability in patient outcomes following therapy [2]. More recent reviews have reported TE estimates in the range of 5% to 10% [6,18]. This wide variability across studies raises questions about the relative importance of TE in psychotherapy and the possible explanations for such variability.

Potential explanations for this variability can be broadly divided into three areas: methodological characteristics (study design and analysis), patient and therapist characteristics, and treatment characteristics. Possibly the most contentious issue in this field concerns the methods used to estimate TE. Many authors have argued that the type of statistical modelling applied in these studies can directly influence the estimated therapist effects (e.g. [8,14,19,20]. A good example of this is the re-analysis of the NIMH TDCRP data conducted independently by two research groups, where significant TE of approximately 8% were shown by one group [6], whilst the other group reported little to no evidence of therapist effects [7]. Although both groups analysed data using hierarchical linear modelling (HLM), they differed in how this method was applied. Kim and colleagues (2006) applied a two-level HLM method (patients nested within therapists) which analyses pre-treatment and post-treatment outcome scores only [6], and Elkin and colleagues (2006) used a three-level HLM method (session scores nested within patients, nested within therapist) which analyses longitudinal outcome data to include the effect of change over time [7].

Some authors have argued that the magnitude of TE may vary according to the study design, and can only be reliably estimated from large-scale naturalistic studies [14,19]. Many TE studies have been conducted within the confines of well-controlled efficacy studies, using a more homogenous patient population and smaller numbers of therapists and patients (e.g. [1,6,7,21]. Such studies have tended to produce mixed results (e.g. [6,7]). On the other hand, naturalistic studies often include heterogeneous patient populations with larger numbers of both patients and therapists, thus more closely representing routine clinical practice (e.g. [9,10,14,15]). Nevertheless, naturalistic studies have also produced mixed results to date. Although three studies report TE of between 4% and 8% [9,14,15], one recent study reported only minimal TE of between 0% and 2% [10]. An additional and potentially important methodological characteristic of these studies concerns the outcome measure used to estimate TE. Some authors have argued that the magnitude of TE estimates may depend on whether the outcome is a generic measure of psychological distress or a disorder-specific measure, and whether outcomes are self-reported or therapist-rated [7,10]. However, a recent meta-analytic review demonstrated mixed findings for studies that used both the same disorder specific measures (e.g. BDI), more generic measures of distress (e.g. OQ-45) or therapist-rated measures (e.g. GAF) [18].

Besides methodological characteristics, it is possible that the characteristics of the patients and therapists included in a particular study may determine the size and significance of observed therapist effects. Kim and colleagues (2006), for example, found that the magnitude of TE in the NIMH TDCRP was correlated with baseline level of severity [6]. In a meta-analytic investigation, Crits-Christoph and colleagues (1991), found that the use of a treatment manual and more experienced therapists were associated with small TE, whereas more inexperienced therapists and no treatment manual were associated with larger TE [2]. Other studies suggest that the existence of outlier therapists can influence the size of TE, with TE being attenuated or eliminated when outlier therapists are removed (e.g. [6,21]. Similarly, it is possible that outlier patients may influence the magnitude of TE in a given sample. Saxon and Barkham (2012), for example, argue that very impaired, complex cases inflate TE [22], which may result in smaller therapist effects in samples without this level of case complexity.

Although there is still uncertainty about the extent to which TE are important determinants of therapeutic outcomes, some clear methodological lessons can be drawn from the literature. The magnitude of observed TE is likely to be dependent on a number of factors including the heterogeneity of the patient population (e.g. case-mix), differences in baseline severity of the disorder, the number of therapists involved and patient sample size [20,22]. Precise TE estimates are more likely to be derived from large naturalistic samples including at least 30 therapists [20]. In addition to controlling for factors that may influence TE, researchers have argued that the use of statistical methods such as multilevel modelling is more appropriate for such data, since they better reflect the natural structure of variability in outcomes (e.g. patients nested within individual therapists) and allow for a partitioning of outcome variance at the patient and therapist levels [22]. In addition, random effects (or mixed) analyses (rather than only fixed effects analyses) better facilitate the computation of standardised therapist variance estimates and the generalisation of findings as relevant to the wider population of therapists [18].

While the current literature provides some insight into the relevance of methodological and patient-therapist characteristics, what has been less studied is the influence of treatment characteristics. Nearly all previous therapist-effect studies have focused on conventional psychotherapeutic interventions, such as cognitive-behaviour therapy (e.g. [4,6,7,10]), interpersonal therapy [6,7] and psychodynamic therapy (see [2]). Only one previous study has examined therapist effects in brief low-intensity psychological interventions. Almlőv et al. (2011) found little evidence for TE in a study involving low-intensity guided internet-delivered Cognitive Behaviour Therapy [23]. The authors suggest that this is partly explained by similarity of therapists in terms of level of experience and therapeutic orientation. The interpretation of these results, however, is limited by the small patient sample size (119 patients drawn from three individual studies) and small therapist numbers (N = 8).

Brief low-intensity psychological interventions have a number of broad features that differentiate them from more traditional, high-intensity psychotherapeutic interventions [24,25]. Low-intensity interventions are typically less complex, involve a reduced level of contact with the person receiving treatment, and often use novel forms of delivery (e.g., telephone delivery, computerised Cognitive Behaviour Therapy, provision of self-help material, group treatment) [25]. In addition to the nature of the treatment itself, low-intensity interventions are likely to differ from high-intensity treatments in terms of who provides and who receives the treatment. Low-intensity treatments are typically intended for patients with mild to moderate symptoms and less complex presentations; they are also designed to be delivered by professionals or para-professionals with less extensive training who are likely to have similar level of experience [26]. These characteristics of low-intensity therapy may influence the size and significance of therapist effects. However, there is paucity of evidence on therapist effects in low-intensity psychotherapy. Therefore, the main aim of the current study is to estimate TE in a large naturalistic treatment sample of brief low-intensity treatments for people presenting with common mental health problems such as depression and anxiety.

Methods

Ethics statement

Use of anonymous clinical records for this study was approved by an English National Health Service (NHS) research ethics committee, on 15 September 2010, reference 10/H1306/68. Patients provided verbal consent at the earliest contact point with the service which was over the telephone, hence verbal consent was appropriate. Patients were asked whether they agreed to allow their anonymous clinical records to be used for research and audit purposes. Verbal consent was then recorded in the electronic patient clinical record. Anonymous datasets were extracted from electronic clinical records for audit/research purposes, which excluded non-consenting patients. This method was approved by the reviewing NHS ethics committee.

Study population

This study was based on routinely collected session-by-session patient reported outcome measures (PROMS) for patients accessing treatment for depression and anxiety disorders in a primary care mental health service in Leeds, England. These data are specifically drawn from a cohort of patients who received low intensity (LI) evidence-based interventions recommended by national guidelines [27,28] and delivered as part of the English Improving Access to Psychological Therapies (IAPT) programme [29]. These interventions included guided self-help based on cognitive behavioural therapy (CBT) principles, one-to-one and group based psycho-education about common mental disorders, and computerised CBT with support by a mental health professional. Such interventions are considered 'low intensity' given their brief length (typically under 8 sessions, although a small proportion of patients may have more sessions), and because they are delivered by qualified therapists whose training is briefer and less extensive than that of psychotherapists or clinical psychologists. Therapists in this service completed a standard, 1-year post-graduate qualification specific to the delivery of low intensity treatments and following a national curriculum (e.g. see [26,30]).

Patients in this cohort were either directly referred to the service by general medical practitioners or encouraged to self-refer. Following referral, all patients attended a 45 minute screening interview with a qualified mental health practitioner. ICD-10 based primary diagnoses were derived from these interviews supplemented by validated case-finding questionnaires. This assessment was used to determine suitability for LI interventions on the basis of a positive screen on depression and/or anxiety measures (described below), and on idiographic data gathered to assess the presenting problem, patient goals and risk factors. Following national guidelines [27,28], those patients with mild-to-moderate symptoms and functional impairment were deemed suitable for LI interventions and were sequentially allocated to the first available therapist. Although for a minority of patients, their preferences did influence the location of treatment and gender of therapist, there was virtually no selection on the part of therapists. Patients who did not meet criteria for LI interventions (e.g. those with severe, chronic and/or complex conditions) and those who did not improve after LI treatment were 'stepped up' to more intensive and lengthier psychotherapy in the service; however, this study only focuses on the sample of patients who received treatment with a therapist qualified to deliver low intensity interventions (including those who were later stepped-up).

Outcome measures

Data on two commonly used PROMS was available. The Patient Health Questionnaire (PHQ-9) is a nine item self-completed questionnaire commonly used to screen for major depression [31]. This measure is reported to have adequate sensitivity (88%) and specificity (88%) using a cut-off score ≥ 10 [31]. The Generalized Anxiety Disorder scale (GAD-7) is a seven item questionnaire originally developed to detect GAD, although adequate sensitivity (77%) and specificity (82%) estimates have been reported for its capacity to screen for other anxiety disorders including social phobia, post-traumatic stress disorder and panic disorder using a cut-off ≥ 8 [32]. Both measures have been extensively validated and widely used in primary care settings across several countries [33]. Each item in these questionnaires is scored on a 0-3 scale and the scores are summed to give an overall score (range for PHQ-9 = 0-27; GAD-7 = 0-21) with a higher score indicating more severe symptoms.

Statistical analysis

Hierarchical structure. The IAPT data structure is hierarchical and consists of three-levels: level 1 is the 'visit-level' for session-by-session PHQ-9 and GAD-7 scores for each patient (with visit 1 being the baseline session), level 2 is the 'patient-level' representing scores nested within patients, and level 3 is the 'therapist-level' representing patients nested within therapists.

Three-level hierarchical linear mixed (HLM) models were used for primary analysis to evaluate longitudinal variation in patient-reported outcomes based on PHQ-9 and GAD-7 scores. HLM models decompose total variation in health outcomes into variance components attributable to each level, in particular, the therapist-level (level 3). We used unconditional and conditional HLM models for this purpose; the unconditional HLM model is a random intercept model that does not include any covariates (explanatory variables) while the conditional model includes patient-level covariates and decomposes the remaining variation into variance components. For the primarily analysis, data from all patients who had completed therapy was used. A sensitivity analysis included full sample of treatment completers and non-completers (i.e. those who dropped out or were stepped-up to more intense and lengthier psychotherapy). HLM models were separately implemented for PHQ-9 and GAD-7 outcome measures. The analysis was conducted in Stata version 13.1 (Stata Corporation, College Station TX, USA). The statistical models used in the analysis are described in detail below.

Unconditional model. Following Raudenbush and Bryk (2002), we present a three-stage formulation of the unconditional HLM model [34].

Visit-level model: The level-1 model for PHQ-9 or GAD-7 scores can be specified as:

$$y_{ijk} = \pi_{0jk} + \varepsilon_{ijk} \quad (1)$$

Here y_{ijk} represents the PHQ-9/GAD-7 score for visit i for patient j who is treated by therapist k. The term π_{0jk} is the patient-level random intercept or the mean PHQ-9/GAD-7 score of patient j in therapist k. The error term ε_{ijk} represents the visit-level random deviation of visit ijk's score from the patient-level mean, i.e. the random 'occasion effect'. ε_{ijk} is assumed to be normally distributed with mean 0 and variance σ^2, i.e. $\varepsilon_{ijk} \sim N(0, \sigma^2)$.

Patient-level model: The patient-level random intercept π_{0jk} can in turn be modelled as an outcome that varies randomly around the mean score of therapist k. This level-2 model can be specified as:

$$\pi_{0jk} = \beta_{00k} + r_{0jk} \quad (2)$$

Here β_{00k} is the mean PHQ-9/GAD-7 score for therapist k, and r_{0jk} represents the random deviation of patient jk's mean from the therapist mean, i.e. the random 'patient effect'. As before, r_{0jk} is assumed to be normally distributed with mean 0 and variance τ_π.

Therapist-level model: The level-3 model is for the therapist-level intercept β_{00k} which can be specified as:

$$\beta_{00k} = \gamma_{000} + u_{00k} \quad (3)$$

Here γ_{000} represents the grand mean of PHQ-9/GAD-7 scores in the sample and β_{00k} vary randomly around the grand mean which is the only fixed effect in the three-level unconditional model. u_{00k} is the therapist-level random effect, i.e. therapist k's random deviation from the grand mean. This random effect is also assumed to be normally distributed with mean 0 and variance τ_β.

Combined model: Using the above equations, the combined three-level model can be represented as:

$$y_{ijk} = \gamma_{000} + u_{00k} + r_{0jk} + \varepsilon_{ijk} \quad (4)$$

This is a mixed model as it contains both fixed effect γ_{000} and random effects $u_{00k}, r_{0jk}, \varepsilon_{ijk}$.

Variance components and intra-cluster correlation coefficient. The three-level model partitions the total variance of the PHQ-9 scores in three components. These are: level-1 variance (σ^2) attributable to visit-level variability within individuals; level-2 variance (τ_π) attributable to variability between individuals and within therapists; and level-3 variance (τ_β) between therapists. The total variance is the sum of these three components:

$$var(y_{ijk}) = \sigma^2 + \tau_\pi + \tau_\beta \quad (5)$$

The proportion of total variance explained by each component can be interpreted as the correlation among observations in each given cluster, also known as the intra-cluster correlation (ICC). In a three level model as the one described above there are three different ICCs:

$$\rho_{(v,p)} = \frac{\sigma^2}{\sigma^2 + \tau_\pi + \tau_\beta} \quad (6)$$

$$\rho_{(p,t)} = \frac{\tau_\pi}{\sigma^2 + \tau_\pi + \tau_\beta} \quad (7)$$

$$\rho_{(th)} = \frac{\tau_\beta}{\sigma^2 + \tau_\pi + \tau_\beta} \quad (8)$$

where $\rho_{(v,p)}$ $\rho_{(p,t)}$ and $\rho_{(th)}$ represent the proportion of total variance explained by within patient variability, within therapist variability and between therapists variability respectively. For the current analysis, we are primarily interested in the therapist-level ICC $\rho_{(th)}$.

Conditional model. The unconditional model (described earlier) allows estimation of the variance associated with each level. Part of this variance in PHQ-9/GAD-7 scores can be explained by covariates. Hence, we estimate two conditional models:

a) Conditional model with quintiles of baseline PHQ-9/GAD-7 score (lowest quintile used as the reference category), age (centred on mean) and gender as covariates.
b) The above model plus the following fixed effects variables: visit number for each outcome score (continuous variable); and time since the baseline visit in weeks (continuous variable).

The conditional model can be represented as:

$$y_{ijk} = \gamma_{000} + \sum_{p=1}^{p=q} \gamma_p W_{pijk} + u_{00k} + r_{0jk} + \varepsilon_{ijk} \quad (9)$$

Here γ_p represents the coefficients on covariates p nested within patients. The models were estimated using fixed effects at level one and random intercepts for levels 2 (patients) and 3 (therapists). The ICC was calculated to estimate the variance explained at each level.

Sensitivity analysis. Three sensitivity analyses were conducted. Firstly, the three-level unconditional HLM analysis for PHQ-9 and GAD-7 was repeated using full sample, including treatment completers and non-completers (i.e. those who dropped out or were stepped-up). Secondly, the three-level unconditional HLM analysis was conducted using only the patients with baseline PHQ-9 score ≥10 (criteria for depression) and baseline GAD-7 score ≥8 (criteria for generalised anxiety disorder) respectively. This was done to evaluate whether the variance attributable to the therapist level is different in the subsample that screened positive for a clinically significant depressive or anxiety disorder (defined based on PHQ-9/GAD-7 thresholds). Finally, following the argument by Wampold and Bolt (2006) [8], we evaluated the robustness of our results by using two-level unconditional and conditional HLM models whereby level-1 was defined as the change score for each patient (i.e. baseline score minus final score for PHQ-9 or GAD-7) and level-2 represented patients nested within therapists. The conditional model included age, gender, baseline severity, total number of visits and total weeks in therapy as covariates. As explained above, the focus is on estimating the variance attributable to the therapist-level.

Results

Descriptive statistics

There were 26,177 patients referred to the service during 2008–2010 of which 6,583 patients were allocated to low-intensity psychological interventions based on initial screening. Of these, 2,210 patients had at least one follow-up measure available (either PHQ-9 or GAD-7) after the initial (screening) consultation. Of these, 1,376 patients had completed treatment. There were 38 practitioners who provided low-intensity therapy with mean number of patients per therapist equal to 36.2 (SD = 25.5; range 1–109, with five therapists with <10 patients).

The mean age of patients in the sample was 39.5 (SD = 14.6), the proportion of females was 36.4% and the ethnicity was predominantly white (white: 71.1%; non-white: 5.4%; not known: 23.5%). At patient-level, the mean baseline score (an indicator of symptom severity) in the sample was 11.4 (SD = 5.7) on the PHQ-9 scale and 10.5 (SD = 5.1) on the GAD-7 scale (see Table 1). Based on the commonly used clinical threshold scores of ≥10 for PHQ-9 and ≥8 for GAD-7, 51% patients could be classed as depressed at baseline and 59% as having an anxiety disorder (note: the two conditions often co-existed). Clinical assessment data indicated that the three most commonly recorded primary diagnoses in this sample were depression (37.4%), generalised anxiety disorder (22.7%) and mixed anxiety and depressive disorder (27.9%), with other conditions being less prevalent. At therapist-level, the mean baseline score was 11.4 (SD = 1.1) on the PHQ-9 scale and 10.5 (SD = 0.9) on the GAD-7 scale. The small standard deviation in relation to the mean suggests little variation in baseline severity between therapists [PHQ-9 ($p = 0.31$) and GAD-7 ($p = 0.43$)]. This descriptive evidence suggests that allocation of patients to therapists was quasi-random; in other words, there was little evidence of systematic selection of patients at therapist-level.

Patients attended, on average, 5.2 sessions each (SD = 2.2) and at the end of the therapy had a mean PHQ-9 score of 5.9 (SD = 5.5) and GAD-7 score of 5.4 (SD = 4.7). Figure 1 presents a scatterplot of session-by-session PHQ-9 scores (up to 10 sessions) of a randomly selected sub-sample from the dataset. The figure shows that scores within individuals are highly correlated. A similar clustering pattern was observed in GAD-7 scores (not presented here).

As described above, we also evaluated the patient-level change score (on PHQ-9 and GAD-7 scales separately) over therapists. In the overall sample, the mean patient-level change score on PHQ-9 was 5.5 (SD = 5.5) and on GAD-7 was 5.2 (SD = 5.1). At therapist-level, the mean change score for patients was 5.4 (SD = 1.1) on PHQ-9 and 5.2 (SD = 1.0) on GAD-7. Figure 2 presents a box plot to explore the distribution of change scores in PHQ-9 within and between therapists. The figure shows that, on average, all therapists had improvement in patient-level PHQ-9 scores, although a small number of patients within most therapists had worse scores at the time of discharge. Crucially, the interquartile range of change scores for all therapists overlapped with each other, which denotes little variation between them. A similar distribution of change scores was observed for GAD-7 scores (not presented here).

Three-level unconditional analysis

The unconditional HLM model decomposed the total variation in patient-level health outcomes (i.e. PHQ-9 and GAD-7 scores) into variation explained by therapists (i.e. between therapist variance τ_β), variation explained by patients (i.e. between patient variance,τ_π) and the residual variance (i.e. within patient varice, σ^2). Table 1 reports the variance explained at each level and the associated ICC coefficients (i.e. the proportion of variance at each level). The analysis found that of the total variation in patient reported outcomes only around 1% was explained by the therapist level (ICC: PHQ-9 = 1.0%; GAD-7 = 0.9%). The largest share of the total variance was explained at patient level, i.e. between-patient heterogeneity accounted for 57% and 54% of the total variance in PHQ-9 and GAD-7 respectively). This compliments the observation in Figure 1 which showed that scores within individuals were highly correlated. This analysis suggests that, in this cohort of low intensity interventions, only a small proportion of the variation in outcomes can be attributed to therapists. In

Table 1. Results of unconditional variance components analysis using patient-level PHQ-9 and GAD-7 scores.

Unconditional model	PHQ-9 analysis (patients = 1,359; therapists = 38)				GAD-7 analysis (patients = 1,366; therapists = 38)			
	Estimate	SE	95% CI		Estimate	SE	95% CI	
Fixed effect: intercept	8.13	0.17	7.80	8.46	7.29	0.14	7.02	7.56
Random-effects								
Therapist-level	0.57	0.20	0.29	1.12	0.45	0.18	0.21	0.97
Patient-level	4.24	0.11	4.04	4.45	3.55	0.09	3.37	3.73
Residual	3.72	0.04	3.64	3.80	3.32	0.04	3.25	3.39
Intracluster correlation (ICC%)	Estimate	SE	95% CI		Estimate	SE	95% CI	
Therapist-level	1.0%	0.7%	0.3%	3.8%	0.9%	0.7%	0.2%	3.9%
Patient-level	57.0%	1.4%	54.2%	59.7%	53.7%	1.4%	50.9%	56.5%

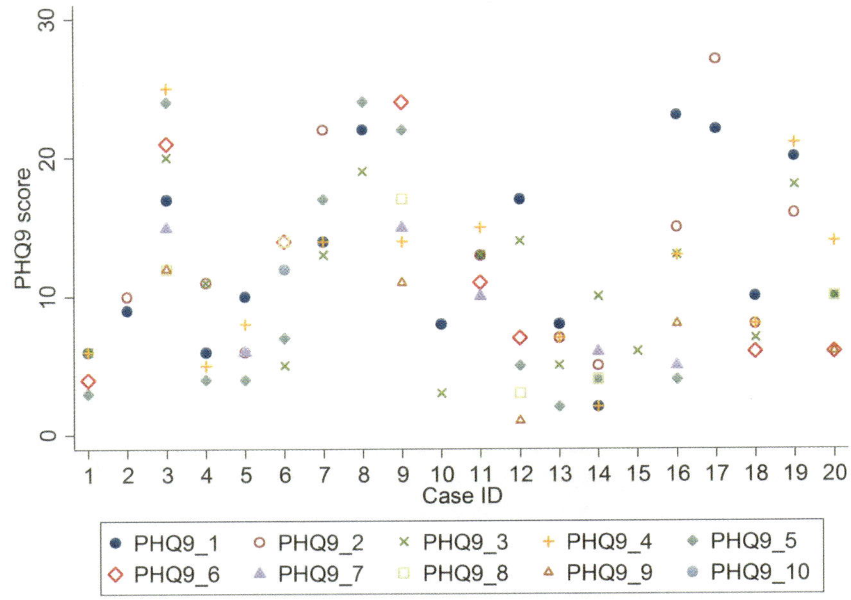

Figure 1. Scatterplot of session-by-session PHQ-9 scores of randomly drawn patients.
doi:10.1371/journal.pone.0099658.g001

other words the therapist effect is very small, which would indicate comparable and fairly uniform average outcomes between different therapists.

Bayesian empirical predictions were used to predict values of random intercepts for each therapist. The random intercepts represent the relative effectiveness of each therapist in improving health outcomes (either PHQ-9 or GAD-7) compared to the

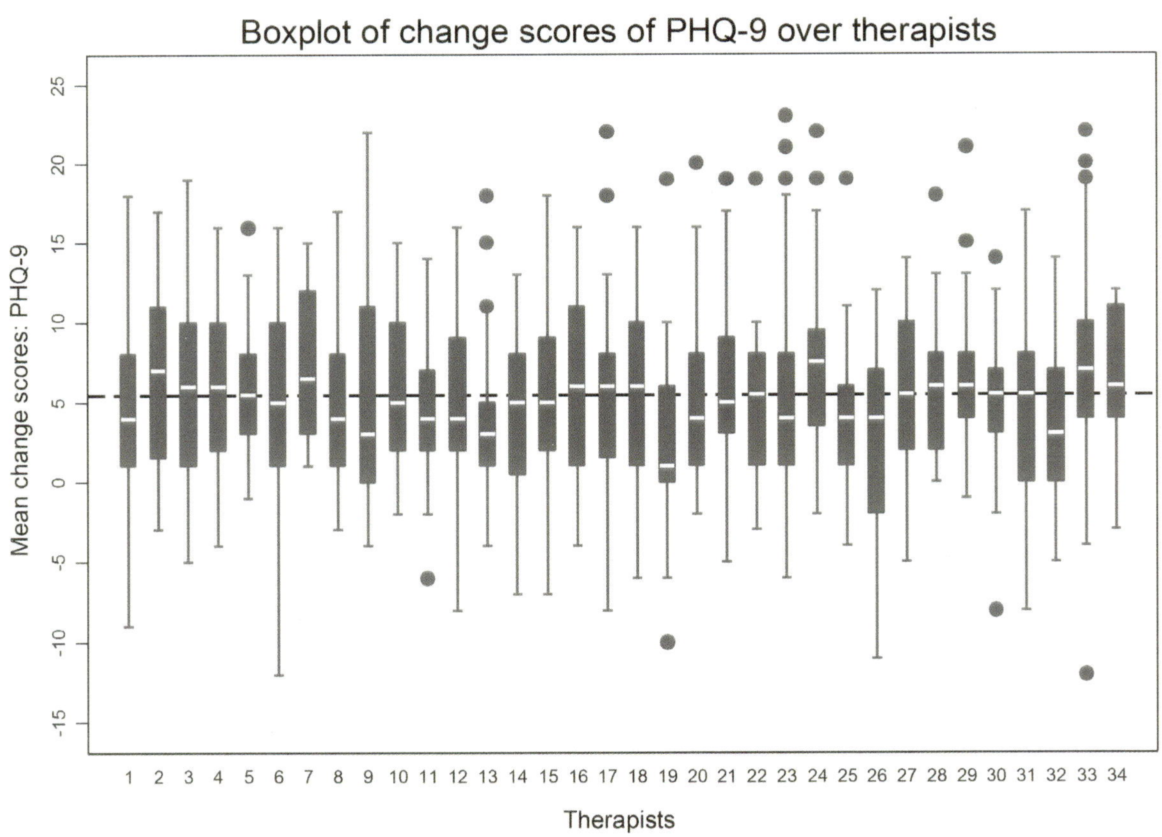

Figure 2. Boxplot of patient-level change scores (difference between baseline and final scores) on the PHQ-9 scale across therapists.

average therapist in the sample. The therapist random intercepts are ranked and presented with their 95% CI in Figure 3 (caterpillar plot). Therapists with better than average outcomes have negative intercepts and hence are in the bottom left corner of the plot and the lowest performing therapists in the sample have positive intercepts and are in the top left. The 95% CI of all random intercepts cross zero which suggests that therapists are not statistically significantly different from the average therapist in the group. Moreover, all therapist-level random intercepts overlap which corroborates the finding that there was no evidence of statistically significant differences in performance between therapists.

Three-level conditional analysis

The conditional multilevel models control for imbalance in patient-level covariates and attribute the remaining variance to the three levels. The first conditional model included fixed effects variables representing quintiles of baseline PHQ-9/GAD-7 scores, age and gender. As expected, patients in quintiles with higher baseline scores (or more severe symptom severity) were found to have higher scores at successive visits (compared to patients in lower baseline quintiles). Patient's age and gender were not found to have a statistically significant relationship with health outcomes. More importantly, the ICC for therapist-level was 0.4% and 0.6% in PHQ-9 and GAD-7 analyses respectively (Table 2), and most of the remaining variance was attributable to between-patient heterogeneity and within-patient random error. Notice, however, that the therapist random effect is statistically non-significant at 5% in the PHQ-9 model but significant in the GAD-7 model.

In the second conditional model, we added (in addition to the covariates in the above model) fixed effects dummy variables for each visit, except the first therapy visit (reference category) to explicitly control for changes in outcomes over the course of treatment. The results were similar to earlier models and the ICC was found to be <1% for therapist level in both models (Table 2).

Sensitivity analyses

To evaluate the robustness of our findings, three types of sensitivity analyses were conducted [Tables 3 and 4]. The first analysis included full sample of patients (including non-completers of treatment) and the second analysis included only those patients with PHQ-9 scores ≥10 or GAD-7 score ≥8 (i.e. patients with baseline scores above the thresholds for depression or anxiety disorders). These analyses found that the variance explained at the therapist level was only between 0.2% and 1.2%. A further sensitivity analysis explored variance attributable to therapists in two-level unconditional and unconditional analyses (i.e. patient-level change score nested within therapists) and found therapist-level ICC to be between 0% and 1.3% for the PROMs.

Discussion

This is the first large study in a naturalistic low-intensity psychotherapy setting that evaluated the contribution of therapists in variability of patient-reported outcome measures. The study had a sample size of 1,376 primary care patients treated by 38 therapists (an average of 36 patients per therapist). The study used three-level hierarchical linear model to estimate therapist effects, but also evaluated two-level model in a sensitivity analysis. The analysis was conducted using the overall sample, and, to assess the robustness of results, using a sub-sample with initial severity above

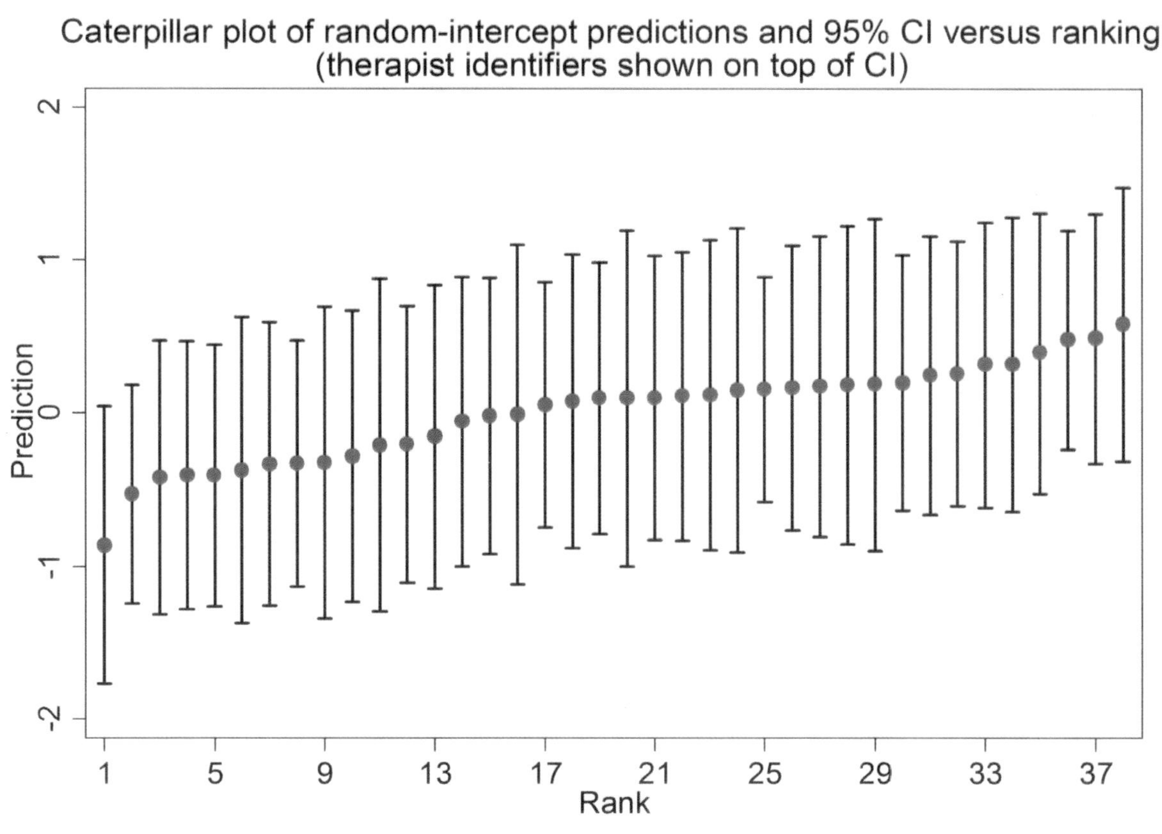

Figure 3. Caterpillar plot of predicted therapist-level random intercept and 95% CI versus average performance benchmark.

Table 2. Results of conditional multilevel analysis using patient-level PHQ-9 and GAD-7 scores.

Conditional model 1	PHQ-9 analysis (patients = 1,174; therapists = 37)				GAD-7 analysis (patients = 1,190; therapists = 37)			
	Estimate	**SE**	**95% CI**		**Estimate**	**SE**	**95% CI**	
Fixed effects								
Baseline PHQ-9/GAD-7 quintiles								
Baseline quintile 2	1.94	0.33	1.29	2.59	2.00	0.28	1.45	2.54
Baseline quintile 3	3.78	0.31	3.18	4.37	3.02	0.28	2.47	3.56
Baseline quintile 4	6.32	0.32	5.69	6.95	4.51	0.29	3.94	5.08
Baseline quintile 5	9.69	0.33	9.03	10.34	7.29	0.27	6.76	7.83
Age of the patient	0.00	0.01	−0.01	0.02	0.00	0.01	−0.01	0.02
Gender (Female = 1)	0.11	0.21	−0.31	0.53	0.03	0.19	−0.34	0.40
Intercept	3.90	0.27	3.38	4.43	4.07	0.23	3.63	4.51
Random effects								
Therapist-level	0.29	0.18	0.08	0.97	0.33	0.15	0.14	0.78
Patient-level	2.86	0.09	2.69	3.04	2.53	0.08	2.38	2.69
Residual	3.61	0.04	3.53	3.70	3.28	0.04	3.20	3.36
Intracluster correlation (ICC%)	Estimate	SE	95% CI		Estimate	SE	95% CI	
Therapist-level	0.4%	0.5%	0.0%	4.3%	0.6%	0.6%	0.1%	3.5%
Patient-level	38.7%	1.6%	35.5%	41.9%	37.7%	1.6%	34.5%	40.9%
Conditional model 2	**PHQ-9 analysis (patients = 1,174; therapists = 37)**				**GAD-7 analysis (patients = 1,127; therapists = 37)**			
	Estimate	**SE**	**95% CI**		**Estimate**	**SE**	**95% CI**	
Fixed effects								
Baseline PHQ-9/GAD-7 quintiles								
Baseline quintile 2	2.05	0.35	1.36	2.75	2.16	0.30	1.56	2.75
Baseline quintile 3	4.03	0.33	3.38	4.68	3.20	0.30	2.62	3.79
Baseline quintile 4	6.68	0.35	6.00	7.36	4.83	0.31	4.21	5.44
Baseline quintile 5	10.26	0.36	9.54	10.97	7.67	0.30	7.09	8.26
Age of the patient	0.00	0.01	−0.02	0.01	0.00	0.01	−0.01	0.01
Gender (Female = 1)	0.26	0.23	−0.19	0.72	0.18	0.21	−0.23	0.58
Visits (continuous)	-0.66	0.06	−0.78	−0.55	−0.54	0.05	−0.65	−0.44
Time since first visit (in weeks)	0.04	0.02	−0.01	0.09	0.01	0.02	−0.03	0.05
Intercept	5.64	0.31	5.04	6.24	5.60	0.26	5.10	6.11
Random effects								
Therapist-level	0.36	0.19	0.13	0.99	0.35	0.16	0.15	0.85
Patient-level	3.10	0.09	2.92	3.29	2.74	0.09	2.57	2.91
Residual	3.19	0.04	3.10	3.27	2.95	0.04	2.87	3.03

Table 2. Cont.

Conditional model 2	PHQ-9 analysis (patients = 1,174; therapists = 37)			GAD-7 analysis (patients = 1,127; therapists = 37)		
	Estimate	**SE**	**95% CI**	**Estimate**	**SE**	**95% CI**
Intracluster correlation (ICC%)	Estimate	SE	95% CI	Estimate	SE	95% CI
Therapist-level	0.7%	0.7%	0.1% 4.8%	0.8%	0.7%	0.1% 4.3%
Patient-level	49.0%	1.8%	45.6% 52.5%	46.6%	1.8%	43.1% 50.2%

the threshold scores for depression or anxiety based on PHQ-9 or GAD-7 scores, respectively.

This analysis of therapist effects in routine low intensity psychological interventions found TE estimates in the region of 0% to 1.3%. While statistically significant, these estimates were substantially smaller than those typically reported in more traditional high-intensity psychotherapeutic interventions (e.g.,5% average TE estimate reported by Baldwin & Imel, 2013 [18]. The results are, however, consistent with the only previous study of therapist effects in low-intensity treatments [23]. Our results suggest that TE are less prominent in brief low intensity interventions.

However, as outlined in the introduction, TE estimates can be influenced by a range of methodological and sample characteristics. It is therefore important to first examine if study design and data analysis methods may account for the small observed therapist effects in this study. While the main analysis used a three-level hierarchical model (consistent with previously published studies), the analysis was repeated using a two-level model (using only pre- and post-treatment scores) in a sensitivity analysis; this analysis also resulted in small (<1%) though statistically significant TE estimates. Therefore the results seem robust to analytical methods and are unlikely to be an artefact of the type of HLM used.

The current study used data from a large, naturalistic cohort. A number of authors have recommended this design as the most appropriate one to identify therapist effects (e.g.[10,14,19] and large effects have been found in a number of such designs (e.g. [9,10,14,15]. The review by Baldwin and Imel (2013), in fact, found that naturalistic cohorts reported significantly larger therapist effects compared to tightly controlled randomised controlled trials (7% vs. 3%) [18]. This aspect of the design, therefore, is also unlikely to account for the small TE estimates.

This study used depression and anxiety outcome measures which broadly matched the clinical diagnosis of patients in the sample. It could be speculated that these measures may not be sensitive enough to capture important variations in effect across caseloads. However, the existing literature reveals large TE estimates using much more generic measures of effect such as the Global Assessment of Functioning, Global Distress Scale, etc [18]. Furthermore, the measures applied in this study have been shown to be sensitive enough to reveal considerable variations in outcome when comparing outcome estimates clustered by specific psychological services (e.g. see [35]). It therefore seems unlikely that the choice of outcome measures entirely provides an alternative explanation for the small therapist effects found in this study.

Although the present results are unlikely to be artefacts of data analysis methods, alternative explanations for the modest TE may include the influence of patient, therapist and treatment characteristics in a low-intensity psychotherapy setting. Consistent with Kim et al. (2006) [6], our sensitivity analyses provide some evidence that baseline severity is modestly associated with the magnitude of TE, since these estimates increased marginally once we excluded cases with sub-clinical baseline scores. Saxon and Barkham (2012) offer a potential clinical interpretation for this association [22]. In an analysis of a large naturalistic cohort of more than 10,000 patients treated by over 100 therapists, they found that greater severity of symptoms was associated with increased TE, such that higher severity and risk was associated with poorer outcomes. Since low intensity treatments are usually offered to patients with mild-to-moderate mental health problems with relatively low risk factors this may naturally attenuate the extent of TE. Besides initial case severity, other characteristics of

Table 3. Sensitivity analysis I: multilevel analysis using [1] full sample and [2] patient with PHQ-9≥ 10 and GAD-7≥8.

[1] Full sample analysis (both treatment completers and non-completers)	**PHQ-9 analysis (patients = 2,190; therapists = 38)**				**GAD-7 analysis (patients = 2,197; therapists = 38)**			
	Estimate	**SE**	**95% CI**		**Estimate**	**SE**	**95% CI**	
Fixed effect: intercept	9.33	0.14	9.05	9.61	8.32	0.11	8.11	8.53
Random-effects								
Therapist-level	0.45	0.17	0.21	0.95	0.22	0.20	0.04	1.242
Patient-level	4.82	0.09	4.64	5.01	4.04	0.08	3.89	4.204
Residual	3.67	0.04	3.60	3.74	3.32	0.03	3.25	3.384
Intracluster correlation (ICC%)								
Therapist-level	0.5%	0.4%	0.1%	2.4%	0.2%	0.3%	0.0%	5.4%
Patient-level	63.5%	1.1%	61.4%	65.6%	59.8%	1.1%	57.6%	62.0%
[2] Patients with PHQ-9≥10/GAD-7≥8	**PHQ-9≥ 10 (patients = 703; therapists = 37)**				**GAD-7≥8 (patients = 811; therapists = 37)**			
	Estimate	**SE**	**95% CI**		**Estimate**	**SE**	**95% CI**	
Fixed effect: intercept	10.29	0.21	9.87	10.71	8.54	0.17	8.21	8.88
Random-effects								
Therapist-level	0.63	0.27	0.28	1.45	0.53	0.22	0.23	1.198
Patient-level	4.06	0.15	3.78	4.36	3.37	0.12	3.15	3.613
Residual	4.10	0.06	3.98	4.22	3.57	0.05	3.47	3.670
Intracluster correlation (ICC%)								
Therapist-level	1.2%	1.0%	0.2%	6.0%	1.1%	0.9%	0.2%	5.7%
Patient-level	50.2%	2.0%	46.2%	54.1%	47.8%	1.9%	44.0%	51.6%

Table 4. Sensitivity analysis: two-level analysis of change scores using [3] unconditional model and [4] conditional model.

[3] Unconditional two-level analysis using change scores	PHQ-9 analysis (patients = 1,194; therapists = 37)				GAD-7 analysis (patients = 1,206; therapists = 37)			
	Estimate	SE	95% CI		Estimate	SE	95% CI	
Fixed effect: intercept	5.44	0.18	5.08	5.80	5.17	0.15	4.88	5.461
Random-effects								
Therapist-level	0.51	0.26	0.19	1.38	2.16E-07	8.79E-07	7.51E-11	0.001
Residual	5.44	0.11	5.22	5.66	5.12	0.10	4.92	5.33
Intracluster correlation (ICC%)								
Therapist-level	0.9%	0.9%	0.1%	6.1%	1.8E-15	0.0E+00	1.8E-15	1.8E-15
[4] Conditional two-level analysis using change scores	**PHQ-9 analysis (patients = 1,184; therapists = 37)**				**GAD-7 analysis (patients = 1,196; therapists = 37)**			
	Estimate	**SE**	**95% CI**		**Estimate**	**SE**	**95% CI**	
Fixed effects								
Baseline PHQ-9/GAD-7 quintiles								
Baseline quintile 2	2.67	0.42	1.85	3.49	1.99	0.36	1.28	2.70
Baseline quintile 3	4.54	0.39	3.77	5.31	4.28	0.36	3.57	4.99
Baseline quintile 4	6.49	0.41	5.68	7.30	6.46	0.39	5.69	7.22
Baseline quintile 5	8.21	0.43	7.38	9.05	7.68	0.36	6.97	8.38
Age of the patient	0.00	0.01	−0.02	0.02	0.00	0.01	−0.02	0.01
Gender (Female = 1)	−0.23	0.28	−0.77	0.31	0.17	0.25	−0.32	0.66
Total number of visits	0.31	0.08	0.16	0.46	0.27	0.07	0.13	0.41
Total weeks in therapy	−0.02	0.02	−0.06	0.02	−0.02	0.02	−0.05	0.02
Intercept	0.11	0.59	−1.05	1.27	0.29	0.53	−0.75	1.33
Random effects								
Therapist-level	0.51	0.21	0.22	1.15	0.47	0.20	0.20	1.10
Residual	4.55	0.09	4.37	4.74	4.13	0.09	3.97	4.30
Intracluster correlation (ICC%)								
Therapist-level	1.2%	1.0%	0.2%	6.0%	1.3%	1.1%	0.2%	6.7%

case complexity (e.g., level of co-morbidity, axis II difficulties) or changes in medication use may influence TE estimates. However, because IAPT routine data does not include measures of case complexity or medication use, we could not explore the influence of these characteristics. Therefore, it is possible that both the low initial severity and case complexity of the low-intensity sample have contributed to the small TE observed in this study.

As described earlier, there was substantial heterogeneity in terms of the diagnoses and presenting problems of clients in this sample. As others have argued [18], it is likely that large within-therapist variability resulting from clinical heterogeneity may overshadow between-therapist variability. In other words, outcome differences between therapists are found to be less significant compared to the wide variation in outcomes within therapists. In this study, the within-therapist (patient-level) variability accounted for most of variance in final treatment outcome (54–57% in the unconditional model, 37–39% in the conditional model).

Another plausible explanation for the modest TE in this sample relates to the level of standardisation of clinical practice that is typical of this cohort of low intensity therapists. Low intensity therapists in the English IAPT programme are trained to offer brief, structured and highly standardised interventions based on common bibliographic materials, and typically work under considerable levels of case-management scrutiny [30,36]. This, in turn, reduces heterogeneity of clinical practice. High levels of standardisation of treatment such as adherence to treatment manuals have been shown to attenuate TE [2,10], and TE estimates from tightly controlled efficacy studies also tend to be smaller [18]. The only other study examining TE in low intensity treatments [23] also applied highly standardised interventions relying on computerized CBT. It remains to be seen whether the accumulation of future studies examining TE in low intensity therapy confirm the standardisation of treatment as an important determinant of between-therapist variance.

Clinical implications

This study concurs with prior evidence on low-intensity psychotherapy that a small proportion of variation in patient outcomes can be attributed to the therapist level, and that between-therapist variability is very modest by comparison to that observed in conventional high-intensity psychotherapies. The findings of this study suggest that when therapists have similar level of training, work under regular supervision and follow pre-specified treatment protocols to deliver low-intensity interventions, there is likely to be less variability in outcomes between therapists. However, it is quite possible that TE estimates could be larger in other services due to variability in experience, supervision and monitoring procedures. Moreover, the findings of low-intensity psychotherapy for patients with less severe common mental health conditions may not apply to outcomes in severe mental health conditions where there tends to be greater variability in baseline severity. Therefore, the well-established practice of systematic collection and monitoring of patient outcomes at therapist-level as means of quality control is still likely to be important, especially in less standardised services. Lessons from the wider literature in this field suggest that quality control strategies should pay particular attention to cases with high baseline severity and risk, since these cases seem more liable to poor outcomes and may require matching to highly skilled 'outlier' therapists [22]. Providing feedback about such 'risk cases' to the relevant therapists may in itself be a useful method to improve the quality of treatment and outcomes for some patients [37,38].

It is clear that not every patient benefits from treatment (this applies equally to low and high intensity treatments); however, this study has shown that patient-level variability is the key factor that explains variation in outcomes. This implies that low-intensity therapists should be interested in understanding patient heterogeneity to reduce variability in outcomes. Future studies could, for example, investigate which patient characteristics (besides the ones investigated here) can explain within-therapist variability to allow more patient-centred therapeutic approaches to emerge.

Author Contributions

Conceived and designed the experiments: JD DM SA EL SG. Analyzed the data: SA AM TC. Wrote the paper: SA EL TC JD DM AM SG.

References

1. Luborsky L, Crits-Christoph P, McLellan AT, Woody G, Piper W, et al. (1986) Do therapists vary much in their success? Findings from Four Outcome Studies. Am J Orthopsychiatry 56: 501–512.
2. Crits-Christoph P, Baranackie K, Kurcias J, Beck A, Carroll K, et al. (1991) Meta-Analysis of Therapist Effects in Psychotherapy Outcome Studies. Psychother Res 1: 81–91.
3. Wampold BE (2001) The great psychotherapy debate: Models, methods, and findings. Mahwah, NJ: Erlbaum.
4. Huppert JD, Bufka LF, Barlow DH, Gorman JM, Shear MK, et al. (2001) Therapists, therapist variables, and cognitive-behavioral therapy outcome in a multicenter trial for panic disorder. J Consult Clin Psychol 69: 747.
5. Beutler LE, Mailk M, Harwood TM, Talebi H, Noble S, et al. (2004) Therapist variables. In: Lambert MJ, editor. Bergin and Garfield's Handbook of Psychotherapy and Behaviour Change. New York: John Wiley and Sons, Inc. pp. 227–306.
6. Kim D-M, Wampold BE, Bolt DM (2006) Therapist effects in psychotherapy: A random-effects modeling of the National Institute of Mental Health Treatment of Depression Collaborative Research Program data. Psychother Res 16: 161–172.
7. Elkin I, Falconnier L, Martinovich Z, Mahoney C (2006) Therapist effects in the national institute of mental health treatment of depression collaborative research program. Psychother Res 16: 144–160.
8. Wampold BE, Bolt DM (2006) Therapist effects: Clever ways to make them (and everything else) disappear. Psychother Res 16: 184–187.
9. Lutz W, Leon SC, Martinovich Z, Lyons JS, Stiles WB (2007) Therapist effects in outpatient psychotherapy: A three-level growth curve approach. J Couns Psychol 54: 32.
10. Cella M, Stahl D, Reme SE, Chalder T (2011) Therapist effects in routine psychotherapy practice: An account from chronic fatigue syndrome. Psychother Res 21: 168–178.
11. Elkin I (1999) A major dilemma in psychotherapy outcome research: Disentangling therapists from therapies. Clin Psychol (New York) 6: 10–32.
12. Crits-Christoph P, Mintz J (1991) Implications of therapist effects for the design and analysis of comparative studies of psychotherapies. J Consult Clin Psychol 59: 20.
13. Wampold BE, Serlin RC (2000) The consequence of ignoring a nested factor on measures of effect size in analysis of variance. Psychol Methods 5: 425.
14. Wampold BE, Brown GSJ (2005) Estimating variability in outcomes attributable to therapists: a naturalistic study of outcomes in managed care. J Consult Clin Psychol 73: 914.
15. Okiishi J, Lambert MJ, Nielsen SL, Ogles BM (2003) Waiting for supershrink: An empirical analysis of therapist effects. Clin Psychol Psychother 10: 361–373.
16. Blatt SJ, Sanislow III CA, Zuroff DC, Pilkonis PA (1996) Characteristics of effective therapists: further analyses of data from the National Institute of Mental Health Treatment of Depression Collaborative Research Program. J Consult Clin Psychol 64: 1276.
17. Luborsky L, McLellan AT, Diguer L, Woody G, Seligman DA (1997) The Psychotherapist Matters: Comparison of Outcomes Across Twenty-Two Therapists and Seven Patient Samples. Clin Psychol (New York) 4: 53–65.
18. Baldwin SA, Imel ZE (2013) Therapist Effects: Findings and methods. In: Lambert MJ, editor. Bergin and Garfield's handbook of psychotherapy and behavior change. 6th edition ed. New Jersey: John Wiley and Sons, Inc.
19. Crits-Christoph P, Gallop R (2006) Therapist effects in the National Institute of Mental Health Treatment of Depression Collaborative Research Program and other psychotherapy studies. Psychother Res 16: 178–181.
20. Soldz S (2006) Models and meanings: Therapist effects and the stories we tell. Psychother Res 16: 173–177.
21. Project MATCH Research Group (1998) Therapist effects in three treatments for alcohol problems. Psychother Res 8: 455–474.
22. Saxon D, Barkham M (2012) Patterns of therapist variability: Therapist effects and the contribution of patient severity and risk. J Consult Clin Psychol 80: 535.

23. Almlöv J, Carlbring P, Källqvist K, Paxling B, Cuijpers P, et al. (2011) Therapist effects in guided Internet-delivered CBT for anxiety disorders. Behav Cogn Psychother 39: 311.
24. Bennett-Levy J, Richards DA, Farrand P (2010) Low intensity CBT interventions: a revolution in mental health care. In: Bennett-Levy J, Richards DA, Farrand P, Christensen H, Griffiths KM, et al. editors. Oxford guide to low intensity CBT interventions. Oxford: Oxford University Press.
25. Rodgers M, Asaria M, Walker S, McMillan D, Lucock M, et al. (2012) The clinical effectiveness and cost-effectiveness of low-intensity psychological interventions for the secondary prevention of relapse after depression: A systematic review. Health Technol Assess 16: 28.
26. Richards DA, Whyte M (2009) Reach Out: National Programme Educator Materials to Support the Delivery of Training for Psychological Wellbeing Practitioners Delivering Low Intensity Interventions. London: Rethink.
27. NICE (2007) Anxiety (amended): Management of anxiety (Panic disorder, with or with agoraphobia, and generalised anxiety disorder) in adults in primary, secondary and community care. London: National Institute for Health and Clinical Excellence.
28. NICE (2010) Depression: The treatment and management of depression in adults (Updated Edition). London: The British Psychological Society & The Royal College of Psychiatrists.
29. Clark DM, Layard R, Smithies R, Richards DA, Suckling R, et al. (2009) Improving access to psychological therapy: Initial evaluation of two UK demonstration sites. Behav Res Ther 47: 910–920.
30. NHS Improving Access to Psychological Therapies (IAPT) Programme (2011) National curriculum for the education of psychological well-being practitioners (PWPS).
31. Kroenke K, Spitzer RL, Williams JB (2001) The PHQ-9. J Gen Intern Med 16: 606–613.
32. Kroenke K, Spitzer RL, Williams JB, Monahan PO, Löwe B (2007) Anxiety disorders in primary care: prevalence, impairment, comorbidity, and detection. Ann Intern Med 146 317–325.
33. Kroenke K, Spitzer RL, Williams JB, Löwe B (2010) The patient health questionnaire somatic, anxiety, and depressive symptom scales: a systematic review. Gen Hosp Psychiatry 32: 345–359.
34. Raudenbush SW, Bryk AS (2002) Hierarchical linear models: Applications and data analysis methods (Advanced Quantitative Techniques in the Social Sciences). London: Sage Publications.
35. Delgadillo J, McMillan D, Leach C, Lucock M, Gilbody S, et al. (2012) Benchmarking Routine Psychological Services: A Discussion of Challenges and Methods. Behav Cogn Psychother 1: 1–15.
36. Turpin G, Wheeler S (2011) IAPT Supervision Guidance (Revised March 2011). University of Sheffield, University of Leicester.
37. Lambert MJ, Whipple JL, Smart DW, Vermeersch DA, Nielsen SL (2001) The effects of providing therapists with feedback on patient progress during psychotherapy: Are outcomes enhanced? Psychother Res 11: 49–68.
38. Slade K, Lambert MJ, Harmon SC, Smart DW, Bailey R (2008) Improving psychotherapy outcome: The use of immediate electronic feedback and revised clinical support tools. Clin Psychol Psychother 15: 287–303.

Permissions

All chapters in this book were first published in PLOS ONE, by The Public Library of Science; hereby published with permission under the Creative Commons Attribution License or equivalent. Every chapter published in this book has been scrutinized by our experts. Their significance has been extensively debated. The topics covered herein carry significant findings which will fuel the growth of the discipline. They may even be implemented as practical applications or may be referred to as a beginning point for another development.

The contributors of this book come from diverse backgrounds, making this book a truly international effort. This book will bring forth new frontiers with its revolutionizing research information and detailed analysis of the nascent developments around the world.

We would like to thank all the contributing authors for lending their expertise to make the book truly unique. They have played a crucial role in the development of this book. Without their invaluable contributions this book wouldn't have been possible. They have made vital efforts to compile up to date information on the varied aspects of this subject to make this book a valuable addition to the collection of many professionals and students.

This book was conceptualized with the vision of imparting up-to-date information and advanced data in this field. To ensure the same, a matchless editorial board was set up. Every individual on the board went through rigorous rounds of assessment to prove their worth. After which they invested a large part of their time researching and compiling the most relevant data for our readers.

The editorial board has been involved in producing this book since its inception. They have spent rigorous hours researching and exploring the diverse topics which have resulted in the successful publishing of this book. They have passed on their knowledge of decades through this book. To expedite this challenging task, the publisher supported the team at every step. A small team of assistant editors was also appointed to further simplify the editing procedure and attain best results for the readers.

Apart from the editorial board, the designing team has also invested a significant amount of their time in understanding the subject and creating the most relevant covers. They scrutinized every image to scout for the most suitable representation of the subject and create an appropriate cover for the book.

The publishing team has been an ardent support to the editorial, designing and production team. Their endless efforts to recruit the best for this project, has resulted in the accomplishment of this book. They are a veteran in the field of academics and their pool of knowledge is as vast as their experience in printing. Their expertise and guidance has proved useful at every step. Their uncompromising quality standards have made this book an exceptional effort. Their encouragement from time to time has been an inspiration for everyone.

The publisher and the editorial board hope that this book will prove to be a valuable piece of knowledge for researchers, students, practitioners and scholars across the globe.

List of Contributors

Antoni Sicras-Mainar
Directorate of Planning, Badalona Serveis Assistencials, S.A., Badalona, Barcelona, Spain

Pablo Guijarro and Beatriz Armada
Pfizer, Madrid, Spain

Milagrosa Blanca-Tamayo
Department of Psychiatry, Badalona Serveis Assistencials, S.A., Badalona, Barcelona, Spain

Ruth Navarro-Artieda
Medical Documentation, Hospital Germans Trias i Pujol, Badalona, Barcelona, Spain

Steven Bell, Annie Britton and Martin Bobak
Research Department of Epidemiology and Public Health, University College London, London, United Kingdom

Ruzena Kubinova
National Institute of Public Health, Prague, Czech Republic

Sofia Malyutina
Institute of Internal and Preventive Medicine, Novosibirsk, Russia
Novosibirsk State Medical University, Novosibirsk, Russia

Andrzej Pajak
Institute of Public Health, Jagiellonian University, Krakow, Poland

Yuri Nikitin
Institute of Internal and Preventive Medicine, Novosibirsk, Russia

Shinn-Won Lim and Hong-Hee Won
Center for Clinical Research, Samsung Biomedical Research Institute, Seoul, Korea

Hyeran Kim, Woojae Myung and Doh Kwan Kim
Department of Psychiatry, Samsung Medical Center, Sungkyunkwan University School of Medicine, Seoul, Korea

Seonwoo Kim
Biostatistics Unit, Samsung Biomedical Research Institute, Seoul, Korea

Ka-Kyung Kim and Jong-Won Kim
Department of Laboratory Medicine and Genetics, Samsung Medical Center, Sungkyunkwan University School of Medicine, Seoul, Korea

Bernard J. Carroll
Pacific Behavioral Research Foundation, Carmel, California, United States of America

Jörg Wiltink, Matthias Michal and Manfred E. Beutel
Department of Psychosomatic Medicine and Psychotherapy, University Medical Center of the Johannes Gutenberg-University Mainz, Mainz, Germany

Philipp S. Wild
Center for Thrombosis and Hemostasis, University Medical Center of the Johannes Gutenberg-University Mainz, Mainz, Germany
Department of Medicine 2, University Medical Center of the Johannes Gutenberg-University Mainz, Mainz, Germany
German Center for Cardiovascular Research (DZHK), partner site RhineMain, Mainz, Mainz, Germany

Astrid Schneider, Jochem König and Maria Blettner
Institute of Medical Biostatistics, Epidemiology and Informatics, University Medical Center of the Johannes Gutenberg-University Mainz, Mainz, Germany

Thomas Münzel and Andreas Schulz
Department of Medicine 2, University Medical Center of the Johannes Gutenberg-University Mainz, Mainz, Germany

Matthias Weber and Christian Fottner
Department of Medicine 1, University Medical Center of the Johannes Gutenberg-University Mainz, Mainz, Germany

Norbert Pfeiffer
Department of Ophthalmology, University Medical Center of the Johannes Gutenberg-University Mainz, Mainz, Germany

Karl Lackner
Institute of Clinical Chemistry and Laboratory Medicine, University Medical Center of the Johannes Gutenberg-University Mainz, Mainz, Germany

Aylin Cimenser
Harvard Medical School, Boston, Massachusetts, United States of America
Department of Physics, Boston University, Boston, Massachusetts, United States of America

Kenneth D. Miller
Center for Theoretical Neuroscience, College of Physicians and Surgeons, Columbia University, New York, New York, United States of America
Department of Neuroscience, College of Physicians and Surgeons, Columbia University, New York, New York, United States of America
Swartz Program in Theoretical Neuroscience, College of Physicians and Surgeons, Columbia University, New York, New York, United States of America

Giannis Lois, Julia Linke and Michèle Wessa
Department of Clinical Psychology and Neuropsychology, Institute of Psychology, Johannes Gutenberg-University Mainz, Mainz, Germany

Shaoyuan Li
Department of Physiology, Institute of Acupuncture and Moxibustion, China Academy of Chinese Medical Sciences, Beijing, China
Department of Anatomy, Xinxiang Medical University, Xinxiang, Henan Province, China

Xu Zhai, Peijing Rong, Jingjun Zhao and Hui Ben
Department of Physiology, Institute of Acupuncture and Moxibustion, China Academy of Chinese Medical Sciences, Beijing, China

Michael F. McCabe
Department of Anesthesia, Critical Care, and Pain Medicine, Massachusetts General Hospital, Harvard Medical School, Boston, Massachusetts, United States of America

Xing Wang
Department of Anatomy, Xinxiang Medical University, Xinxiang, Henan Province, China

Shuxing Wang
Department of Physiology, Institute of Acupuncture and Moxibustion, China Academy of Chinese Medical Sciences, Beijing, China
Department of Anatomy, Xinxiang Medical University, Xinxiang, Henan Province, China
Department of Anesthesia, Critical Care, and Pain Medicine, Massachusetts General Hospital, Harvard Medical School, Boston, Massachusetts, United States of America

Colin Green and David A. Richards
University of Exeter Medical School, University of Exeter, Exeter, United Kingdom

Jacqueline J. Hill
Mood Disorders Centre, University of Exeter, Exeter, United Kingdom

Adwoa Hughes-Morley, Linda Gask and Peter Bower
Centre for Primary Care at the Institute of Population Health, University of Manchester, Manchester, United Kingdom

Karina Lovell
School of Nursing, Midwifery, and Social Work, University of Manchester, Manchester, United Kingdom

Carolyn Chew-Graham
Primary Care and Health Sciences, Keele University, Keele, United Kingdom

John Cape and Stephen Pilling
Research Department of Clinical, Educational, and Health Psychology, University College London, London, United Kingdom

Ricardo Araya and David Kessler
School of Social and Community Medicine, University of Bristol, Bristol, United Kingdom

J. Martin Bland
Department of Health Sciences, University of York, York, United Kingdom

Simon Gilbody
Department of Health Sciences at Hull York Medical School, University of York, York, United Kingdom

Glyn Lewis
Mental Health Sciences Unit, University College London, London, United Kingdom

Chris Manning
Upstream Healthcare, Teddington, United Kingdom

Michael Barkham
Department of Psychology, University of Sheffield, Sheffield, United Kingdom

Shu-Li Wang
Department of Dental Laboratory Technology, Central Taiwan University of Science and Technology, Taichung, Taiwan

Cheng-Ho Chang and Li-Yu Hu
Department of Psychiatry, Kaohsiung Veterans General Hospital, Kaohsiung, Taiwan

Shih-Jen Tsai
Department of Psychiatry, Taipei Veterans General Hospital, Taipei, Taiwan

School of Medicine, National Yang-Ming University, Taipei, Taiwan

Albert C. Yang
Department of Psychiatry, Taipei Veterans General Hospital, Taipei, Taiwan
School of Medicine, National Yang-Ming University, Taipei, Taiwan
Center for Dynamical Biomarkers and Translational Medicine, National Central University, Chungli, Taiwan

Zi-Hong You
Division of Nephrology, Department of Internal Medicine, Taichung Veterans General Hospital, Chia-Yi Branch, Chia-Yi, Taiwan
Institute of Medicine, Chung Shan Medical University, Taichung, Taiwan

Julián Alfredo Fernández-Niño, Betty Soledad Manrique-Espinoza and Aarón Salinas-Rodríguez
Center for Evaluation Research and Surveys, National Institute of Public Health, Cuernavaca, Morelos, Mexico

Ietza Bojorquez-Chapela
Department of Population Studies, El Colegio de la Frontera Norte, Tijuana, Baja California, Mexico

Rachel H. Jacobs, Lisanne M. Jenkins, Laura B. Gabriel, Alyssa Barba, Alvaro Verges, Amy T. Peters and Natania A. Crane
Department of Psychiatry, University of Illinois at Chicago, Chicago, Illinois, United States of America

Kelly A. Ryan and Amanda M. Baker
Department of Psychiatry, University of Michigan, Ann Arbor, Michigan, United States of America

Sara L. Weisenbach
Department of Psychiatry, University of Illinois at Chicago, Chicago, Illinois, United States of America
Department of Psychiatry, University of Michigan, Ann Arbor, Michigan, United States of America
Research and Development Program, Jesse Brown VA Medical Center, Chicago, Illinois, United States of America
VA Ann Arbor Healthcare System, Ann Arbor, Michigan, United States of America

Ian H. Gotlib
Department of Psychology, Stanford University, Stanford, California, United States of America

Jon-Kar Zubieta
Department of Psychiatry, University of Michigan, Ann Arbor, Michigan, United States of America
Department of Radiology, Molecular and Behavioral Neuroscience Institute, Ann Arbor, Michigan, United States of America

K. Luan Phan
Department of Psychiatry, University of Illinois at Chicago, Chicago, Illinois, United States of America
Departments of Psychology and Anatomy and Cell Biology, University of Illinois at Chicago, Chicago, Illinois, United States of America
Mental Health Service Line, Jesse Brown VA Medical Center, Chicago, Illinois, United States of America

Scott A. Langenecker
Department of Psychiatry, University of Illinois at Chicago, Chicago, Illinois, United States of America
Department of Psychiatry, University of Michigan, Ann Arbor, Michigan, United States of America
Department of Radiology, Molecular and Behavioral Neuroscience Institute, Ann Arbor, Michigan, United States of America

Robert C. Welsh
Department of Psychiatry, University of Michigan, Ann Arbor, Michigan, United States of America
Department of Psychology, Stanford University, Stanford, California, United States of America

Eva Haastrup and Henrik Ullum
Department of Clinical Immunology, the Blood bank, Rigshospitalet, University Hospital of Copenhagen, Copenhagen, Denmark

Katrine Grau
Department of Epidemiology Research, Statens Serum Institut, Copenhagen, Denmark

Jesper Eugen-Olsen and Christian Thorball
Clinical Research Centre, Hvidovre Hospital, University Hospital of Copenhagen, Copenhagen, Denmark

Lars Vedel Kessing
Psychiatric Centre, Rigshospitalet, University Hospital of Copenhagen, Copenhagen, Denmark

Kerina H. Jones, Philip A. Jones, Rodden M. Middleton, David V. Ford, Katie Tuite-Dalton, Hazel Lockhart-Jones, Jeffrey Peng, Ronan A. Lyons, Ann John and J. Gareth Noble
College of Medicine, Swansea University, Swansea, Wales, United Kingdom

Hugh MacPherson, Stewart J. Richmond, Harriet Lansdown, Sara Perren, Ann Hopton and Karen Spilsbury
Department of Health Sciences, University of York, York, United Kingdom

Liz Newbronner
Department of Health Sciences, University of York, York, United Kingdom
Firefly Research and Evaluation, North Yorkshire, United Kingdom

Ruth Chamberlain
Firefly Research and Evaluation, North Yorkshire, United Kingdom

Ruth Chan and Jean Woo
Department of Medicine and Therapeutics, The Chinese University of Hong Kong, Shatin, Hong Kong

Dicken Chan
The Jockey Club School of Public Health and Primary Care, The Chinese University of Hong Kong, Shatin, Hong Kong

Kim L. Felmingham
School of Psychology, University of New South Wales, Sydney, Australia
Brain Dynamics Centre, Westmead Millennium Institute, Westmead Hospital, Sydney, Australia
School of Psychology, University of Tasmania, Hobart, Australia

Erin M. Falconer
Brain Dynamics Centre, Westmead Millennium Institute, Westmead Hospital, Sydney, Australia

Leanne Williams
Brain Dynamics Centre, Westmead Millennium Institute, Westmead Hospital, Sydney, Australia
Western Clinical School, University of Sydney, Sydney, Australia

Andrew H. Kemp
School of Psychology, University of Sydney, Sydney, Australia

Adrian Allen and Richard A. Bryant
Brain Dynamics Centre, Westmead Millennium Institute, Westmead Hospital, Sydney, Australia
School of Psychology, University of Tasmania, Hobart, Australia

Anthony Peduto
MRI Unit, Department of Radiology, Westmead Hospital, Sydney, Australia

Barbara Baldo, Rachel Y. Cheong and Åsa Petersén
Translational Neuroendocrine Research Unit, Department of Experimental Medical Science, Lund University, Lund, Sweden

Paula Kuivasaari-Pirinen, Maritta Hippeläinen, Kaisa Raatikainen and Seppo Heinonen
Department of Obstetrics and Gynaecology, Kuopio University Hospital, Kuopio, Finland
Institute of Clinical Medicine, University of Eastern Finland, Kuopio, Finland

Heli Koivumaa-Honkanen
Institute of Clinical Medicine, University of Eastern Finland, Kuopio, Finland
Clinic of Child Psychiatry, Oulu University Hospital, Oulu, Finland
Department of Psychiatry, Kuopio University Hospital, Kuopio, Finland
Department of Psychiatry, South-Savonia Hospital District, Mikkeli, Finland
Department of Psychiatry, North Karelia Central Hospital, Joensuu, Finland
Department of Psychiatry, SOSTERI, Savonlinna, Finland
Department of Psychiatry, SOTE, Iisalmi, Finland
Department of Psychiatry, Lapland Hospital District, Rovaniemi, Finland
Department of Psychiatry, Institute of Clinical Medicine, University of Oulu, Oulu, Finland

Zhan-Zhan Li and Lizhang Chen
Department of Epidemiology and Health Statistics, School of Public Health, Central South University, Changsha, China

Ya-Ming Li
Department of Nursing, Central South University, Changsha, Hunan Province, China
The Second Affiliated Hospital, Xiangya Medical School, Central South University, Changsha, Hunan Province, China

Xian-Yang Lei
The Second Affiliated Hospital, Xiangya Medical School, Central South University, Changsha, Hunan Province, China

Dan Zhang, Li Liu and Si-Yuan Tang
Department of Nursing, Central South University, Changsha, Hunan Province, China

Malin Wennström, Shorena Janelidze and Lennart Minthon
Lund University, Department of Clinical Sciences, Clinical Memory Research Unit, Wallenberg Laboratory, Malmö, Sweden

Cecilie Bay-Richter
Aarhus University, Department of Clinical Medicine, Translational Neuropsychiatry Unit, Risskov, Denmark

Lena Brundin
Michigan State University, College of Human Medicine, Department of Psychiatry and Behavioral Medicine, Grand Rapids, Michigan, United States of America
Van Andel Research Institute, Laboratory of Behavioral Medicine, Grand Rapids, Michigan, United States of America

Shehzad Ali
Department of Health Sciences, University of York, York, United Kingdom
Centre for Health Economics, University of York, York, United Kingdom

Elizabeth Littlewood, Dean McMillan, Tim Croudace and Simon Gilbody
Department of Health Sciences, University of York, York, United Kingdom

Jaime Delgadillo
Primary Care Mental Health Service, Leeds Community Healthcare NHS Trust, Leeds, United Kingdom

Alfonso Miranda
Centro de Investigación y Docencia Económicas, Mexico City, Mexico

Index